Conception to Birth

Monographs in Epidemiology and Biostatistics
edited by Brian MacMahon

Monographs in Epidemiology and Biostatistics
Volume 14

Conception to Birth

Epidemiology of Prenatal Development

Jennie Kline

Adjunct Associate Professor of Public Health (Epidemiology)
in the Sergievsky Center, Columbia University,
and Senior Research Scientist, New York Psychiatric Institute

Zena Stein

Professor of Public Health (Epidemiology)
in the Sergievsky Center, Columbia University,
and Director, Epidemiology of Developmental Brain
Disorders Department, New York Psychiatric Institute

Mervyn Susser

Gertrude H. Sergievsky Professor of Epidemiology,
and Director, the Sergievsky Center, Columbia University

New York   Oxford
OXFORD UNIVERSITY PRESS
1989

Oxford University Press

Oxford   New York   Toronto
Delhi   Bombay   Calcutta   Madras   Karachi
Petaling Jaya   Singapore   Hong Kong   Tokyo
Nairobi   Dar es Salaam   Cape Town
Melbourne   Auckland

and associated companies in
Berlin   Ibadan

Copyright © 1989 by Oxford University Press, Inc.

Published by Oxford University Press, Inc.,
200 Madison Avenue, New York, New York 10016

Oxford is a registered trademark of Oxford University Press

Library of Congress Cataloging-in-Publication Data
Kline, Jennie.
Conception to birth : epidemiology of prenatal development /
Jennie Kline, Zena Stein, Mervyn Susser.
p. cm. — (Monographs in epidemiology and biostatistics ; v. 14)
Bibliography: p.
ISBN 0-19-504286-7
1. Fetus—Diseases—Epidemiology. 2. Fetus—Growth.
3. Pregnancy, Complications of—Epidemiology. I. Stein, Zena.
II. Susser, Mervyn. III. Title. IV. Title: Epidemiology of
prenatal development. V. Title: Prenatal development. VI. Series.
[DNLM: 1. Abnormalities—occurrence. 2. Epidemiology of prenatal
development. 3. Fetal Disorder—occurrence. 4. Pregnancy Outcome.
W1 MO567LT v. 14 / WQ 210 K65f]
RG627.K53 1989
614.5'992—dc19
DNLM/DLC   for Library of Congress   88-38168   CIP

9 8 7 6 5 4 3 2 1

Printed in the United States of America
on acid-free paper

Preface

Many fields contribute to an understanding of prenatal development. The scientific disciplines include developmental biology and physiology, embryology and teratology, auxology, genetics, and demography; the medical specialties include obstetrics, pediatrics, and, in particular, the subspecialties perinatology and neonatology. Our book aims to convey the unique contribution of epidemiology through a systematic treatment that it has so far been denied.

What is special about this contribution stems from a combination of features, none in itself unique. One of these features is the demarcation of the territory of epidemiology, among population sciences, as the study of health states in human beings. Another feature is the focus of epidemiology on environmental factors and the consequent requirements for quantitative, population-based data; these are the necessary foundation for inference about the causes of health disorders. A third feature is the public health concern for the prevention and control of disease, from which the discipline originates.

Our intent is to illuminate, under the critical light of epidemiology, the existing and evolving knowledge of prenatal development, through all of gestation from conception to birth. We have tried to be scientifically constructive. Whatever the issue, we do not hesitate to present our own formulations and reformulations. In this way we wittingly open ourselves to criticism, in the hope that we might stimulate the scientific imagination as well as the critical faculties of our readers.

Such a book must be a synthesis, not merely a review. Much effort has nonetheless been expended in ensuring that what we assert as facts are facts in modern understanding, that what has been cited will be found in the original sources, and that the interpretations we offer are as robust as the contending minds of the three authors can make them. We also have paid close attention to nomenclature, terms, and definitions. As in any growing field of study, terminology grows as well. Usage tends to be changeable, idiosyncratic, and ill-defined as a result. We have provided many definitions as props and guides and have assumed authority where lack of sense, or conflicts with sense, left no other recourse.

In following our particular construction of this field, readers uniniti-ated in epidemiology should acquire appreciation of the epidemiological approach and of population data. Fresh perspectives and new materials on prenatal development should reward them. Epidemiologists, for their part, should acquire some insight into prenatal development. In addition, as they read, they will find the principles of their craft being exercised, some of the time in new ways and much of the time on new subject matter. In these exercises, both acolytes and the ordained might reinforce their epidemiological understanding.

The book is divided into five sections:

I. Disorders of development: Weighing the evidence for environ-mental causes.
II. Conception and early gestation.
III. Later gestation.
IV. Age and parity.
V. The physical environment, reproduction, and surveillance.

The first section guides readers in evaluating observed associations between suspected teratogens and developmental outcomes. We discuss a number of established criteria by which the quality of causal inferences might be judged—time order, strength, consistency, specificity, and co-herence. For each of these criteria, real and potential teratogens are used to illustrate their salience and the related problems of interpretation.

After laying this groundwork for causal thinking we turn, in the sec-ond and third sections of the book, to draw an epidemiological map of development. Conceptions are followed from the initiating events of fertilization to birth as the endpoint. To describe the progress of cohorts of conceptions through time requires a recasting of most of the available material. Virtually all prenatal observations at a population level are cross-sectional; they cannot capture directly those losses, observed and unobserved, that occur unevenly in the course of the developmental process; most often, observation depends solely on data obtained at the termination of the reproductive process. These data will frequently yield numerators but no denominators. Population rates, normally the epi-demiologist's standby, are in such circumstances not to be had. In the face of potentially large losses and in the absence of rates, great care is necessary for an accurate rendering of longitudinal growth and development.

To accomplish this mapping of early development in the second sec-tion of the book, we devote three consecutive chapters to the proba-bilities of conception and of loss, to the interpretation of frequency measures, and to actual frequencies observed. Another three chapters are devoted to miscarriage data in which normal and aberrant karyotypes have been differentiated. These chapters deal with variations and regularities in chromosomally normal and aberrant miscarriages, with environmental influences on patterns of loss, and with recurrence in individuals and aggregation in families.

The third section of the book, on later gestation, was written by only two authors (Z.S. and M.S.). This section turns to fetal growth and the duration of that growth, subjects by now familiar in reproductive epidemiology. The first of these chapters does the still necessary work of distinguishing among the three conceptual entities of preterm delivery, retarded growth and immaturity, and of disentangling their historical conflation. Preterm delivery is covered in two further chapters: one considers the types of indices used for enumeration; another considers possible causes. The next two chapters pose questions about existing concepts of fetal growth and birth weight. One chapter deals with indices of fetal growth and with factors that influence growth. The other elaborates on norms appropriate for different groups and on thresholds appropriate under different conditions.

A chapter on familial resemblances in birth weight aims to resolve the apparent contradiction between the predominant maternal and environmental effects on prenatal growth and the known genetic contribution to individual postnatal growth. The last chapter of this section analyzes maternity and birth in less developed countries. Scattered and scanty material on maternal mortality, and on fetal growth and its significance for infant mortality, is brought together and discussed in terms of epidemiological concepts selected for their relevance to the less developed world.

Section IV explores two major issues in the analysis of reproductive outcomes, namely maternal age and gravidity. The first of two chapters on maternal age extends and clarifies the original synthesis of Z.S. on this subject. The second deals with the powerful influence of maternal age on trisomies. The last chapter of this section contributes to the analysis of gravidity, a perilous area for interpretation. This chapter (with the help of Bruce Levin) extends and clarifies an earlier contribution of J.K.

Section V takes up the public health challenge of detecting and controlling environmental hazards to reproduction. The section provides a systematic analytic treatment of surveillance. The penultimate chapter, devoted to the rationale for undertaking surveillance and the techniques of monitoring, makes a clear distinction between activities encompassed by surveillance and by monitoring. In discussing monitoring techniques, we develop (again with help from Bruce Levin) an overall analytic framework not hitherto available. The last chapter considers what epidemiological and public health action might follow the discovery, through surveillance, of suspicious leads. Appropriate research strategies as well as social, economic, and political questions are discussed.

Beyond the foretaste of content outlined here, readers may be curious as to how this book was written and how it came about. This work is truly conjoint. An intense effort spanning several years has produced its content, framework, and style. Predecessors of the chapters of the book can of course be found in earlier publications, often jointly authored with other colleagues whom we have not singled out for special mention. From the previous description, it will be evident that all three of us engaged with two-thirds of the book, and two of us with the remaining third. The alphabetical ordering of the authors' names conforms with our long-sustained practice in intimate collaborations; by this means we have hoped to avoid invidious allocations of priority. We agreed, however, that one of us (M.S.) should accept editorial responsibility.

When the concern of the authors with prenatal development began, few epidemiological forerunners had paid attention to the whole of gestation, early as well as late. In Britain, Thomas McKeown and his colleagues, Dugald Baird and Angus Thomson and their colleagues, and Alan Stephenson had opened the field; in the United States, Theodore Ingalls, Brian MacMahon (a student of McKeown), and Samuel Shapiro had made a beginning. In the mid-1960s two of the authors (Z.S. and M.S.) had their interest provoked by the hypothesis that prenatal nutrition was a critical factor in postnatal mental development. They then sought to conduct epidemiological analogues of the "crucial experiment" (in Thomas Huxley's phrase) to test the hypothesis.

That focus was broadened in the course of a sabbatical leave in London in the academic year of 1972–73. We take this opportunity to assure academic administrators that sabbatical leaves often do produce the intended results of allowing for scholarly reflection and summation and for the stimulation that leads in new directions. Z.S., interested in Down's syndrome, was charged by the possibilities that had emerged for prenatal karyotyping. A particular stimulus was renewed contact with the work of Eva Alberman, epidemiologist, and Paul Polani, geneticist, who had combined to study the aberrant karyotypes so heavily concentrated in miscarriages. In France, too, the epidemiological studies of karyotypes at miscarriage of André and Jouelle Boué were just beginning to appear. In New York, Z.S. had already consulted on some of these matters with our colleague Dorothy Warburton, human geneticist at the Columbia-Presbyterian Medical Center, and had been at once impressed by her expertise, scientific imagination, and generous collegiality. At about the same time, J.K. had become the first student in the Ph.D. Program in Epidemiology at Columbia University, and her interest too was sparked.

In these circumstances, the decision was easily made to embark on a major long-term epidemiological program to study abnormal prenatal development by karyotyping miscarriages. Dorothy Warburton joined to form the triumvirate that headed the project; J.K. joined as project director. The core directorate was enlarged to include J.K. when she completed her dissertation, and in 1982 she became the principal investigator.

While the conjunction of three authors follows naturally from this history, it was through accidents of circumstance that Dorothy Warburton is not a fourth. Concurrently she, with two others, has been writing what can be considered a companion volume to this one, on morphological maldevelopment in the prenatal period. She has always been free and informed in her advice, and we know how much more she could have added to our understanding and subtracted from our labor in this work.

New York   M.S.
August 1988

Acknowledgments

Dorothy Warburton and Bruce Levin have afforded us continuous and extensive help. John Kiely has generously provided unpublished analyses from his ongoing studies of perinatal mortality in New York City. Allen Wilcox, too, provided fresh data before publication and commented on the chapters relevant to these data in the second section of the book. Neil Risch has been invaluable as an adviser on issues of genetic epidemiology. Stephen Ng has reviewed some of our analytic concepts. The typing of this volume, from often contorted handwritten scripts and revisions, has been steadily and uncomplainingly carried out in the main by Aureau Pupo, with assistance from Mani Sengupta, Leslie Dwelle, and others in the Sergievsky Center. Andrea Versenyi was a mainstay in compiling the bibliography.

An additional acknowledgment must be made for the use of unpublished material of wide scope. A number of citations to unpublished data on miscarriages from the New York City Study of Early Reproductive Loss are made in the text. In all such cases, the citations refer not only to the three authors of this text but also to Dorothy Warburton.

The Sergievsky Center of the Faculty of Medicine, Columbia University, and the Epidemiology of Developmental Brain Disorders Department, New York Psychiatric Institute provided necessary resources. Part of the work reported here was carried out with support from Public Health Service grants, in particular NIH grant R01-HD-15909.

Contents

Disorders of Development: Weighing the Evidence for Environmental Causes

1 Criteria for Teratogenesis: I. Time Order, Strength of Association, Consistency on Replication

The man-made environment poses hazards to reproduction. In the eighteenth century, Peter Johann Frank (1790) recognized poverty as the "mother of disease" and passionately asserted the social and medical obligation to improve the environment. In our time, industry, agriculture, and medicine itself have brought new dangers. To identify and evaluate the existence and extent of dangers to the public health is a role that falls to epidemiology.

In this book, we apply the logic of epidemiology to the assessment of adverse reproductive effects. We intend to bring out both the strengths and the weaknesses of the discipline for this task. We begin with the questions of inference raised by teratogenesis. Many agents have been suspect, and some have been indicted. Exposure to the physical environment of soil, water, air or the workplace; ingestion of food, drink and drugs; specific infections; and body states such as hyperpyrexia and diabetes are all under suspicion. To establish guilt by demonstrating the effects of environmental factors on the developing organism is another matter. As always with sound epidemiology and sound science, we need, first, to be clear about terms and their meanings.

TERMS, DEFINITIONS AND LIMITS

A *teratogen*, for our purposes, is a factor extrinsic to the developing organism that acts in the interval between conception and birth to injure the progeny or provoke abnormal development. *Teratogenesis* describes the fact and the manner of the injuries and developmental provocations caused by teratogens. *Teratology* has been more narrowly or broadly defined, according to the preference of different authors. Teratology began as "a discourse or narrative concerning prodigies; a marvelous tale, or collection of such tales" (*Oxford English Dictionary*). Medicine adopted the term for the study of monstrosities or anomalies of organization (although skeptics may believe that the original sense of "marvelous tales" still applies). Thus in its first medical usage, teratogenesis meant the production at birth of a monster or misshapen organism (from the Greek *tera*). Some modern lexicographers, for instance Dorland (1981), adhere to a usage that limits teratogenesis to the production of anatomical defects.

One problem in defining terms is how inclusive the definition should be. Our definition, following the lead of others (World Health Organization 1967; Wilson 1973), encompasses a range of effects broader than physical defects. Besides malformations thought to arise from dysmorphic organogenesis, we include effects arising prenatally that manifest only postnatally after variable latent periods. Disturbances in growth and gender, neoplasms, deficits in intelligence, and disordered behavior fall into this group. Growth, function and survival are basic to development; they lead us to a grouping of disordered development into five classes: deranged growth, retarded growth, deranged function, retarded function, and death. *Deranged growth* is expressed mainly in malformations, but also in neoplasms. *Deranged function* can be physical, as in endocrine disorders, or mental, as in autistic and certain cognitive disorders. *Retarded growth* can manifest either prenatally or postnatally; *retarded function* is generally, although not necessarily, manifest postnatally.

Besides differences in inclusiveness and domain, the definition of teratogenesis is clouded by our ignorance of etiology and pathogenesis. Whether or not a disorder is of prenatal origin is not always clear. The same type of manifestation may take origin either before conception, during pregnancy, or after birth.

While our usage conforms to a broad concept of teratogenesis, we do not deal with all the possible classes. To explicate the procedures of causal inference central to this section, we have chosen malformations as our chief examples. Fetal death and prenatal growth are dealt with in other chapters. Also, we have chosen in the main not to deal with the class of disorders and derangements that, while they may originate in the prenatal period, manifest only in later life.

Teratogenesis is a process confined by definition within the narrow developmental time frame of gestation. Usually the initiating exposure occurs and the outcome becomes apparent within these limits, but the definition does not insist on this coincidence in time. The process must begin, although it need not be completed, between conception and birth. Indeed, the prenatal pathogenetic process may be dissociated from the initial exposure to a causal factor as well as from the appearance of an adverse outcome. A child can be affected by maternal exposure to polychlorbiphenyls that occurred years before conception. On the other hand, the cancers consequent on prenatal exposure to diethylstilbestrol and possibly to hepatitis B virus (adenocarcinoma of the vagina and liver cancer, respectively) may not be expressed until adulthood.

The strength of the presumption that a factor has acted between conception and birth therefore hinges on biological understanding of the processes that lead to a particular outcome. Understanding is invariably less than perfect. Shadowed areas and imprecise knowledge—about the timing of exposure, latent periods, and onset—are not peculiar to teratogenesis; rather they emphasize the continuity of human development. The discrete entrances and exits of conception and birth mark critical developmental events, but these thresholds are crossed by many continuing developmental processes.

Teratogenesis refers only to abnormal development. For heuristic purposes, this defined boundary should not be allowed to exclude normal development from attention. Discoveries about what underlies abnormal development further our understanding of the collateral processes that underlie normal development. The converse holds also: the understanding of normal development and its mechanisms furthers our ability to identify factors that interfere with development.

To describe what may instigate teratogenesis, we choose the word *factor*. Mundane, overused and worn as it is, the word suits our need for a term that covers a broad range of possibilities. We designate as a factor anything that may influence the development of the conceptus and its course during pregnancy. Some factors, deficits as well as excesses, reside in the external environment; these may be physical like polluted air and water and radiation, or social like poverty, or psychological like some types of stressful life events. Measures or indices that aim to capture physical factors are generally external to the maternal–fetal dyad, but not invariably so: thus, they include "biological markers of exposure," such as blood lead levels detectable in maternal body fluids or tissues (Stein and Hatch 1987), as well as occupational histories and suspect substances detectable in ambient air, water and soil.

Other environmental factors are acquired through the woman's voluntary or involuntary activity: ingested substances such as alcohol and drugs, and such transmitted microorganisms as the rubella or human immunodeficiency viruses, may reach the conceptus by invading the maternal environment that secludes and nurtures it. Measures and indices to capture these exposures may rely on the reports of the woman or on detection in her body fluids of the microorganisms or of the substances she has incorporated and their breakdown products. Use may also be made of the intermediate effects of exposure in the woman; these are "biological markers of effect." They can include cytological reactions and other precursors of pathology, and immunological responses such as antibody formation and immune cell reactions. Later, frank clinical signs of toxicity or infection in the mother can betray the exposure.

Still other factors are attributes the woman already has at the moment of conception. Maternal age, ethnicity and family history may point to a raised risk of certain anomalies, and maternal biochemical states—such as an excess of phenylalanine or a deficit of iodine—may indicate specific dangers. In a model that includes multiple causes, maternal susceptibilities also need to be considered as causal factors. Thus an absence of immunity to such infections as rubella or cytomegalovirus, or other "biological markers of susceptibility", indicate conceptions at risk.

When we turn from the causes to the consequences of teratogenesis, our broad grouping of outcomes leaves questions about what specific outcomes will be admitted as relevant. Malformations, deformities, fetal death and growth retardation before birth, and mental and physical dysfunction and congenital neoplasms after birth, can safely be included as adverse outcomes resulting from factors acting between conception and birth. Developmental abnormalities determined in the parental germ cells by preexisting point mutations or chromosomal aberrations or by genetic errors at fertilization can safely be excluded. These same genetic causes are similarly excluded when they lead to fetal deaths or disturbances in mental and physical growth and development.

Associations with a diversity of reproductive outcomes have been reported for a multitude of factors (reviewed in Brent 1977; Kurent and Sever 1977; Wilson 1977; Strobino et al. 1978, 1979; Kalter and Warkany 1983; Gal and Sharpless 1984; Shepard 1986). Few of these associations compel a causal interpretation. Before we proceed with our main topics, we can draw the battle lines, so to speak, by tabulating factors among those we know that merit inclusion as "definite" human teratogens, which is to say "without doubt in our judgment." These 20 factors fall into five groups: (1) medications, (2) physiological dysfunction, (3) chemical and physical agents abroad in the environment, (4) substances voluntarily ingested, absorbed or inspired by the woman, and (5) maternal infection. The individual factors are listed in Table 1-1.

Our discussion concentrates on the deployment of some of the criteria epidemiologists apply in their efforts to judge causality (U.S. Public Health Service Report of Advisory Committee to Surgeon General 1964; Hill 1965; Susser 1973, 1987). In so organizing our material, we do not seek to be comprehensive. Our examples are chosen for their bearing on teratogenesis as a causal process, rather than to lead us through a systematic exposition of the means for establishing causality. In what follows, then, evidence that seals the classification of a teratogen as definite, or fails to do so, is tested against those criteria of judgment that seem most relevant to reaching a causal inference in that instance.

In this discussion, a *cause* is something that makes a difference to an outcome. This broad usage encompasses any determinant, whether active or passive (some definitions confine causes to active determinants). If active, a determinant brings about change. If passive, the determinant is an attribute or condition—say sex or heritage or geography—under which outcomes change as the attribute or condition is varied. Teratogens are active determinants; our discussion is organized around

Table 1–1 Some definite teratogens and their effects

Teratogen	Effects	References
Medication		
1. Thalidomide	Phocomelia, amelia, defects of the radius and abnormalities of the ear	Weicker et al. 1962; Lenz and Knapp 1962; McBride 1963
2. Androgenic hormones (androgens and certain progestins)	Masculinization of the female fetus	Zander and Muller 1953; Jacobson 1962; reviewed in Schardein 1980
3. Tetracycline	Discoloration of the teeth	Rendle-Short 1962; Harcourt et al. 1962; Genot et al. 1970
4. Aminopterin	Multiple malformations	Thiersch 1952; Goetsch 1962
5. Diethylstilbestrol	Cervical adenosis, clear cell adenocarcinoma of the vagina	Herbst et al. 1971, 1974, 1975; Greenwald et al. 1971
6. Isotretinoin	Craniofacial, cardiac, thymic, and central nervous system abnormalities	Lammer et al. 1985
Physiological dysfunction		
7. Hyperphenylalaninemia	Intrauterine growth retardation, microcephaly, congenital heart defects	Reviewed in Lenke and Levy 1980
8. Iodine deficiency	Cretinism, cerebral palsy, motor and mental retardation	Pharoah et al. 1971; Hetzel and Pharoah 1971; reviewed in Pharoah et al. 1980
9. Starvation	Intrauterine growth retardation*	Smith 1947; Antonov 1947; Stein et al. 1975a
10. Diabetes	Multiple malformations, growth and metabolic disorders	Bennett et al. 1979; Mills 1982; Mills et al. 1988; Pettit and Bennett 1988
Physical environment		
11. Irradiation	Microcephaly, mental retardation	Reviewed in National Research Council (BEIR) 1980
12. Polychlorinated biphenyls	Stained skin, gingiva and nails, conjunctival hypersecretion	Miller 1971; reviewed by Rogan 1982
13. Methylmercury	Minamata disease	Harada 1968; Amin-Zaki et al. 1979
Substances voluntarily ingested or inspired		
14. Cigarette smoking	Intrauterine growth retardation*	Simpson 1957; reviewed in U.S. Public Health Service 1971, and by Abel 1980

(*continued*)

Table 1–1 *(Continued)*

Teratogen	Effects	References
15. Alcohol	Fetal alcohol syndrome (usually dysmorphic facies, growth retardation, central nervous system involvement)	Lemoine et al. 1968; reviewed by Abel 1984; Vitez et al. 1984; Ernhart et al. 1985
Maternal infection		
16. Syphilis	Congenital syphilis	Hutchinson 1887; reviewed in Ingall and Norins 1976
17. Rubella	Cataracts, congenital heart disease, deafness	Gregg 1941
18. Cytomegalovirus	Sensory and mental deficit, cytomegalovirus inclusion disease	Reynolds et al. 1974; Hanshaw et al. 1976
19. Toxoplasmosis	Hydrocephalus, chorioretinitis, calcification	Eichenwald (1959) Koppe et al. (1974, 1986)
20. Human immunodeficiency virus	Immunodeficiency syndrome, neurologic impairment	MMWR 1982

*Perinatal mortality rates increase with both prenatal starvation and smoking. In both cases, an intermediary factor may be intrauterine growth retardation, but other mechanisms cannot be excluded.

them, although passive determinants are not ignored. Causes have three essential properties: association, time order and direction.

Association requires that a causal factor must occur in conjunction with the putative effect. Association is judged by the criterion of probability; for this purpose, we turn to the conventions of statistical inference. If no association exists, we need proceed no further; refutation settles the question. Uncertainty or affirmation allows testing to continue.

Time order requires, in a given association, that the suspect causal factor must precede the effect. If the reverse holds, refutation has again settled the question, while failure to refute allows testing to continue.

Direction is an attribute that, given appropriate time order, describes an asymmetrical association. In such an association, a determinant brings about an outcome, and does not merely coexist with it as in a symmetrical association. The outcome must be shown to change in consequence of a change in the causal factor.

To say a cause has direction is a tautology of a sort, for this property subsumes the others. All other relevant criteria and the whole procedure of causal inference must be brought to bear to prove the presence of consequential change. Thus a sound judgment that asserts the presence of direction depends virtually always on the evolution of a process; the evidence must unfold through time.

Besides the property of time order, four additional criteria—strength of association, consistency on replication, specificity of association, coherence—weigh heavily in these judgments. Some contribute most to verification, others to falsification of the claim to teratogenicity. These and some other issues of method are illustrated with examples drawn from the literature on both definite and doubtful teratogens.

Because specificity and coherence find extensive and complex application in interpreting teratogenic effects, these two criteria each occupy a chapter on their own. We open with a discussion of time order, an elementary property, but one that is crucial in assessing teratogenesis.

TIME ORDER

Time order requires that the supposed cause is consistently antecedent to the supposed effect. This prerequisite is sometimes established from simple observation, but this is seldom the case with teratogenesis. All case-control and cross-sectional study designs simultaneously collect the data that will contribute both the suspect causal variable and the outcome variable. In these designs, both variables refer to the past; the cause has operated and the effect has eventuated before any observation is made. The temporal relationship of the variables, therefore, escapes direct observation. Cohort studies, whether historical or prospective, usually afford epidemiologists better insight into the time order of relevant events.

Some difficulties related to time order are special to the study of teratogenesis. In human teratology, the interpretation of associations rests heavily on the correspondence between time of exposure and the conjectured initiation of pathogenesis. Yet indirect inference about time order has been a historical necessity that follows from the inaccessibility of prenatal development to direct observation. The brilliant and minutely detailed images of structure and function afforded by several new techniques can be expected to give access to much that is obscured. It remains true, though, that virtually all observations of the state of development of an individual organism come from terminations of pregnancy in births, stillbirths and miscarriages. In these circumstances, even in pregnancies in which knowledge about the incursion of a noxious factor is precise, direct knowledge of its relation to the initiation of a maldevelopment is not to be had. This uncertainty beclouds and renders indeterminate many inferences about teratogenesis.

Our examination of the classic studies of Hertig et al. (1959) (to be discussed in Chapter 4) underlines the point. No more precise and exquisitely timed observations of the very early stages of development could be hoped for than to retrieve—from an excised uterus and its appendages—ova fertilized by coition at the time of ovulation. These circumstances still leave us unable to penetrate the secret early developmental phase of a majority of conceptions. The manner of retrieval used in that study yields a cross-sectional and not a longitudinal view, leaving the true probabilities of maldevelopment, attrition and survival hidden. We must rest content with estimates founded on assumption.

Although the time sequence between a causal factor and its consequence is a fundamental property of causality, once established it has little further to contribute to verification for the causal analyst. On the other hand, time order is crucial as a falsifying criterion. For instance, a report of the early 1960s (Stott 1961) indicated that in Down's syndrome prenatal maternal exposure to stressors was reported more frequently than in other pregnancies. The causal explanation offered for this association could be decisively rejected from existing knowledge of time order: known facts were sufficient to deduce that the underlying disorder must have arisen before the postulated stresses of a recognized pregnancy. Yet it is an indication of the quicksands into which faulty knowledge of time order can lead that this inference could pass muster for publication almost 30 years ago. In a more recent report (Shapiro et al. 1983), a reduced frequency of congenital anomalies at birth was considered as a possible result of improved perinatal health services. This idea, too, is incompatible with the known facts, which are sufficient to deduce that nearly all such anomalies arise before most women enter health care for their pregnancies.

STRENGTH OF ASSOCIATION

The stronger the association between a suspect factor and a reproductive outcome, the more likely it is that the association is causal. This follows from the scarcity of strong associations and the frequency of weak ones (Susser 1987). If we are mistaken in designating the independent variable in any association as the causal factor, then some other related factor must be the true cause. To produce such confounding, the factor wrongly suspected as causal in the initial observation must be associated with the outcome no less strongly than is the true cause. The stronger an observed association, the less this is likely to be the case, and hence the less the likelihood of confounding.

On the other hand, associations that appear to be weak cannot be ignored for that reason alone; some are certainly causal. Other associations are not truly weak; their measured strength underestimates their true strength. An underestimate could result from imprecision in the specification of a factor or outcome, as we discuss later. It could also result from the incomplete elaboration of a causal model, when more variables are closely involved in the causal process than just the supposed cause and outcome included in the analysis. Thus, a third variable might specify a condition of the causal relationship—for instance, the susceptibility of the host to infection—or it might suppress or distort the relationship (Susser 1973).

The strength of an association is measured by the relative risk, odds ratio, correlation coefficient, or regression coefficient, depending on the method of data collection and on whether the exposure and/or outcome variables are categorical or continuous. The relative risk compares the frequency of a specific outcome among those exposed with that among those not exposed to a factor. The odds ratio compares the odds of exposure among those identified as having a particular outcome (cases) with the odds of exposure among a comparison group unaffected by the outcome under study (controls).

The strength of an association between continuous variables expressed quantitatively—say birth weight as outcome and the number of cigarettes smoked as exposure—can be described by a correlation coefficient. Better, they can be described by a simple linear regression coefficient that estimates the average change in outcome that accompanies a unit of change in the exposure. A multiple regression coefficient describes the concomitant changes in outcome and exposure with other factors held constant. In either instance, one needs to keep in mind the variability in these coefficients under different circumstances; the values obtained are particular to frequency distributions of relevant variables in the study population and not safely generalized.

Although no reason compels a causal factor to give rise to more than a modest association (e.g., less than a twofold relative risk), nearly all definite teratogens have had large relative risks. For instance, mothers of infants with phocomelia, amelia and defects of the radius had an odds ratio for thalidomide exposure 220 times greater than mothers of unaffected infants (Weicker et al. 1962; Lenz and Knapp 1962). A relative risk of 144—which we calculate from the one reported cohort study of thalidomide effects (McBride 1963)—is compatible with and fortifies the risk estimate.

In other instances, the risk estimates are smaller but still substantial. Young women exposed to diethylstilbestrol (DES) in utero, compared with unexposed women, have had relative risks of cervical adenosis estimated in the range 18 to 35 (Herbst et al. 1975; Bibbo et al. 1977). The risks of adenosis among stillbirths and neonatal deaths are of similar magnitude (Johnson et al. 1979). The relative risk of masculinization in female fetuses exposed to androgens—estimated from a study of the use of norethindrone, a progestin that is converted to an androgen (Jacobson 1962)—was 18, although some other reports suggest this could be an overestimate (Bongiovanni and McPadden 1960; Ishizuka et al. 1962; Schardein 1980). The estimated relative risk of discolored teeth after prenatal exposure to tetracycline, again from only one study (Genot et al. 1970), was "infinite"; more than 80 per cent of those exposed and none of the unexposed were affected. The risk of major malformations with exposure to isotretinoin early in gestation, observed in only 28 prospectively studied deliveries (Lammer et al. 1985), appears to be from 9 to 26 times higher than expected. One notable exception to the rule of large risks is the relatively small risk for low birth weight with cigarette smoking, which is about twofold for birth weights of less than 2500 grams.

Misclassification of Exposure

Estimates of risk often vary substantially from one study to another. A number of circumstances influence the stability of such estimates; one of importance is the accuracy and precision with which exposure is measured, coded, and hence classified. Exposure is misclassified when exposed persons are classed as unexposed, or vice versa. Such misclassifications may be either nondifferential and random (i.e., independent of the outcome under study) or differential and nonrandom (i.e., biased systematically toward or against the study outcome). With differential misclassification, that is, the rates of misclassifying true exposure among those affected and among those unaffected are unequal.

Nondifferential misclassification, since it is unbiased in relation to the outcome, ordinarily leads to an underestimation of the true strength of association, but without change in the true direction of the association. Change in the direction of the association accompanying the misestimation cannot be ruled out entirely. Such reversals are possible when the sum of the proportions misclassified among those truly exposed and those truly unexposed is more than 100 per cent. They are also possible when a third confounding variable is randomly misclassified (Greenland and Kleinbaum 1983).

Differential misclassification artifactually links the exposure to the outcome. With such systematic misclassification, the estimated strength of association between exposure and outcome may be either too high or too low (Copeland et al. 1977). Unlike nondifferential misclassification under ordinary circumstances, differential misclassification on sufficient scale may produce a spurious association when in truth none exists; at the extreme, the direction of an association may be reversed.

Nondifferential misclassification of exposure certainly occurred in early studies of the congenital rubella syndrome (reviewed by Hardy 1973). Precise classification requires a sensitive and specific indicator of rubella virus infection, at least in the mother, and preferably in the fetus. After Gregg (1941) had discovered the association of rubella with a cluster of congenital cataracts in his ophthalmic practice, infection could still be defined only by a woman's report of a typical illness and rash or, at best, by direct clinical observation.

In all those studies, previous to the availability of antibody tests, both exposed and unexposed pregnancies must sometimes have been misclassified. Subclinical maternal infection is common and has been shown to place the fetus at risk (Avery et al. 1965). In epidemics, infected women with neither signs nor symptoms (Green et al. 1965; Brody 1966) will be assigned to the unexposed group. Conversely, some pregnant women with exanthemata difficult to distinguish from rubella may be mistakenly assigned to the exposed group (reviewed by Hardy 1973; Benenson 1975). Rubella tends to occur in epidemics. During any epidemic of an infectious disease such misclassification of exposure is typical: the number misclassified tends to be greater than when no epidemic is known to be active, although the proportion of all cases misclassified tends to be smaller.

Once rubella virus was isolated (Weller and Neva 1962; Parkman et al. 1962) and an antibody test was developed (Stewart et al. 1967), it became possible to assess immune reaction to the virus and to diagnose infection with precision. Fetal infection, we are now sure, does not always follow maternal infection; when it does, malformation does not always follow the fetal infection. The stage of gestation during which maternal infection occurs is one condition for the occurrence of rubella-related malformations (Miller et al. 1982). This is first a matter of the stage of organogenesis at which infection supervenes, but apparently also of the varying frequency of transmission of infection from pregnant woman to fetus. Transmission appears to be most frequent in the first trimester and again shortly before delivery (Miller et al. 1982); only first-trimester transmission is relevant to malformations. The immune state of the mother is another condition affecting transmission: fetal infection seems to be rare with repeat maternal infection (Cradock-Watson et al. 1981).

In the presence of demonstrated fetal infection, the risk of malformation rises sharply. Among all the infants of mothers infected during pregnancy, 8.5 per cent had typical congenital rubella syndrome malformations. Among those infants known to be infected from the presence of immunoglobulin antibodies—IgM in the newborn period or persisting IgG after the first year of age—20 per cent had typical malformations (Miller et al. 1982). Clearly not all infections that mothers transmit, indeed it appears only a minority of them, are damaging to their fetuses.

Differential misclassification of exposure probably occurred in studies of the thalidomide disaster. In at least one study (Weicker et al. 1962), such biased misclassification is to be expected because the procedures for obtaining a history of exposure appeared to differ among affected and among unaffected pregnancies. Among "cases" (154 infants with phocomelia), exposure of mothers in early pregnancy was determined from medical records, from searches for medicines in the home, and from four consecutive interviews. At the third and fourth interviews, specific inquiry was made about the use of the drug. The estimate of exposure frequency at the first interview was only 24 per cent; at the end of all these procedures, the frequency had risen to 70 per cent. Among the 314 controls, no similar ascertainment procedure is described. If, as it appears, the controls were less fully investigated, the 1 per cent among them who supposedly used thalidomide is bound to be an underestimate. It would follow that the odds ratio of 243 relating thalidomide to phocomelia is a biased overestimate.

Misclassification of Outcome

Errors in assigning outcome are of the same two types as are found in misclassification of the exposure: if the errors do not vary with exposure status, the misclassification is nondifferential; if they do vary with exposure status, the misclassification is differential. As with exposure, the nondifferential misclassification of outcome status ordinarily leads to underestimates of the strength of an association, although the same exceptions hold. When misclassification is differential, say because the method of ascertaining pregnancy outcome differs for exposed and unexposed, then again the estimated association may be strengthened, or weakened, or even reversed in direction.

With fetal alcohol syndrome, for example, overestimation is probable in early studies. In most of the studies, with only a few exceptions (Vitez et al. 1984; Ernhart et al. 1985), the diagnosis was made with knowledge of maternal alcohol consumption and therefore subject to ascertainment bias (Susser 1984). In general, as in particular with the fetal alcohol syndrome, when initial reports prove startling and subsequent observers are not blind to the exposure, differential misclassification is likely to lead to overestimates of the strength of association. In more usual circumstances, misclassification is often nondifferential and leads to underestimates.

To sum up the matter of *strength of association* and its accurate estimation, it is in teratology as in other fields a powerful affirmative criterion for causal inference. Although single studies are seldom definitive, enormous relative risks such those found with rubella and thalidomide exposures are not easily overturned. Weak associations must generally be regarded as indeterminate unless buttressed by the additional criteria that favor a positive causal inference, including some to be discussed. In other words, weak associations are not falsifying any more than they are persuasive until the ever-continuing process of testing brings in sufficient evidence to guide judgments about causality.

CONSISTENCY ON REPLICATION

The consistency of an association on repeated test depends on its replicability across a variety of samples and with a variety of research strategies. A consistent association, even one that is neither strong nor specific, is less likely to be spurious than an association observed on one or few occasions (Susser 1973).

In any single study an association may emerge that is owed to an unmeasured confounding variable or to unrecognized bias in the design of the study. The replication of an association under different conditions makes the possibility of these sources of error less likely. Thus, the degree of consistency of association contributes heavily to the judgment that an observation is true. Consistency evenhandedly verifies or refutes; inconsistency renders judgment indeterminate. When consistency is unattainable, as in a single set of observations, a firm causal inference usually cannot be made unless the association is very strong, highly specific, and backed by its coherence with collateral evidence. The corollary is that, if an association is modest, consistency in repeated studies weighs the more heavily.

The contribution of consistency in assessing whether an association is real, and if real whether it is causal, is seen with cigarette smoking. Evidence for its effects on birth weight on the one hand contrasts with that for effects on congenital malformations on the other. Birth weight exemplifies the way in which consistency leads to a firm causal judgment. Malformations exemplify the way in which inconsistency detracts from such a judgment.

With regard to birth weight, cigarette smoking has been examined in at least 50 studies carried out over more than three decades and in a variety of geographic areas (reviewed in: U.S. Public Health Service 1971; Abel 1980). In virtually every study, a decrement in birth weight among offspring of smokers has been observed, and in the majority the decrement is in excess of 150 grams. This decrease corresponds to an increase in the risk of low birth weight (under 2500 grams) among smokers of 1.3 to 2.2 times that in nonsmokers. The effect of smoking is seemingly modest, since it amounts to less than half a standard deviation of birth weight. Yet the association has held for women from varying ethnic and socioeconomic strata, for women of large and small build, and for offspring of all birth orders and of both sexes.

Most studies did not assess the effects of such possible confounding exposures as alcohol and coffee drinking and marijuana smoking, each of which tends to correlate with cigarette smoking. The consistency of the result alone, however, in many populations of diverse origins and habits, virtually rules out any single confounding factor. In the event, the link of each of these three substances to birth weight is equivocal, and the smoking effect persists with adjustments for them (Kaminski et al. 1978, 1981; Tennes and Blackard 1980; Hingson et al. 1982; Linn et al 1982b, 1983; Kuzma and Sokol 1982; Wright et al. 1983; Marbury et al. 1983; Olsen et al. 1983; Mills et al. 1984; Hatch and Bracken 1986; Kline et al. 1987; Martin and Bracken 1987).

The consistency of this association with birth weight over time is remarkable in the face of the marked changes in the types of cigarettes smoked, especially with filters and reductions in suspect chemicals. For example, although the nicotine and the tar contents of cigarettes have declined markedly in the last decade, in a New York City sample from the period 1975–1980 the magnitude of the association found between smoking and birth weight (adjusted for several factors) is nearly identical to that observed in the same setting between 1959 and 1965 (Kline et al. 1981b). Although constancy over time supports the causal inference, it also points to our ignorance about what constituents of cigarette smoke or what aspects of smoking behavior are responsible.

In the association of maternal smoking with congenital malformations, as noted, inconsistency is a feature. With malformations overall, the risk ratios have ranged from 0.5 to 1.3 (reviewed by Stein et al. 1984a). Such variable findings are compatible with any causal interpretation, whether a null, an adverse, or a protective effect, and they yield little support for any one interpretation. The ambiguity may reside in the use of unrefined or poorly defined variables—notably, combining all malformations when effects might be specific to only one. Studies that grouped malformations anatomically did no better, however. Groupings—of congenital heart diseases, neural tube defects, and cleft lip and/or cleft palate—have each been associated with smoking at least twice, and for each there are also several null or negative findings. In the face of variable results, the causal inference is rendered indeterminate.

Inconsistencies between studies may arise from true differences between populations or from differences related to sampling or method, including study design. To begin with, response rates must be considered. Low response rates threaten the validity of any study, whether cohort or case control in design. The exposed and unexposed or the cases and controls who do respond may have different characteristics from those who do not. The extent of selective ascertainment can be measured and weighed in interpretations, but low response rates, whether the same or different in the two study groups, can render any bias that results irremovable.

Imprecision in the specification of exposure and outcome variables also nurtures inconsistency. With congenital malformations, this problem is ever-present. The problem of precision is connected with the state of knowledge and the quality of the information collected. It is also connected with the design of the study. Depending on design, either the exposure or the outcome variables may be the more affected. Thus case-control designs must often use impoverished measures of exposure, and cohort designs must often use impoverished measures of outcome.

Case-control studies are uniquely threatened by differences in the accuracy of reports of exposure between cases and controls. If they do differ, a high response rate is no protection against the reporting bias and spurious estimates of exposure and risk that can result. For instance, women who have borne malformed infants might differ from those with unaffected infants in their inclination to respond to questions about "undesirable" habits such as smoking and drinking, or about factors they perceive as carrying a potential risk, such as the use of medications (see Mitchell et al. 1981; Bracken 1984). Cohort studies, which have an advantage in ascertaining exposure without bias before the outcome is known, are more liable to threats from bias in the ascertainment of outcome for a number of reasons. Foreknowledge of a suspect exposure, for example, may influence the assessment of outcome, whether it is based on reports of the subjects themselves or on the observations of examiners. Cohort studies are perhaps most vulnerable to follow-up that differs in degree of completeness for exposed and unexposed.

To conclude, the power of consistency as a verifying criterion is seen in the modest association of cigarette smoking with birth weight, a finding entrenched by the consensus of a large number of studies. The finding also gains from the realization that the size of the effect on birth weight turns out not to be so modest relative to the effect of other factors. Inconsistency, seen in the association of cigarette smoking with congenital malformations, leads to a judgment of indeterminacy. Although we lean toward rejecting a causal relationship, the force of these inconsistent results carries less conviction and leaves more room for studies to overturn the current stalemate than does the consistency of the results for birth weight. This balance between consistency and inconsistency holds generally in the application of the criterion. That is, consistency is a forceful verifying or falsifying criterion, but inconsistency alone is a weak criterion that leaves the questions at issue unanswered.

2 Criteria for Teratogenesis: II. Specificity of Association

Specificity refers to the singularity of the association between factor and outcome. In its ideal form, one factor to the exclusion of others is associated with one outcome to the exclusion of others. The more causes that contribute to a single outcome, or the more outcomes that follow from a single cause, the less specific is the association. Complete specificity, when outcome and factor only and always occur together, is seldom if ever found in the absence of contrivance. In its common usage, specificity conceals an ambiguity. Every association is two-sided in that it can be scrutinized separately from the side of the independent and from that of the dependent variables. Such scrutiny adds to complexity but also to comprehension. Thus, departures from specificity in causes and outcomes need to be treated separately. In either case, one must recognize that specificity is based on induction and is highly vulnerable to Hume's inductive fallacy: it is never definitive and the existence of other causes or other outcomes cannot be ruled out.

Complete *specificity-in-the-effect* is present when a factor has only one outcome; the more outcomes of a given cause, the less specific the association is. In terms of clinical manifestations, specificity-in-the-effect is not common. One example, admittedly at a refined level of interpretation, is provided by the synthetic hormone diethylstilbestrol (DES), which was once widely used to treat threatened miscarriage and to prevent repeated miscarriages. Adverse effects take several forms. These include underdevelopment and maldevelopment of the reproductive organs and both benign and malignant neoplasia of the cells lining the vagina. All of these effects are confined to the reproductive tract, however, and seem ultimately to be the result of a single disorder of cell development or histiogenesis (Walker 1984).

Complete *specificity-in-the-cause* is present when an outcome has only one cause; the more the number of factors connected with a given outcome, the less singular and specific they are. One example of an apparently specific cause is found with cola-coloring of infants, which so far occurs only in the offspring of mothers exposed to polychlorbiphenyls (PCB) (Rogan 1982).

Refinement of the Outcome Variable

In searching for specificity of either type, we need to be aware that uncertainties may pervade the classification of effects that appear to be distinct but may or may not be so. For example, to group neural tube defects is common practice. This single grouping is not likely to be homogeneous; it comprises an assembly of manifestations—anencephaly, craniorhachischisis, encephalocele, meningocele, myelocele and combinations of these (Leck 1977). Several of these might relate to different causes or combinations of causes. Compression of all these manifestations even into two classes—anencephaly and spina bifida—somewhat refines analysis, but it still does not eliminate potential heterogeneity.

Cruder classifications than this are commonly used. Operational definitions of pregnancy outcomes have often been governed less by biological understanding than by the needs of research strategy and sample size. On occasion, particularly in case-control studies, each clinical manifestation has been treated as a separate entity. More commonly—especially because of the notably low frequency of malformations encountered with the cohort design—refined categories have been grouped to form cruder ones. Such grouping may obscure relationships, especially when a factor poses risk for an outcome that is but a minor constituent of a larger group of outcomes unrelated to the factor. The relevant outcome may be overshadowed by the other constituents of the group and the risk could go undetected. On the other hand, a factor capable of producing a number of effects that are severe and distinct but also rare may go undetected because individual effects of the related set are treated separately; ungrouped, they may not form samples of sufficient size to demonstrate an association with the factor. Here we meet the hoary taxonomic problem of "splitting and lumping."

In the search for causes, then, the question is what are the advantages of treating outcomes separately or of aggregating them? The question revolves around the three issues of plausible theory, existing knowledge, and research design. Theories of pathogenesis invoke, mandate, or proscribe the particular effects; what is known about the natural history of the conditions under study imposes a logical requirement for classification compatible with that existing knowledge; and research design poses practical requirements that limit choice.

Pathogenesis   In the field of teratogenesis, pathogenetic theory for the most part gives little positive guidance in classifying conditions in the search for unknown causes. On the other hand, pathogenetic theory often gives decisive guidance, in a negative sense, in excluding certain conditions from a category. Obviously, any condition owed to a major gene is not the consequence of teratogenesis and must be excluded. If a hypothesis invokes exposure in the latter half of pregnancy, malformations resulting from disordered organogenesis in the early weeks of pregnancy must also be excluded, and vice versa.

When theory is well-grounded, its contributions are greater. In our study of the Dutch famine, which aimed to test whether acute prenatal malnutrition depleted brain cells and thus depressed subsequent mental performance, pathogenetic theory made strong contributions that were both affirmative and negative (Stein et al. 1975a). Effects on brain size could be placed firmly in the second half of pregnancy or later, after the brain cells had begun to proliferate and then grow in size. This entailed critical exposure that could also be expected to act in the second half of pregnancy. Further, theory contributed on the negative side of excluding certain outcomes. In line with theory, the main postulated outcome was mild mental retardation resulting from a depleted number of brain cells. Since structural central nervous system damage was not at issue, it followed that severe mental retardation, nearly always accompanied by structural brain impairment, was not a key outcome. Other outcomes arising in the first half of pregnancy could also be treated as irrelevant to the central hypothesis.

Weakly grounded pathogenetic theory can as easily spawn error as produce a salient classification. From an observation that malformations of different organ systems occur in the same individual more often than would be expected by chance, some authors have argued for a common cause of all malformations (Roberts and Powell 1975). The theory that individuals carry a general predisposition to malformations requires a model that takes aggregation to an extreme and places all malformations in a single group with no very evident biological basis. Similarly, a common genetic predisposition has been postulated to explain the apparently excessive familial aggregation of several types of malformation (Fraser et al. 1972).

In line with this idea of a common cause, another theory reversed the general understanding about fetal growth retardation, arguing that it underlies (rather than follows) a variety of malformations (Spiers 1982). Although it is true that malformations cluster in individuals and families and also occur in conjunction with low birth weight more often than would be expected by chance (Leck 1975; Heinonen et al. 1977), the distinct epidemiologic characteristics of specific malformations and their several patterns of familial aggregation count against a single common cause (Leck 1975). Thus, while these theories are all subject to test—and may deserve testing—they are not theories to be used in creating pragmatic classifications from existing knowledge.

Weak theory, combined with a paucity of fact, allows one to entertain a great variety of pathogenetic hypotheses. The large number of possibilities leaves open the choice of an appropriate classification. At first sight, the diversity of teratogenic effects that are characteristic of successive stages of gestation seems to argue for the separation of outcomes by stage of gestation, as in the Dutch famine study cited earlier. Organ defects can be attributed to disordered organogenesis in early gestation and distinguished from effects that appear later such as small body size, slow growth and so-called deformations (anatomical deformities possibly resulting from intrauterine physical forces).

These manifest differences in pathology do not dispose of the case for grouping. At least two good grounds for grouping remain. First, a common cause capable of acting at different stages of gestation might result in a different pathogenesis at each stage and produce different effects. Second, a common pathogenesis might proceed at a fundamental molecular, cellular, or tissue level, and produce seemingly diverse effects at higher levels of organization. Under both these conditions, a single environmental cause could produce multiple outcomes, whether syndromes affecting single individuals or constellations of different malformations affecting populations.

Prenatal rubella infection illustrates the first case. Here a common cause, in the form of single pathogen, acts at different stages of gestation to produce multiple effects. Congenital heart defects, nerve deafness, and cataracts all arise at different stages of gestation. Singly or in combination, depending on timing, all can result from prenatal rubella infection (Miller et al. 1982).

Maternal diabetes also produces multiple disorders in offspring. At least some of these can be attributed to the same underlying metabolic derangements acting at different stages of gestation. Hyperglycemia appears to be a major factor in pathogenesis, although the protopathic bias of insulin treatment and resultant hypoglycemia cannot be entirely ruled out. Offspring of women with diabetes during pregnancy face two to four times the risk of a major congenital malformation as do the offspring of nondiabetic women, prediabetic women, and diabetic fathers. Findings have been consistent whether the populations under study were Pima Indians in Arizona (Comess et al. 1969) or the cohorts of white, black and Hispanic women enrolled at 12 different sites across the United States in the National Collaborative Perinatal Project (Chung and Myrianthopoulos 1975). The disorders found in the offspring of diabetic women involve multiple organ systems more often than do malformations in the offspring of women who are not diabetic; in addition, the malformations appear in excess in many individual organ systems (reviewed in Bennett et al. 1979). The malformations can be attributed to very early stages of gestation (Mills 1982). At the same time, the long-range postnatal manifestations of excessive growth rate, stature and obesity are foreshadowed in the fetus in the later stages of gestation

(Pettit et al. 1983; Pettitt and Bennett 1988) and are most likely attributable to disturbances during that stage.

Prenatal starvation also illustrates the multiple effects of a common
cause—this time in the form of a complex pathogen with many social
connotations—again acting at different stages in development. Cohorts
exposed to the Dutch famine in the earlier months of pregnancy experienced an excess of central nervous system abnormalities, of preterm
births and first-week neonatal deaths, and of obesity in adult male survivors. Cohorts exposed at the same time to exactly the same set of
circumstances, but in the later months of pregnancy, experienced
lowered birth weight, an excess of deaths in the first 3 months of life,
and a deficiency of obesity in adult males (Stein et al. 1975a; Ravelli et al.
1976). The complexity of the pathogen is patent in a situation in which
the ravages of famine were accompanied by the brutalities of the Nazi
occupation, and some of the historical factors bound up with exposure
to starvation are unmeasurable and remain uncontrolled. Nonetheless,
the observations demonstrate sharp distinctions between effects of a
common complex of causes acting at different stages of gestation.

The second case—common pathogenesis at a fundamental level that
produces diverse effects at higher levels of organization—might be illustrated by thalidomide and other drugs and also by the effects of the
metabolic defects of hyperphenylalaninemia. With thalidomide, the developing organism has proved susceptible only through the narrow win-
dow of time from 34 to 50 days after the last menstrual period (Lenz
1964). Effects vary even within these bounds. Besides the typical limb
defects, reported defects affect the ear, the eye, the cranial nerves, and
the cardiovascular, gastrointestinal, and renal systems (Kajii 1965; Takemori et al. 1976; reviewed by Khera 1984). These multifarious clinical
defects might well originate, at the cellular or molecular level, in a common pathogenetic process. Thus, one proposition is that a single underlying mechanism—damage to the neural crest—produces both skeletal
and visceral abnormalities (McCredie 1974).

In discussing diethylstilbestrol earlier, we referred to the apparently
common histiogenic origin of reproductive tract anomalies ranging
from anatomical defects to benign vaginal adenosis and malignant adenocarcinoma of the vagina (Walker 1984). With isotretinoin, a single
defect in neural-crest activity common to the craniofacial, cardiac, thy-
mus, and central nervous system defects can be inferred from animal
studies (Lammer et al. 1985). With prenatal hyperphenylalaninemia,
too, effects are diverse. They include congenital cardiac anomalies, microcephaly and mental retardation, and all these are products of a single
inherited metabolic abnormality (reviewed in Lenke and Levy 1980).

Natural History   Attention to the natural history of reproductive outcomes can aid in decisions about classification, especially if knowledge of

pathogenesis is also brought to bear. On the one hand, dissimilarities in the population distributions of congenital defects—including those of the same as well as different organ systems—suggest that their causes are likely to differ (Leck 1977). Thus, the risk factors for the various positional foot deformities are not the same, nor are those for the various types of congenital heart disease. Thalidomide did not produce every kind of limb reduction deformity but only certain specific ones.

On the other hand, similarities in natural history might justify "*lumping*" no less than dissimilarities might justify "*splitting.*" The concomitant variations found with anencephaly and spina bifida give grounds for grouping besides their common anatomical origin. The two conditions share a number of features including high frequencies in Ireland and the United Kingdom and similar secular trends within geographic areas (Leck 1974, 1977; Elwood and Elwood 1980). In the same fashion, two other conditions—isolated cleft lip and cleft palate combined with cleft lip—share anatomical origins as well as a male preponderance that can justify grouping. On the contrary side, with isolated cleft palate, natural history favors separation from cleft palate combined with cleft lip, because in isolated cleft palate females are preponderant (Leck 1977).

Familial recurrence is an aspect of the natural history of anomalies that can be a telling criterion in classification. Justification for grouping can be found in the occurrence within the same families of different anomalies, especially when the same organ system or a common pathogenesis may be involved. For instance, after a woman has had either an anencephalic or spina bifida birth, she is at greater risk for both defects in subsequent births (Elwood and Elwood 1980). At the same time, some underlying differences between the two types of anomaly coexist with their similarities. With both defects the propensity for the same defect to recur is greater than for the other to occur.

Another example of the recurrence of related events that on a strict definition are dissimilar involves late miscarriage and premature birth. Although these two outcomes have seldom been examined together, as might be anticipated they appear to share mechanisms related to premature onset of labor. Thus, women who experience repeated late miscarriages also have higher rates of viable preterm births (Strobino et al. 1980b).

Practical Issues   In examining the pragmatic issues of research design, rhyme or reason are not at once evident in the practice of researchers. Reasons for grouping are seldom made explicit. Unrelated effects may come to be grouped together inappropriately on the basis of false theory, false assumptions, or inadequate observations or recording. Sometimes grouping aims to increase numbers and statistical power, for doubtful gain if the outcomes do not have common origins. At other times, manifestations recognized as heterogeneous may be grouped out of simple necessity, because the detail that would allow the entity to be divided into its constituents is not on the record.

Miscarriage is a striking example of heterogeneous outcome that is usually treated as homogeneous for lack of information. Later chapters emphasize the dichotomy between miscarriages with normal and those with aberrant chromosomes. Forty to fifty per cent are chromosomally aberrant and these, depending on the type of aberration, can be attributed to factors operating before or at conception. Factors operating during pregnancy, however, have their predominant impact on the chromosomally normal fraction. Even this fraction is not homogeneous. In some miscarriages with normal chromosomes, the conceptus is morphologically abnormal and in others apparently normal, and again their causes can be expected to differ.

In practice, approaches to grouping malformations are far from uniform. Sometimes all malformations are grouped together in a single class on the ground that they all arose during organogenesis. Sometimes all those of a single organ system are grouped on the presumption that teratogens are organ-specific. Sometimes, with less theoretical but some practical justification, malformations are grouped by severity as major or minor. Grouping by severity partly protects against inconsistent or irregular ascertainment and variable detection and recording of minor malformations.

At the stage of data collection, splitting is almost always the prudent approach. Data collected and preserved in a refined form leave open the option of grouping or separating entities on analysis. Aside from this practical reason, the weakness and paucity of theory enjoin caution in grouping before specific effects have been sought.

Refinement of the Exposure Variable

Often an exposure can be measured only in a crude and unrefined manner. Merely to designate individuals as exposed to a factor is insufficient to capture the exact risk that attends exposure. Even were the designation to be entirely accurate and without misclassification, only a part of the exposed group might experience the factor in a way that increased the risk of a particular outcome. Low doses, lack of individual susceptibility, and timing asynchronous with critical developmental phases might all block the emergence of an effect.

The chances for discovering a new association improve if the exposure is neither rare in the population targeted for study, nor ubiquitous in the general population; they are best where those exposed constitute a sizeable subgroup, identifiable by social, occupational or other experience. Chances also improve if the exposure has a large, striking effect or an unusual effect. Should the consequences of such an exposure approach specificity-in-the effect, or seeming specificity-in-the-cause for a particular outcome, chances further improve. The rubella epidemic of 1940 met some of these conditions: exposure was widespread but not ubiquitous, and its teratogenic effects were strong, unusual and fairly specific. The teratogenic properties of rubella virus nevertheless had waited long to be discovered; it was only the clustering of one of its more unusual effects, congenital cataracts, that revealed its cryptic role to a practicing ophthalmologist (Gregg 1941). By comparison, the discovery that thalidomide was teratogenic in about 18 months was rapid indeed. The association of the new drug with phocomelia was strong and specific and the defect striking and unusual. Thus, the connection emerged even in study populations diluted by exposed women not at risk, such as those who used the drug after the critical period of organogenesis.

In meeting conditions that favor detection, the rubella and thalidomide episodes were not typical. Chance and fortune outside the control of the researcher favored discovery. On the other hand, the specification of exposure (as well as of the outcome, as discussed previously) is, to a variable degree, within the grasp of the researcher. By refining the exposure variable, the researcher can improve specificity in general and, in turn, enhance the measured strength of association. Refinement of the exposure variable is achieved by precisely defining the constituents of the factor itself, precisely estimating the dose of exposure, and taking account of susceptibility to the factor, for instance, in terms of developmental phase of the organism at the time of exposure.

The Nature of the Factor   When individuals or communities have been exposed to a particular factor, it is not unusual to find on investigation that they have encountered not one but many suspect substances. Although at the Love Canal toxic dump site in Niagara, New York, the actual number of chemicals present was unknown, scores were detected in unusually high concentrations (Vianna 1980). Such cases engender severe problems of inference because no truly comparable multifarious exposure will ever recur. There is no way of telling which if any of the congeries of chemicals at Love Canal was responsible for the adverse outcomes reported.

More typical problems arise with cigarette smoking. Exposure to cigarette smoke has generally been defined in one of three ways: present or absent (smoker, nonsmoker), amount smoked in a given time, or total amount and duration of smoking. Cigarettes expose the smoker to numerous constituents, some of which vary with the brand smoked and some with the style of smoking (Stedman 1968; U.S. Public Health Service 1979). The evidence on maternal smoking is, as noted earlier, sufficient to support a firm causal connection to intrauterine growth retardation. For this and the many other outcomes studied, however, the strength of the associations might have been undermined by an unrefined index of exposure to smoking. Thus, the usual definitions of exposure may not capture the relevant constituents of tobacco smoke or the dose involved. Refinement may strengthen the estimated association by focusing on the elements of exposure as well as outcome that are most germane to the hypothesis under study.

Dose   Refinement achieved by specifying the dose of the exposure usually strengthens estimates of association. This holds whether the likelihood of a particular outcome increases in parallel with dose or is raised only when exposure rises above a threshold level. Common problems in measuring any exposure include the difficulties of estimating the amounts emitted by the source of exposure, the intimacy and duration of contact, and selective losses from the exposed cohort, especially among those affected. Measures in the pregnant woman have the added problem that they are at a remove from measures of exposure of the conceptus which, were they attainable, would be more to the point in teratogenesis.

Dose can be described in terms of the amount of exposure either during the whole of pregnancy or during a presumed critical period in gestation; in each case the index can be the total, the average, or the maximum dose. Which of these six different ways of characterizing dose is most relevant to the outcome under study will seldom be clear at the outset. When exposure is episodic, a precise estimate may require the determination of the frequency of episodes and of the amount and duration of exposure on each occasion. A continuous exposure will need to be checked for constancy. All these determinations depend on the reliability and accuracy of memory, of records, or of clinical observations and biochemical indices at various points in time. If biological markers of effect are used to indicate exposure, then additional questions of validity arise; a marker of effect in the woman is not necessarily an indicator of the dose that will produce an effect in the fetus.

In practice, it may be difficult to distinguish between effects resulting from a cumulative dose and effects resulting from exposure during a critical period of gestation. That is, if exposure is continuous and the stage of gestation is a condition for an effect of exposure, effects may be incorrectly attributed to cumulative dose rather than to dose during a critical period—and vice versa. An example of this difficulty in discriminating between the timing and the total amount of exposure is found in two studies of vaginal adenosis in women exposed prenatally to diethylstilbestrol (Herbst et al. 1975; Sonek et al. 1976). The stage of gestation at which treatment begins limits the possible dose. In both series, however, stage of gestation also dictated the dosage schedule prescribed. The potential confounding of the amount of the treatment with the timing of the treatment makes it difficult, without collateral evidence, to distinguish a critical-period effect from a cumulative-dose effect.

In the event, the earlier treatment began, the more serious and common disorders of the vagina and cervix in the offspring appeared to be. For adenocarcinoma of the vagina, risk was highest when treatment began at 5 to 6 weeks; treatment begun at 9 to 16 weeks carried a lower risk. For the milder form of cellular dysplasia seen as adenosis, risks were also higher with early treatment. Strictly, from these data risk cannot be attributed to a critical period. On the other hand, the fact that the very large range of dosage showed no relation to cancer risk does favor a critical-period rather than a dose-effect hypothesis (Walker 1984).

The duration of the pregnancy itself needs to be taken into account in assessing exposure, since the longer the pregnancy, the greater is the opportunity for exposure. Confounding as a result of the censoring of opportunities for exposure is an especial hazard with teratogens that themselves affect duration of pregnancy. Hence, in case–control studies in which the cases are pregnancies that end early and the controls are births, the longer duration of gestation in controls can lead to inadvertent overestimates of accumulating exposures among them and, as a result, to underestimates of risk ratios. Appropriate measures of exposure limit comparisons to the length of gestation through which miscarriages endure.

In studies of continuing prenatal exposures and birth weight, also, early deliveries may lead to contradictory effects. The longer the pregnancy, the greater the opportunity for exposure but the larger the birth weight will be. At the same time, an adverse factor may itself lead to early termination and may lower birth weight on that account. With a beneficial factor that raises birth weight, effects might be overestimated if length of gestation is not controlled. An increase in birth weight attributed to nutritional supplementation in a large-scale study in Central America (Habicht et al. 1974) could be overestimated in just this way. The longer pregnancy continues, the higher the birth weight, but also the more supplement a woman can take; hence supplementation might spuriously appear to raise birth weight. Clearly the effects of any exposure during pregnancy are likely to be misestimated if length of gestation is not taken into account.

Teratogenic effects may differ depending on the dose. In the experimental animal, large doses early in gestation tend to be lethal to the embryo, which allows no opportunity to observe effects in survivors. On the other hand, surviving offspring may have experienced smaller doses, and only in them is it possible to observe nonlethal effects such as malformations or growth disturbances. For example, in pregnant Wistar rats, large doses of tumor-inhibiting chemicals such as chlorambucil were associated with complete resorption of the litter. Smaller doses of the same chemicals were associated with increased rates of various malformations (Murphy 1960).

This finding has a moral for human studies. Without close monitoring of effects from conception on, the conflation of different doses with different effects can mislead. For instance, early embryonic death may never be detected simply because pregnancy itself cannot be detected at and just after conception. Thus, with high levels of exposure only intact survivors might be available for observation so that no effects are seen while with lower levels later in gestation teratogenic effects might appear. An example of this kind is found in cohort studies in the aftermath of the atomic bombing of Hiroshima. Microcephaly and mental retardation were most strongly associated with heavy exposures from the eighth through the fifteenth week of gestation (Wood et al. 1967a; Miller and Mulvihill 1976; Otake and Schull 1984). A deficiency of births among women exposed to heavy doses, however, suggested that embryonic attrition had occurred in the first 3 weeks of gestation (Miller and Blot 1972). It might be relevant that, at later stages of gestation, an excess of fetal deaths was in fact observed when the radiation dose had been sufficient to cause radiation sickness in the woman (Yamazaki et al. 1954).

With such gaps in observation discounted, the more typical human experience is that the severity of effect is consistent with the size of the dose. Thus with alcohol exposure during pregnancy, chronic heavy drinking is needed to produce the embryopathy of the fetal alcohol syndrome (reviewed in Neugut 1981 and Abel 1984). Moderate drinking has been linked with lesser effects such as lowered birth weight or with no effect at all (reviewed by Stein and Kline 1983; Mills et al. 1984; Kline et al. 1987; Sulaiman et al. 1988).

Stage of Gestation   In characterizing organogenesis, embryologists proposed the idea of the critical period, a stage in gestation when a disturbance or a noxious factor may cause a disorder of development that is irreversible (Stockard 1921). In this light, the timing of events assumes particular importance for teratogenesis. A reasonable criterion for a teratogen is that the nature of the outcome corresponds to the timing in gestation of an appropriate mechanism that could produce the outcome. This criterion poses the difficulty that many pathogenetic mechanisms remain in doubt. For example, competing ideas about anencephaly and spina bifida postulate, on the one hand, that the neural tube fails to close (von Recklinghausen 1886) and, on the other hand, that the neural tube closes but later reopens (Morgagni 1762). If the first and now favored mechanism operates, exposure must occur before day 27 after conception (Elwood and Elwood 1980). Thus, a reported association between hormonal pregnancy tests and spina bifida (Gal et al. 1967; Gal 1972) could be questioned because exposure in some cases occurred after the likely time of pathogenesis (Sever 1973).

Exposure to a single teratogen that persists throughout gestation, we have noted, might produce different effects at successive stages. If the exposure variable is refined, therefore, by excluding as irrelevant exposures after the affected organs have developed, specificity and consequently estimated strength of association are enhanced. The thalidomide disaster affords an example. In 112 mothers of infants with phocomelia and 188 mothers of unaffected infants (Lenz and Knapp 1962), for thalidomide taken at any time during pregnancy the odds ratio is 215; for thalidomide taken only during early pregnancy the odds ratio rises to 380.

Evidence of various kinds can aid us in fixing the time of exposure. In diabetic women, for instance, one analyst used existing knowledge of organogenesis to attribute malformations in their offspring to critical periods of development at 3 to 6 weeks of gestation (Mills 1982). In another approach to timing in diabetes, preconception and periconception blood sugar levels have been inferred from measurements of glycosylated hemoglobin levels (HbA_1) taken at the first prenatal visit before the fifteenth week of gestation. Women with high levels had offspring with higher rates of malformations than women with lower levels. From such data, teratogenic effects have been attributed to uncontrolled hyperglycemia in the period immediately following conception (Leslie et al. 1978; Miller et al. 1981; Ylinen et al. 1984; Stubbs et al. 1987).

Extrapolations backward from blood sugar levels for periods of up to 2 months to average levels at conception and in early pregnancy cannot pinpoint peaks and valleys over that time, nor the exact levels that obtained during the successive stages of organogenesis. A multicenter cohort study was therefore mounted among diabetic women, on the hypothesis that strict control of blood sugar levels in the periconception phase prevents malformations (Mills et al. 1988). Diabetic women intending to conceive were recruited and followed through their pregnancies. The results gave the hypothesis ambiguous support. The rate of malformations in diabetic women recruited and monitored from the beginning of pregnancy remained higher (4.9 per cent) than that in a comparison group of conceptions among nondiabetic women (2.1 per cent). At the same time, a beneficial effect attributable to early treatment did appear: within the group of diabetic women, those who entered the closely controlled regimen of prenatal care early in pregnancy had a lower rate of malformations (4.9 per cent) than those who entered later (9.0 per cent). The ambiguity in this apparent benefit is that the rate of malformations did not correlate with the degree of control of diabetes.

To sum up our discussion of specificity, this criterion is often less easily met in creating an index of exposure (the independent variable) than one of outcome (the dependent variable). Environmental exposures tend to be ill-defined, invisible, poorly observed if observed at all, and dispersed or diffused in uncertain ways. In planned studies it may sometimes be possible to specify the nature of the factor, the exact dose, and the precise time of exposure. More often such precise information about the independent variable is not at hand. In these circumstances, specificity and estimates of strength of association may still be enhanced when the dependent variable can be refined and precisely specified. In choosing specific outcomes and creating dependent variables to measure them, the investigator generally has the advantage of direct observation and a store of clinical experience in describing disorders. In teratology, specificity-in-the-effect bolsters causal inference. Obfuscations of causal relationships may ensue from the use of variables that are either too crude or overrefined. An appropriate degree of refinement and correct classification may be essential to detecting associations.

3 Criteria for Teratogenesis: III. Coherence

Coherence is an ultimate criterion, one in which the observed association is weighed against all previously existing theory and knowledge. Its function is synthetic, to place the result in the context of the current paradigm that governs the theory and constructs of a particular field. Compatibility is sought with the concepts and data of all seemingly relevant domains, for instance with biological theory, with known facts, and with clinical reports. If the association is coherent with preexisting understanding, a causal inference is supported. If it is incoherent, then the hypothesis must be rejected or new theory developed.

The coherence of an association with other clinical and pathological facts and with observations in animals creates a complex with numerous dimensions. Among these, one may separate theoretical, factual, biological, and statistical coherence. Several issues raised under the headings of other criteria can also be subsumed under the criterion of coherence. Thus, the falsification of a causal inference because of incompatibility with the time order of the associated variables rests on factual or theoretical incoherence; and the discovery of a critical developmental stage during which a factor is efficient may not only enhance the specificity of an association but endow it with theoretical coherence in the light of our understanding of prenatal development.

By the logic of this criterion, the focus must include evidence collateral to epidemiology, much of it not based on human observations. Although epidemiological evidence is crucial to establishing environmental causes of abnormal development, biologic and experimental evidence can contribute materially to judgments of causality. Human data which consist only of case reports can also contribute something, as in such examples as exposure to androgenic hormones and tetracycline.

STATISTICAL COHERENCE

Expectations of coherence generated by statistical notions or by the statistical form of observed data, are of many kinds. In considering the refinement and specificity of exposure variables, we referred to the set of expectations that has formed around *dose–response relationships*. A monotonic relationship between a suspect factor and an outcome—one in which the outcome becomes more likely as exposure increases—lends the conviction of common sense to causal inference. The absence of a monotonic relationship, however, does not falsify a causal inference. For manifold reasons, in the empirical world causal factors have been found to produce a great variety of dose–response patterns. Thus, effects may appear only with an exposure or dose that rises above a threshold level. With high doses an underlying linear relationship may be distorted. In an example cited in our discussion of specificity, should high doses early in gestation destroy the conceptus, only those exposed to lower doses would survive to manifest effects later in pregnancy.

Expectations of coherence also tend to be generated by associations at the ecological level—those in which the units of observation refer to groups and not to individuals. One type of ecological association is concomitant variation, in the frequency of exposure and of outcome, with time or place. Concomitant variation may support or lead to causal interpretations of observations at the individual level. For example, two such observations bolstered thalidomide studies on individuals: increases in the frequency of limb anomalies were confined to countries in which thalidomide was marketed (Watson et al. 1962; Smithells 1962) and also fluctuated over time with the sales of thalidomide (Lenz and Knapp 1962; Leck and Millar 1962; Smithells and Leck 1963; Lenz 1964). Similarly, the relationship between clear-cell vaginal adenocarcinoma in young women and prenatal diethylstilbestrol exposure was recognized after a cluster of cases was observed in the late 1960s, although previously the condition was virtually nonexistent in youth. The causal role of the synthetic hormone was reinforced by the correspondence in time, more than a decade earlier, of the birth year of reported cases and the marketing of the drug (Herbst et al. 1977; Herbst 1981).

Observations at the ecologic level on their own seldom justify a causal interpretation at the individual level, since exposure and outcome are not measured in the same individual. The *ecological fallacy* (Robinson 1950; Blalock 1964; Susser 1973) is to interpret an association at one level as if it held equally well at the other level. In well-controlled circumstances, however, ecological observations might justify causal interpretations when the group is the unit. Ecological analyses of the Dutch famine of 1944–45 (Stein et al. 1975a) leave little room for doubt about the causal role of periconceptional maternal starvation in reducing fertility. In this instance, although the outcome data referred to individuals, starvation had to be presumed from the documented effects of famine at the group level. The group effects of famine on the number of births in successive months proved sufficiently striking and robust on analytic test to permit extrapolation to the individual effects of maternal starvation.

BIOLOGICAL COHERENCE

The failure of observations in animals to mimic those in humans does not in itself falsify a causal hypothesis or preclude a causal interpretation. Conversely, the congruence of observations in animals with those in humans can corroborate a causal hypothesis that relates to humans. The strength of animal tests rests, in large part, on the specificity conferred by control of conditions in experimental studies. The timing of exposure in relation to developmental stage, the forms of intervention, and the dose can all be varied, and potentially confounding factors can be controlled.

Examples of corroboration by animal experiments are many. With masculinization following prenatal androgenic hormones, even the first few case reports (Zander and Muller 1953; Hoffman et al. 1955; Hayles and Nolan 1957) could reasonably be interpreted as being causal because of their coherence with studies in rodents, insectivores, and monkeys (reviewed by Jost 1955). Tooth discoloration by tetracycline is coherent with animal studies that show tetracycline to be incorporated in bone and to produce fluorescence of bone and teeth (Owen 1963; Lewis 1964). Human pathology also corroborates this effect. Thus, a study of human abortuses and perinatal deaths in which the mother had taken tetracycline showed bone fluorescence as in the animal studies (Totterman and Saxen 1969). Isotretinoin, an effective treatment for acne, is a retinoic acid and a vitamin A analog. The typical pattern of anomalies that was found in the offspring of women treated during pregnancy closely resembles the pattern in offspring of animals exposed to retinoic acid (Lammer et al. 1985).

The association in humans of prenatal diethylstilbestrol with vaginal adenosis and adenocarcinoma is also compatible with animal study results (Walker 1984). Effects vary with species and strain, and in only some are the pathologic changes analogous to those in humans. In rodents, early neonatal diethylstilbestrol exposure leads to anomalies and cancers of the reproductive tract. This postnatal exposure in mice, it can be argued, conforms with prenatal exposure in humans, since in the newborn mouse the reproductive system is at a developmental stage similar to that in the human fetus as 3 to 4 months gestation (Bern et al. 1976).

Causal inference may also find support from coherence with biological evidence on human beings that is drawn from clinical observations or from pharmacological, pathological, and physiological studies. The many case reports of masculinization of the female fetus occurring with androgens and synthetic progestins were coherent with other findings on maternal arrhenoblastoma (a testosterone-secreting tumor of the ovary) and also congenital adrenal hyperplasia (Evans and Riley 1953; Wilkins 1957). Likewise, the case reports of the discoloration of teeth following prenatal exposure to tetracycline (Rendle-Short 1962; Harcourt et al. 1962; Douglas 1963; Kutscher et al. 1963; Swallow 1964) were coherent with the effects of tetracycline postnatally (Shwachman and Schuster 1956; Zegarelli et al. 1961). When epidemiological data are lacking, such observations sometimes bear the entire burden of inference about causes.

The synthetic function of coherence in causal inference is also illustrated with the vaginal clear-cell adenocarcinomas attributable to diethylstilbestrol. The initial human evidence for an association was brought to attention by a case-control study (Herbst et al. 1971) that might ordinarily have been considered preliminary; it was based on a mere eight cases, one of which was the subject whose mother suggested that the cause might have been the diethylstilbestrol she had been treated with for bleeding in early pregnancy (Herbst, personal communication). Further studies taken individually also had problems. A second small case-control study (Greenwald et al. 1971) compared exposure histories for only five cases and eight controls. In three cohort studies of prenatally exposed women, moreover, no case of vaginal adenocarcinoma has been observed (Herbst et al. 1975; Bibbo et al. 1977; Beral and Colwell 1981).

Yet the absence of malignancies in the three cohort studies does not falsify the hypothesis for human beings. Large numbers are needed to exclude a raised frequency of these rare tumors. A causal association is supported by other coherent results. In cohorts exposed prenatally an increased risk for alterations of the genital tract, including vaginal adenosis, has been found (Herbst et al. 1975; Bibbo et al. 1977). The tissue from which both vaginal adenosis and adenocarcinoma originate is the same (Herbst 1981).

Causal interpretations are especially tenuous when data consist entirely of individual case reports, when associations are inconsistent, and when the suspect factor is so highly correlated with other factors that their effects are difficult to separate. Thus far we have implicitly assumed that epidemiological studies provide the human data from which causality is assessed. For some of the teratogens we have classified as definite, however, clinical case reports have been the main source of human data. Case reports draw attention to the possible specificity of an association, since it is the coincidence of a rare outcome and a rare exposure, or a newly arising exposure, that tends to provoke clinical awareness.

Causal inferences cannot be drawn solely on that basis, with the exception of rare instances with a high degree of specifity-in-the-cause. The main problem is that what is almost certain to enter clinical consciousness and to be reported in the journals is precisely the coincidence of supposed cause and supposed effect. What goes unreported by clinicians is, usually, the same effect in the absence of the supposed cause.

Moreover, what naturally goes unremarked by clinicians is the presence of the supposed cause in the absence of the effect. Almost inevitably, such observations are beyond the reach of the clinician and cannot be reported (Susser 1984).

Epidemiological approaches are needed to bring the nonclinical domain within reach. Thus, in the single available study of isotretinoin, exposed pregnancies were reported to the Food and Drug Administration and the drug manufacturer. Among these, 36 were notified before 12 weeks gestation. From this prospective portion of the sample, estimates of the prevalence of malformation could be made and compared with expectations from a surveillance system (Lammer et al. 1985). In the following we illustrate some of the difficulties that arise in interpreting case reports in the absence of useful epidemiologic studies.

A typical approach to evaluating case reports is to consider—as a rough guide to strength of association—whether the number of reported cases in which exposure and outcome coincide exceeds the number expected if exposure and outcome had occurred at random, that is, independently of each other. This approach invokes several doubtful assumptions.

First, we must assume that outcome has been similarly ascertained among exposed cases and the reference population or sample from which the expected frequency of the outcome is derived. Once early reports have associated the suspect factor with the outcome, clinical vigilance is almost bound to raise the reported frequency of the suspected outcome among exposed pregnancies. For conspicuous conditions such as anencephaly, it can be argued that the likelihood of recognition in the reference population would be as high as in exposed pregnancies. With less conspicuous conditions such as developmental delay or even the dysmorphic facial features of fetal alcohol syndrome, overascertainment among the exposed or, conversely, underascertainment in the reference population is almost ensured.

Second, we must assume that the association of the reported cases with the suspect factor is unconfounded by other factors. That is, we assume that the reported cases are similar to those used for comparison in all respects (other than the suspect exposure) that could affect the occurrence of the condition. When medical treatment is under suspicion as the factor, either the condition under treatment, or other treatments given at the same time, might contribute to the outcome under study and confound an association. When suspicion falls on habits such as alcohol drinking—typically fostered within a complex of social situation, behavior, and constitution—other closely associated habits such as smoking may be confounding factors.

Several problems of inference from case reports arise with a syndrome attributed to vitamin K antagonist warfarin given prenatally (Stein et al. 1984a). The syndrome includes hypoplasia of the nose and stippled epiphyses and rests entirely on case reports. In 1966, a first report appeared of an infant with nasal hypoplasia after prenatal administration of warfarin (DiSaia 1966). In 1968, with the second report (Kerber et al. 1968), the causal conjecture was made. Since then, at least 28 cases in liveborn children exposed prenatally to warfarin have been added (Shaul and Hall 1977; Hall et al 1980; Stein et al 1984a). The syndrome, now labeled warfarin embryopathy, is attributed to exposure at 6 to 9 weeks of gestation (Hall et al. 1980).

The first difficulty with this causal conclusion is the absence of a sound basis for the expected incidence of the syndrome. Another syndrome— the inherited Conradi-Hunermann type of chrondrodysplasia punctata (Spranger et al. 1971)—is similar if not identical to warfarin embryopathy, and has an estimated incidence of only 1 per 500,000 births (Fraser and Scriver 1954). The rarity of this preexisting syndrome enhanced the causal attribution (as rarity also did with phocomelia and thalidomide and with adenocarcinoma of the vagina and diethylstilbestrol). The argument has been somewhat weakened, however, by reports suggesting higher frequencies of the combination of nasal hypoplasia with epiphyseal stippling (Sheffield et al. 1976).

A second difficulty that could undermine a causal conclusion is bias in diagnosis. Bias of the same kind, we pointed out previously, beset the earlier attempts to establish the existence of the fetal alcohol syndrome. For virtually all cases of the prenatal warfarin syndrome, it seems likely that the diagnosis was not made blind to knowledge of exposure. Nasal hypoplasia is the main visible clinical feature of the syndrome. Except for severe cases characterized by choanal stenosis or a sunken nose, nasal hypoplasia is a matter of degree, subjectively assessed and not measured, and liable to be influenced by a history of exposure. In at least five cases in which the nose was either normal or mildly affected (Holzgreve et al. 1976; Harrod and Sherrod 1981; Whitfield 1980; Pettifor and Benson 1975; Pauli, cited by Hall et al. 1980), diagnosis of the syndrome in the absence of knowledge of warfarin exposure would have been improbable.

A third difficulty in interpreting the prenatal warfarin case reports is the potential for confounding by other prenatal factors that have been linked with nasal hypoplasia or epiphyseal stippling. Hypoplasia of the nose is a recognized feature of certain congenital conditions; for example, it is a classical feature of congenital syphilis and a prominent one of fetal alcohol syndrome. Both hypoplasia of the nose and epiphyseal stippling have been attributed to maternal use of dephenylhydantoin in occasional case reports (Hanson and Smith 1975; Sheffield et al. 1976). Nevertheless, the possibility of confounding is more a theoretical than a real difficulty. Among those cases of warfarin embryopathy in which potential confounding exposures were reported (13 of 30 cases), one mother had had syphilis, another was a heavy drinker, and none was using hydantoin (Stein et al. 1984a)

From the available data, a causal interpretation is the path of prudence when it comes to using warfarin during pregnancy. From a scientific rather than a practical standpoint, interpretation must be guarded. The argument relies on the assumption of a very low incidence of nasal hypoplasia and stippled epiphyses with a high degree of specifity-in-the-cause. As noted, this specificity itself could be the product of diagnostic bias.

As to strength of association, no useful estimate can be calculated: for this purpose we need to know, but do not know, the expected frequency of the syndrome among all births and among those exposed to warfarin in the first trimester. The risk of adverse outcomes from warfarin and other coumarin derivatives in 418 pregnancies culled from the literature (Hall et al. 1980) is bound to be an overestimate because of selective reporting. Better estimates of frequencies and replications to test consistency cannot be expected, because the use of warfarin during pregnancy is now contraindicated. So far, animal studies give no help (Hirsch et al. 1970), except for one study with a suggestive increase in minor skeletal anomalies produced by warfarin (Kronick et al. 1974). Causal judgment will have to rest on such coherence as emerges from the conjunction of case reports with other nonepidemiological evidence.

Sometimes, one must recognize, it is not possible to determine whether or not an association is causal, a limitation that applies to epidemiologic studies as well as to case reports. The separation of the effects of the factor under study from those of a confounding variable, for example, may defy every kind of ingenuity. The difference between a confounded measure of the strength of association and the true measure will be influenced by both the direction and size of the association between the confounding variable and the factor under study and the direction and size of the association between the confounding variable and the outcome (Susser 1973; Greenland and Neutra 1980). Confounding may be left unanalyzed because the analyst failed to conceptualize the possibility, or failed to operationalize a variable to represent the confounding factor. Sometimes the ability to construct the variable and measure its properties may be beyond available technical capabilities. Sometimes, even when the appropriate variable can be conceptualized, put into operation, and measured, the potential confounder still cannot be separated from the hypothesized cause.

The difficulty of ensuring the separation of variables snares studies of the teratogenic effects of anticonvulsant drugs. Women with epilepsy are at increased risk of bearing offspring with congenital malformations, particularly heart defects and cleft anomalies (reviewed by Annegers et al. 1974; Janz 1975, 1982). Explanations for this excess risk are several.

Genetic theories attribute the raised risk in offspring to transmission from epileptic parent to offspring of a gene or complex of genes that account for both epilepsy and malformation, or to some constitutional abnormality in epileptic women that disturbs normal placentation or embryogenesis. Epileptogenic theories attribute the raised risk of malformation to seizures during pregnancy. Teratogenic theories incriminate a range of anticonvulsants used by epileptic women in the first trimester of pregnancy.

Examination of the teratogenic effects of anticonvulsants has been frustrated because their therapeutic use is confounded by the presence of epilepsy in the mother, by her tendency to have seizures during pregnancy, and also by multiple-drug treatment regimens. One approach to controlling the potential genetic and epileptogenic factors associated with epilepsy is to use untreated epileptic women as the comparison group. Against this comparison it can be argued that the seizure disorders of women who need treatment are unlike those of women who do not need it. Another approach might be to test the effect of anticonvulsants on specific malformations giving special attention to refinements of the potential causes in terms of type of drug, dose, and stage of gestation. Such an undertaking is complicated by the frequently simultaneous use of several drugs and difficult to accomplish because of the low frequencies of both the outcome and of women at risk.

Just such a case has arisen with sodium valproate. This anticonvulsant was introduced in 1964 in France, in the late 1960s and early 1970s in other European countries, and in 1978 in the United States. Before its use, the malformations associated with epilepsy were chiefly cardiac or cleft anomalies. Several case reports of spina bifida after the use of sodium valproate during pregnancy (reviewed by Jeavons 1982) and data from the Lyon monitoring program (Robert and Guibaud 1982; Robert 1982) therefore aroused suspicion. Among women with epilepsy, the ratio of spina bifida to cardiovascular malformations appeared to be greater in those who were treated with sodium valproate than in those who were not. These findings suggested specificity-in-the-effect. Although other birth defect monitoring programs in Europe and in the Americas did not find the association (Bjerkedal et al. 1982; Castilla 1983), with a rare exposure power to detect effects is low, and the later assembly of 13 prospective studies seems to confirm a risk of spina bifida with sodium valproate (Lindhout and Schmidt 1986).

On this basis, a causal effect might be assigned to the drug rather than to the epilepsy for which it was prescribed, and with less concern for the tangles of confounding than there would be with drugs such as hydantoin and phenobarbital. Yet in animal studies, specificity-in-the-effect seems not to obtain. The effects vary among rodent species and with dosage; they include rib and vertebral anomalies, renal defects, encephalocele, and exencephaly (Whittle 1976; Kao et al. 1981; Nau et al.

1981). For the present, then, inconsistent results and a degree of biological incoherence somewhat undermine the support given to a causal interpretation by the apparent specificity-of-the-effect in studies of human beings.

CONCLUSION

In summary, causal inferences in teratology, as well as in the broader sphere of abnormal prenatal development and reproduction, require a weighing of the evidence against all available criteria. Several of the definite teratogens identified have strong associations with one or a few specific outcomes. This fact does not require that all teratogens behave in a similar fashion, and not all do. We have stressed the conditions under which specificity-in-the-effect might not occur. Yet the degree of this specificity that exists for the agents discovered may also attest to the difficulties that attend the detection of agents with modest or nonspecific effects. For weak or nonspecific teratogens, the criteria of consistency and coherence weigh all the more heavily. In the study of malformations in particular, these are formidable criteria to meet: the rarity of the defects often results in small sample sizes, so that failure to detect an effect provides little information, whereas our understanding of the pathogenesis underlying malformations is often incomplete and provides little guidance.

II Conception and Early Gestation

4 Conception and Reproductive Loss: Probabilities

Reproduction underlies every aspect of the continuity of life. The persistence of human societies no less than that of the unicellular amebae, and indeed the evolutionary links between them, are ultimately founded on the endless cycle of the reproductive process. For analysts of the process, repetitive cycling poses the problem of where to begin. In human beings, we might well begin with the societal and individual forces that bring men and women to mate and shape the biological and psychic capacities that allow them to consummate the process in a conception.

Such an approach would take us deep into sociology, demography, psychology and the biology of the reproductive tract, matters well beyond the scope of the modest epidemiological work we intend. Our focus here is not on the antecedents and mechanisms of reproduction, but on the fertilized ovum and its development into a viable human organism. We therefore choose conception as our starting point. Progress from conception through successive phases of prenatal development is our main consideration.

The focus of this chapter is the chance of fertilization after coitus, and the chance of the new organism surviving from fertilization to birth. The chapter has four sections. First, we focus on fertilization and implantation. The object of this section is to estimate the probability of pregnancy when a putatively fecund couple have had intercourse around the time of ovulation. In the second section, drawing on much the same material, we estimate the chances of losing a conception in the earliest phase between fertilization and implantation (about 6 days after ovulation and zygote formation) and then between implantation and the time of the expected menstrual period (about 14 days after zygote formation). In the third section, we weigh the chances of loss of a conception at any time from the first missed menstrual period to term. Finally we set out the range and estimates of the probability of loss overall, from fertilization to term.

THE PROBABILITY OF FERTILIZATION

Fertilization is a process that begins with the fusion of the membranes of sperm and egg and ends with the formation of the zygote. If natural fertilization is to occur, the sperm must arrive in the female genital tract close to the time of ovulation. The time bounds during which either sperm or oocyte can survive and still join in a successful conception are narrow, perhaps no more than 24 hours. When insemination exactly coincides with the release of the oocyte, the chances of conception can be expected to be better than the average achieved under the field conditions of everyday life. In theory, the maximum chance might be obtained when the introduction of sperm can be made to coincide with ovulation, as with artificial insemination, but the degree to which this manipulation is physiologically identical with coitus is uncertain.

A secure estimate of fertility requires knowledge of the adequacy of sperm, of the time of coitus, and of the fact and time of ovulation. None of the in vivo studies discussed later could establish sound data on every one of these parameters. In all, the potential for fertilization is likely to be underestimated, even in couples who report sexual intercourse around the time of ovulation.

Direct observations of fertilization in human beings have never been made; thus, all in vivo estimates are retrospective. They rely on observations made some time after fertilization and, more usually, after implantation. Not all conceptions implant in the uterus. To render precise estimates of the probability of fertilization that take account of such failures, therefore, requires observations made before implantation. Such observations are difficult to achieve. Estimates made from observations after implantation are less tenuous, but these too rest on incomplete data. Their vulnerability to error depends on the accuracy of inferences about preimplantation losses.

In a 28-day menstrual cycle, ovulation—rupture of the ovarian follicle with release of the oocyte—occurs about 14 days after the first day of menstruation, whereupon for about 24 hours the oocyte is susceptible to fertilization. If fertilization ensues, the conceptus moves down the fallopian tube, dividing as it goes. About 3 to 4 days after fertilization the conceptus, now in the eight-cell stage or slightly larger, reaches the uterine cavity. Cell division continues, forming first the many-celled entity of the morula and then the blastocyst, in which the cells surround a cavity and begin to differentiate into embryo and trophoblast.

Soon the embryo is surrounded by a layer of trophoblast. Within 6 to 9 days after fertilization, the trophoblast attaches to the uterine wall and establishes vascular connections between the growing embryo and the maternal circulation. At about this time the trophoblast begins to secrete human chorionic gonadotropin (hCG) in amounts detectable in maternal blood and urine. One effect of circulating hCG is to prolong the production of progestins by the corpus luteum (the follicular structure remaining after the release of the ovum from its follicle), thereby preventing the shedding of the uterine lining that marks menstruation. In a normal pregnancy, hCG begins at a low level; during the first trimester it rises steeply, reaching a peak at about 8 to 10 weeks of gestation (Edwards 1980).

The appearance of measurable hCG in maternal blood or urine provides the foundation for the most sensitive and reliable tests to detect early pregnancy. From the sequence just described, it follows that detectable levels of hCG must be expected to appear, not at fertilization, but at implantation. Efforts have been made to detect fertilization even before implantation occurs. The Early Pregnancy Factor (EPF) is said to be a hormone that indirectly suppresses immune responses to the fertilized ovum and that is detectable as soon as 48 hours after fertilization (Morton et al. 1977; Morton 1984). Mild thrombocytopenia has also been described as an early maternal response to pregnancy (O'Neill et al. 1985). Preimplantation responses are much less well-studied than hCG; their validity and reliability as markers of pregnancy are far from being established.

Figure 4-1 and Table 4-1 designate the time intervals for the preimplantation period and the postimplantation period. Although we would prefer to measure the duration of a pregnancy from ovulation

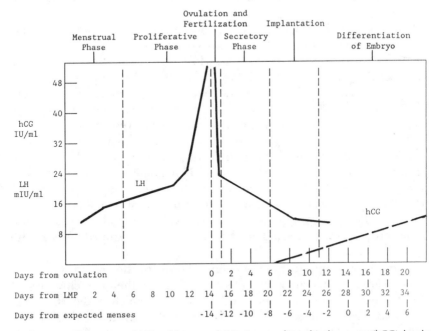

Fig. 4–1 Luteal hormone (LH) and human chorionic gonadotrophic hormone (hCG) levels during one menstrual cycle before and after fertilization (schematic representation).

Table 4–1 Schedule of development and gestation

Stage of conceptus	Days (OV) from ovulation	Days (LMP) from last menstrual period[a]	Clinical signs
Fertilization	0	14	None
Blastocyst	1–6	15–20	None
(Implantation)	(6, 7)	(20, 21)	None
Postimplanta- tion embryo	7–13	21–27	None
Embryo	14–34	28–48	First missed menstrual period
Embryo	35–48	49–62	Conventionally rec- ognized pregnancy
Fetus	49–181	63–195	
Viable infant[b]	182+	196+	

[a]Assuming a 28-day menstrual cycle, counting from the first day of bleeding.

[b]Viability has been variably defined. Some infants are born alive at 20 weeks, although very few survive the newborn period.

(day 0 refers to the day of ovulation), we also give the measure of duration from the last menstrual period (day 0 refers to the first day of the LMP) since the latter measure corresponds to usage in most reports in the literature. The notations "days (OV)" for days from ovulation and "days (LMP)" for days from first day of the last menstrual period avoid ambiguity.

The physiological processes surrounding conception are largely inaccessible to direct observation. For the purposes of estimating the frequencies with which conception and loss occur and when they occur, therefore, operational markers are necessary. The simplest marker—universally available if not always reliable as an indicator of conception—is amenorrhea. Amenorrhea is the earliest reasonably valid symptom of pregnancy any woman can be expected to recognize and report although, of course, it does not always denote a pregnancy. Through the 1970s, the confirmation of a diagnosis of pregnancy invariably followed after the first missed menstrual period. Hormonal tests, first devised by Aschheim and Zondek (Aschheim 1930), were biological not immunochemical, and were insensitive before the advent of amenorrhea. Up to the 1980s, then, pregnancy was inaccessible to epidemiological and clinical studies over a period after conception that spanned 2 weeks and more.

In the 1970s, routine immunochemical tests for the diagnosis of pregnancy were introduced (Vaitukaitis et al. 1972). In their current phase of development, the most refined and sensitive of these can detect a pregnancy as early as one week after conception (Armstrong et al. 1984; Wilcox et al. 1988). As a result, a previously inaccessible phase of pregnancy has become biochemically detectable. We can anticipate that new imaging and immunological techniques will soon open even earlier phases of pregnancy to observation.

The shifting boundaries of accessibility of pregnancies to observation create difficulties in the descriptive terminology for probabilities related to the successive phases of gestation. For instance, we shall have occasion to group pregnancies in relation to their current accessibility to observation, even though in the studies involved pregnancies may have been differently accessible. To deal with this problem, we follow two rules, one more precise than the other. First, whenever timing of observations in relation to gestation seems important, we aim to specify the nature of the observations exactly, so that the reader is not left in doubt. Second, when exactness is of little importance to the argument, we divide pregnancies roughly, in terms of general accessibility to recognition, into subclinical and clinical phases.

The *subclinical* phase of pregnancy endures up to the time of the next expected menstrual period, or about 14 days after conception. *Subclinical* losses are conceptions followed by bleeding within the time limits expected for the next menstrual period and, in practice, are distinguishable from menstrual loss only by refined chemical tests that are still undergoing development and evaluation. Conceptions and losses in the subclinical phase are, therefore, further subdivided into *prerecognition* and *biochemical* phases. *Prerecognition* losses are totally inaccessible to observation; *biochemical* losses are those that have become accessible to observation by means of new sensitive and specific assays for human chorionic gonadotropin (hCG).

The *clinical* phase of pregnancy begins shortly after the expected date of onset of the menstrual period. In this phase, pregnancies can be recognized by amenorrhea and conventional pregnancy tests. Losses after the expected menstrual period are, for the most part, clinically recognizable. Some early losses, particularly those in which bleeding occurs 1 to 2 weeks after the expected menstrual period, escape recognition. We use the term *clinically recognized* loss to refer to losses after a delayed or "missed" menstrual period that are recognized as such by the woman or her physician. By including in this definition losses reported without medical confirmation, we admit some episodes of delayed menstruation in which conception did not occur. On the other hand, to exclude all such reports would underestimate clinically recognized loss. The error produced by inclusion is probably less than that produced by exclusion; in addition, the inclusive count is uncontaminated by variations in the use of medical services, as we discuss later.

Fertilization: Estimates from the Preimplantation Period

For the preimplantation period, three types of published data can be used to estimate the probability of fertilization: (1) direct observations of

Table 4–2 Morphologic abnormality in 34 fertilized human ova

Days since last menstrual period at hysterectomy (ovulation = day 14)	Number of couples with optimum conditions for fertilization	Number of ova found (%)	Number of ova judged abnormal (%)
16–17 (tubal)	9	1 ⎫ (33)	0 ⎫ (50)
18–19 (preimplantation)	15	7 ⎭	4 ⎭
20 (implantation)	5	0 ⎫	—
21–22 (early postimplantation)	25	2 ⎬ (11)	0
23–24 (early postimplantation)	17	3 ⎭	0
25–28 (postimplantation)	31	18 ⎫ (58)	5 ⎫ (29)
29–31 (next menstrual period due)	5	3 ⎭	1 ⎭
Total	107	34 (32)	10 (29)

Source: Adapted from Hertig et al. 1959.

fertilized ova after surgical excision of the uterus and fallopian tubes (Hertig et al. 1956, 1959; Hertig and Rock 1973); (2) prospective studies using the Early Pregnancy Factor (Rolfe 1982; Smart et al. 1982); and (3) observations of in vitro fertilization (Trounson et al. 1982; Edwards et al. 1983, 1984; Testart et al. 1983; Lopata 1983). It must be emphasized that numbers are small in many of these studies. Although we describe the data in detail because they offer the only guide available to this period of pregnancy, a claim of "no significant difference" might easily be sustained against any interpretation proffered. This warning applies to many passages that follow.

Fertilized ova were observed directly in a pioneering study that is unique and likely to remain so (Hertig et al. 1959). Among women slated for hysterectomy, 107 had engaged in sexual intercourse around the presumed time of ovulation. Hysterectomy was carried out thereafter at varying intervals up to 3 days beyond the date of the next expected menstrual period. Fertilized ova were retrieved from the excised reproductive organs. The findings (shown in Table 4-2) have been variously interpreted. The study is well known, and we shall deal with it somewhat briefly.

During the preimplantation period, 24 hysterectomies were carried out. Of the 24 possible fertilizations, only 8 (33 per cent) could be established by retrieving a conceptus. Compared with retrievals in the postimplantation period, in which the conceptions had survived the preimplantation period, this is an underestimate. Postimplantation retrievals indicate success in at least 21 of 36 possible fertilizations (58 per cent).

One should note here that with early hysterectomies, before 24 days (LMP), the fate of a large majority of ova was unknown. In these preimplantation and early postimplantation stages, no trace was found in 82 per cent (58 out of 71). The missing data are sufficient to engender an entirely different result. The minimum fertilization rate would seem to be 58 per cent and the maximum 100 per cent. The maximum estimate takes account of the higher frequency of abnormal conceptions among retrievals in the preimplantation period than in the postimplantation period. Hertig et al. (1959) inferred that fertilization had been effected in most instances but the conceptions were not retrieved because the proportion abnormal was very high and many failed to implant. An alternative inference is that fertilization often failed.

The second source of observations bearing on the probability of fertilization derives from two small prospective studies that used Early Pregnancy Factor to identify fertilizations. The investigators suppose the factor always to be raised in women with clinically recognized pregnancy and never in the absence of pregnancy. The difficulties that attend the measurement of the factor are great enough to call into question this characterization and the supposition of its specificity to pregnancy (Thomson et al. 1980; Cooper and Aitken 1981; Smart et al. 1982; Whyte and Heap 1983; Tinneberg et al. 1984). The two prospective studies (Rolfe 1982; Smart et al. 1982), taken at face value, indicate a probability of fertilization of about two-thirds, within reach of the minimum estimates of 58 per cent from Hertig et al. (1959).

The third source of observations derives from in vitro fertilizations. Ova taken from a woman who ovulates but has been unable to conceive (often because of a tubal disorder) are fertilized to produce zygotes for implantation in the uterus. Hormones given during the follicular stage of the cycle stimulate the ripening of several ova instead of the single ovum expected in a natural cycle. The sperm may also be treated to concentrate their fertilizing capacity. The criterion for fertilization is not always stated and may differ from laboratory to laboratory, although at a minimum all require the formation of at least two pronuclei. At this stage, the sperm has penetrated the ovum but the two nuclei have not yet fused to form a zygote.

The several unknowns in the procedure might prove advantageous or disadvantageous to fertilization, and caution against generalizing too readily from the in vitro to the natural situation. The common sense assumption, still untested, is that in vitro fertilization would succeed less often than would natural fertilization under the most favorable conditions. The techniques are still under development, and many attempts do not result in successful implantation and birth.[1] In experienced laboratories, 70 to 80 per cent of fertilizations reach the pronuclear stage (Trounson et al. 1982; Edwards et al. 1983, 1984; Testart et al. 1983;

[1]In one setting the probability of clinically recognized pregnancy with in vitro fertilization approximates those of natural conception rates (Liu et al. 1988).

Lopata 1983). Of these, 90 per cent or more form a zygote and undergo cleavage (Johnston et al. 1981; Trounson et al. 1982; Marrs et al. 1984).

From these three scanty and diverse sets of observations, we may expect fertilization to result from insemination at the time of ovulation in the range of about 60 per cent to about 80 per cent of the time. The upper limit especially is tentative, and it could approach 100 per cent.

With a process so complex and delicate, it is perhaps surprising that the rates are this high. In the early hours of fertilization, from the penetration of the vestments of the ovum by the sperm until the first cleavage, much might go wrong. Normal fertilization is a process: it includes the blocking of penetration of the ovum by more than one sperm (polyspermy); the completion of maternal meiosis II and the extrusion of the second polar body; the development of the two parental haploid gametes into pronuclei; and zygote formation with the joining of the two pronuclei. Even at that early stage, the presence of certain anomalies in the genome of either ovum or sperm could prevent further development. The impediments to fertilization remain obscure. Studies of in vitro fertilization in human beings offer the hope of advancing understanding because the nature and timing of events can be closely monitored.

Fertilization: Estimates from the Postimplantation Period

We turn now to estimates of the probability of fertilization derived from studies of conceptions that survive to implantation. As noted before, hCG is produced by the trophoblast. The first efforts to detect the low levels of hCG of early pregnancy proved challenging. The assays sensitive to these low levels of hCG were at first liable to cross-reactions with luteinizing hormone.[2] Luteinizing hormone reaches peak levels shortly before ovulation. Thus, to detect early pregnancy, these assays sacrificed specificity and risked false positives. False negatives for pregnancies that persist are, of course, soon recognized; false positives are not. In the absence of more solid criteria of early pregnancy, a false-positive test that reverts to normal cannot be distinguished from a biochemical loss. Inflation of the estimates of loss by false positives, therefore, cannot be avoided.

Studies of early pregnancy that used hCG assays have been reviewed elsewhere (Kline and Stein 1985a). In later studies, more refined assays have superseded them. For early pregnancy, these have proffered more specific and more sensitive tests. Such tests can detect the low levels of hCG that are present close to the time of implantation. Assuming im-

[2]hCG and luteinizing hormone are structurally similar and are each made up of an alpha subunit and a beta subunit. Although the alpha subunits of the two molecules appear to be identical, the beta subunits differ somewhat in their amino acid sequences.

plantation around 6 to 7 days after ovulation, the improved assays have detected pregnancy within a few days of implantation. With one assay, hCG was detected in two artificial insemination cases as early as 9 days after ovulation (Armstrong et al. 1984); among women trying to conceive, hCG was detected not much later—on average at 25.4 days (LMP) (Wilcox et al. 1985).

The greater specificity of the current hCG assays reduces the proportion of false-positive tests and the consequent inflation of conception rates. Their greater sensitivity reduces the proportion of false-negative tests and the consequent deflation of conception rates, but in this regard a gap remains. The preimplantation phase remains inaccessible in epidemiological studies using measures of hCG. Hence, probabilities of fertilization based on hCG levels properly refer not to fertilization only, but to the combined probabilities of fertilization and of survival into the early postimplantation phase. Such estimates must underestimate conceptions if, as the studies of Hertig and colleagues suggest, fertilized ova are lost before implantation.

Four studies so far (Wilcox et al. 1985, 1988; Lippman and Farookhi 1986; Ellish et al. 1986; Kline et al. unpublished) have used the more specific assays that detect the sequence of amino acids unique to the beta subunit of the hCG molecule.[3] These studies enrolled women intending to conceive. One of the four studies (Wilcox et al. 1988), much larger than the others, provides the basis for our discussion. 221 North Carolina women were followed over 707 menstrual cycles. In 30 per cent of first cycles hCG was detected, thus providing an estimate of the combined probabilities of fertilization and survival to the early postimplantation phase.

Demographic data also provide a guide to rates of fertilization. These large-scale studies entail outcome measures of fertilization that are predominantly births or well-established pregnancies and estimates of women's exposure to conception derived from social and mating behavior. In this literature, the language and definitions of reproduction are often at odds. English and French usages, for example, can be directly contradictory. Before we proceed, therefore, we digress to define the terminology we have adopted.

> *Fertility* (as in English demographic usage) is actual reproduction, measured in live births, to an individual, couple or population.
>
> *Fecundity* refers to the physiological capacity of an individual or couple to produce a *live birth*, whether or not this capacity has been fulfilled.

[3]Refined assays are specific to a unique sequence of amino acids of the beta subunit of hCG (the carboxy-terminal peptide region) (Wehmann et al. 1981). Two-site immunoradiometric assays are very sensitive and can detect low levels of hCG (Armstrong et al. 1984; Kondo et al. 1984; reviewed in Armstrong et al. 1986).

Fecundability, a precondition for fecundity, describes the capacity of a woman to conceive. Fecundability can be defined as the probability of conceiving during one menstrual cycle in women who menstruate regularly, who engage in sexual intercourse, and who do not practice contraception.

Total fecundability is a term reserved for all conceptions (Leridon 1977).

Effective fecundability is limited to live births as the indicator of conception; in demography the average interval from marriage to birth in noncontracepting populations is a usual basis for computation (Henry 1957; Leridon 1977). Effective fecundability serves demographers as an operational index. This index underestimates total fecundability by excluding from the count of conceptions not only subclinical losses, but also clinically recognized losses (see Leridon 1977 and Chapter 17 of this text).

Effective fecundability, defined as the likelihood of a live birth resulting from a single cycle for women of about 25 years of age and estimated from various demographic data, is on the order of 20 to 25 per cent (Leridon 1977). This estimate of effective fecundability compares well with the rate for recognized fecundability obtained in a prospective study of a cohort of women trying to conceive: clinically recognized pregnancies occurred in 24 per cent of the first menstrual cycles observed (Wilcox et al. 1988).

The congruence of this refined single-sample estimate and the crude demographic estimates is surprising. One might expect estimates derived from a prospectively followed cohort in which all couples were trying to conceive and clinically recognized losses were enumerated to differ sharply from demographic estimates based on live births. Possibly the differences in the two approaches cancel out in unknown ways. If taken at face value, their similarity suggests that in a volunteer sample of North Carolina women in the 1980s, modal patterns of ovulation and the timing of sexual intercourse, and also the likelihood of survival of the conception to birth, differ little from the modal patterns of the quite different populations on which demographic estimates are founded.

We summarize our estimates thus far for a cycle in which there is sexual intercourse around the time of ovulation: the probability of fertilization resulting in a zygote ranges from 60 to 80 or even 100 per cent; the probability of fertilization resulting in the implantation of the conceptus is equally variable, ranging from 30 to 60 per cent; the probability of a live birth is about 20 to 25 per cent. Live births are easily defined and recognized, unlike early pregnancies. The wide ranges of probabilities for fertilization and implantation compared with the narrow range of live birth probabilities point to the importance, in epidemiological studies, of being able to define a "case" without misclassification and to ascertain all the cases that occur in a study sample.

THE FREQUENCY OF EARLY REPRODUCTIVE LOSS

The probability of survival is the reciprocal of the probability of loss. A number of fresh issues are raised by the change in focus from survival to attrition. A pregnancy may end at any one of several stages (see Table 4-1): between fertilization and implantation; during the time of implantation; and at various stages of gestation after implantation. From what has gone before in our discussion of fertilization and survival, it should be clear that the evidence is scant for estimates of loss before and soon after implantation. To make such estimates, we turn again to the same set of studies.

Loss between Conception and Implantation

Estimates of early loss, as with estimates of fertilization, have relied heavily on the morphology of fertilized ova retrieved at hysterectomy. In these unique studies (see Table 4-2), Hertig and his colleagues (1959) worked under the handicap that karyotyping was not available to them. In their estimates, they made two important assumptions. First, they assumed explicitly that *all* morphologically abnormal conceptions would abort. Second, they assumed implicitly that *only* those conceptions in which the conceptus or trophoblast was anomalous would abort.

The first assumption—that all visibly abnormal conceptions would have aborted spontaneously—is probably correct. The second and implicit assumption—that the only conceptuses lost will manifest abnormalities of the embryos or trophoblast early in pregnancy—is more difficult to judge. The correspondence between pathological observations in the subclinical phase and those in the clinical phase rests on surmise. We know that in some clinically recognized losses an organized embryo or fetus is found. We do not know whether such a pregnancy would appear normal or abnormal in the subclinical phase. For instance, the pathology might or might not correspond to the normal postimplantation embryos with hypoplasia of the trophoblast described by Hertig et al. (1956, 1959).

In any event, prospective studies of unselected pregnancies judged normal by ultrasound in the first trimester suggest that the assumption may not have introduced much error. The rate of loss for conceptions free of detectable morphologic abnormalities is probably low, on the order of 2 to 3 per cent (Gilmore and McNay 1985; Cashner et al. 1987; Simpson et al. 1987). Since defects undetectable by ultrasonography play a role in miscarriages, the rate of loss for genetically and morphologically normal embryos and fetuses may be even lower.

Another unknown in the studies of ova retrieved at hysterectomy is the state of the ova in those participating women from whom conceptions were not retrieved. After coitus around the time of ovulation, hysterectomy interrupted the development of any conception at successive stages up to the time of the next expected menstrual period. Predictions about the number of conceptions that would have been lost before implantation or after implantation rested on comparisons of the proportions of dysmorphic specimens retrieved at each stage. In the face of the formidable technical difficulties, retrieval of pre- and peri-implantation conceptions may well not have been random. The ova in cases in which retrieval did not succeed might have been in any one of several states: fertilized and normal, fertilized and abnormal, unfertilized, or absent. Each of these states would impose different probability estimates of loss as well as fertilization.

The underlying design and analytic problem is that the observations about the type and numbers of surviving conceptions are cross-sectional, but the inferences are longitudinal. The necessary assumptions about expected losses of normal and abnormal conceptions, and about unretrieved ova, weaken these inferences. Observations made at gestational intervals close to attempted fertilization cannot be projected with assurance to the cross-sectional observations made at later gestational intervals. At any gestational interval, early or late, it is always uncertain whether conceptions supposedly not retrieved existed and, if they did, whether they were similar to those that were retrieved. In addition, small numbers render the frequencies unstable and could magnify error. Predictions must therefore be viewed as tentative.

Four of the 8 retrieved preimplantation conceptions (50 per cent) and 6 of 21 postimplantation conceptions (29 per cent) were classified as abnormal because either the conception was dysmorphic or implantation was anomalous (see Table 4-2). If we assume, with the investigators, that in time all abnormal conceptions must abort and only abnormal conceptions abort, then the preimplantation data would indicate that at least 50 per cent of all fertilizations will not result in a live birth. If we assume further that all abnormalities arise at conception, then the probability of loss in the interval between the preimplantation and postimplantation periods alone is 30 per cent.[4] The descriptions of the six abnormal postimplantation conceptions, however, leave open the possibility that at least three became abnormal at implantation or later (Hertig et al. 1956). If that was the case, the estimate of loss in all fertilizations rises from 50 to about 58 per cent. The probability of loss between the preimplantation and postimplantation periods rises from 30 to 42 per cent and could rise at a maximum (if all abnormalities detected before implantation

---

[4]This is estimated from the decrease in anomalies between the preimplantation and the postimplantation periods. Our estimates do not draw on observations in the peri-implantation period (days 20–24 LMP) because a low rate of retrieval and small sample size suggest that those data are less reliable, perhaps because of technical difficulties peculiar to that period.

were also to be lost before implantation) to about 50 per cent. In summary, although unproven assumptions can place an estimate in doubt, estimates of preimplantation and peri-implantation loss on the order of 30 to 50 per cent are compatible with the data.

Postimplantation Losses before the Next Expected Menstrual Period

Among conceptions that survive implantation, the nature of the available data requires that losses be divided into those that occur before and those that occur after the expected time of the next menstrual period. Pregnancies in the phase before the expected onset of menstruation seldom produce symptoms leading to subjective recognition by the woman. Hence both pregnancy and loss remain pervasively subclinical; ascertainment depends on biochemical or other technical means. Early clinical recognition depends heavily on a missed menstrual period.

During the premenstrual interval (days 25–28 LMP and days 1–3 after the next expected onset of menstruation), 21 conceptions were retrieved after hysterectomy and 6 were classified as abnormal, an estimated loss of 29 per cent.

The strongest biochemical data on loss between implantation and the next expected menses are provided by the prospective study of 221 North Carolina women (Wilcox et al. 1985, 1988). Pregnancy was ascertained by immunoradiometric assay (IRMA) for the carboxyterminal peptide region of the beta subunit of hCG. The assay was highly sensitive and specific in biochemical terms. However, diagnosis was entirely biochemical: it was not possible to collect bleeding specimens around the time of the menstrual period to search for pathologic confirmation of pregnancy.

The definition of a test indicating pregnancy rested on two grounds: the biological coherence of the test results with the reproductive cycle in women who were trying to conceive, and the results of a study of women (presumably with intact ovarian function) who were unable to conceive because of bilateral tubal ligation or sterilization (Wilcox et al. 1985, 1988). When a clinically recognized pregnancy (diagnosed by a physician) did not ensue after a positive test, a biochemical pregnancy loss was assumed. Of course, in the absence of another indicator of pregnancy, this definition leaves some room for both false-positive and false-negative diagnoses.

Direct validation of a positive test when the presumed early pregnancy appears to fail requires knowledge that fertilization and implantation have indeed taken place; that is, validation of a failed "biochemical" pregnancy requires another "more valid" indicator. Since the direct evidence of embryonic tissue in the bleeding specimen has been unattainable in practice, one must make do with indirect evidence of specificity and sensitivity. A positive test should never be present in the absence either of ovulation or of coitus at the time of ovulation. In fact, excepting some uncommon malignancies in premenopausal women, false positives seem to be rare (Armstrong et al. 1984; Wilcox et al. 1987).

Before implantation, it is uncertain whether or not hCG is produced. Any production must be at levels below that detectable with the assay employed in the North Carolina study.[5] Hence a pregnancy that fails to implant will go undetected. *After implantation,* the rate of pregnancy loss can be estimated. In the North Carolina study, the probability of biochemical loss by the time of the next expected menses was 22 per cent (95 per cent confidence interval, 16 to 28 per cent). Among 198 cycles in which pregnancy was judged to have occurred, 45 ended with bleeding around the time of the next expected menses, 43 subclinically and two in clinically recognized losses.

In summary, from Hertig et al. (1959) we infer that 50 per cent of fertilizations will not survive to term; perhaps 30 to 50 per cent of these losses will occur before or during implantation. For conceptions that survive to the postimplantation period, the prospective study of Wilcox et al. (1988) suggests that 22 per cent will be lost early, ending with bleeding around the time of the next expected menses.

THE PROBABILITY OF LOSS AFTER THE FIRST MISSED MENSTRUAL PERIOD

After the first missed menstrual period, we are on firmer ground with estimates of pregnancy loss. In many instances, a pregnancy can be confirmed by means other than the measurement of hCG. The pregnancy may be visualized by ultrasound or, with a pregnancy loss, the products of conception can be examined pathologically. In instances of early loss, diagnosis may rest on less definitive criteria: clinical symptoms of pregnancy (in particular, amenorrhea) and loss (in particular, bleeding) or an elevation in hCG sufficient to render a conventional pregnancy test positive followed by symptoms of pregnancy loss.

Most of the literature bearing on attrition after the first missed menses focuses on clinically recognized losses. The criteria for defining loss are not always given and may or may not be comparable across studies. Many investigators include episodes without pathological confirmation in which a conventional pregnancy test is positive. Although many of these may be corroborated by other symptoms of pregnancy or reproductive loss, this important point of definition generally goes unstated. Further ambiguities arise when these same symptoms occur in the absence of a positive pregnancy test: for instance, low hCG levels by

[5]An assay sensitive to levels of hCG as low as 3.0 pg/ml in serum has been reported (Odell and Griffin 1987) but has not been applied in an epidemiologic study of pregnancy.

the time of testing may reflect a decrease following earlier loss; or the woman may not have been tested. In studies that report such episodes, some are enumerated among losses and others are not.

These problems of definition in early pregnancy were made acute, we have noted, when it became possible to detect elevations in hCG before an affected woman herself recognized a pregnancy. Previous research into early loss drew on samples of women who suspected pregnancy, usually after a missed menstrual period. Recent research with the more sensitive assays has recruited women who are trying to conceive.

The distinctions between biochemical and clinically recognized loss may serve to bridge the information gleaned from these different sampling schemes. In early pregnancy, the distinction is murky because it rests in part on variations in perceptions and behaviors of the woman. Clinical recognition nearly always depends first on the woman suspecting she is pregnant, and next on her seeking medical attention. Thus, in women who have sought a pregnancy test and tested positive, loss of the pregnancy is often enumerated as clinically recognized regardless of medical attention at the time of loss and in the absence of pathologic confirmation. On the other hand, in women who have not sought a pregnancy test, loss at the same stage in gestation might be enumerated as subclinical. The North Carolina cohort of women seeking to conceive experienced 45 losses before 7 weeks (LMP): 43 (95 per cent) were biochemical; another 2 had been diagnosed by a physician. At 7 weeks (LMP) and later, all 17 losses were clinically recognized (Wilcox et al. 1988).

The possibilities for error in estimating clinically recognized pregnancy loss vary with the several types of study design as well as with clarity of definition. The soundest in theory are difficult in practice: in cohorts of women attempting to conceive, conception is detected prospectively by early systematic testing, often after coitus timed to coincide with ovulation has taken place. As noted, other prospective cohort studies enroll women already pregnant at variable intervals after conception. Cross-sectional studies identify pregnancies only at their termination. Retrospective studies depend on obstetric histories taken at any convenient point in the life course.

Cohort studies that begin with a fixed population of nonpregnant women and follow them through conception to termination yield rates derived directly from the number of losses. All women are under observation at the time conception occurs, even though the pregnancy is diagnosed later. The probability of loss is simply a cumulative incidence rate, that is, the number of losses divided by the number of recognized pregnancies up to a specified period of gestation. The four largest hCG studies (Miller et al. 1980; Edmonds et al. 1982; Whittaker et al. 1983; Wilcox et al. 1988) all yielded rates of clinically recognized loss of 12 to 14 per cent (Table 4-3).

Table 4–3 Miscarriage in four cohort studies

	Miller et al. (1980)	Edmonds et al. (1982)	Whittaker et al. (1983)	Wilcox et al. (1988)
Sample	"Normal women"	"Normal population"	"Normal women"; enrolled from preconception clinic after 3 cycles using barrier contraceptives	Women with no fertility problems enrolled after stopping contraception
Number of women	197	82	91	221
Number of cycles	623	207	226	707
Per cent clinical pregnancies per woman	52	62	93	70
Per cent clinical pregnancies per cycle	16	25	38	22
Per cent losses (N of clinical pregnancies)	14 (102)	12 (51)	13 (85)	12 (155)
Gestational bound defining losses	<20 weeks	No mention	Second trimester	<28 weeks

In prospective studies of women pregnant at varying stages of gestation on entry to observation, the probabilities of terminations by spontaneous loss, induced abortion or birth can be estimated by life-table or survival analysis. Since the 1960s, a number of reports have provided life-table estimates for the probability of pregnancy loss (French and Bierman 1962; Erhardt 1963; Pettersson 1968; Taylor 1969; Shapiro 1971; Harlap et al. 1980a). Although some pregnancies come under observation early and others later, in these analyses all contribute their experience for each gestational interval in which they are under observation, and only for those intervals. Pregnancies that first become known by the fact of their loss are not enumerated; their inclusion spuriously inflates estimates of loss. Pregnancies in progress, but first observed at later gestation intervals, do not contribute to the denominator of earlier intervals; to include them spuriously underestimates rates of loss in earlier intervals.

In the life-table analysis, the rates of loss within each gestational interval are applied to a hypothetical cohort to give an overall estimate of the probability of loss. A rate of loss is calculated for each gestational interval, taking as denominator all surviving pregnancies identified before

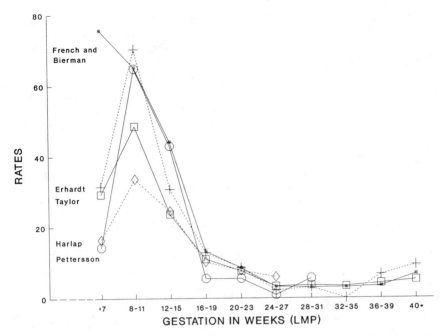

Fig. 4–2 Rates of loss (per 1000 pregnancies) in successive 4-week gestational age intervals recomputed from five life-table studies: French and Bierman 1962 (recomputed excluding ectopic pregnancies); Erhardt 1963; Pettersson 1968; Taylor 1969 (when computed for daily intervals, the probability of loss calculated before 7 weeks of gestation is 61 per 1000); Harlap et al. 1980a

the gestation interval plus half of those pregnancies identified during the interval (Figure 4-2 shows the data in this form).

A hypothetical cohort of, say, 1000 women is then "followed," assuming losses at each stage of gestation occur at the previously obtained rates, to estimate the overall probability of loss and also the probabilities of loss between gestation intervals. An assumption underlies the calculation of the overall probability of loss in these studies—namely, that the characteristics of women identified early in pregnancy are similar to those of women identified at later stages. Indeed, their social and reproductive characteristics are generally not the same (French and Bierman 1962; Taylor 1964; Harlap et al. 1980a). Analyses that do not control for the differences could thus be in error.

In prospective studies, published estimates for loss between the first missed menstrual period and 28 completed weeks of gestation range from 14 to 22 per cent (French and Bierman 1962; Erhardt 1963; Taylor 1969; Harlap et al. 1980a). When losses beyond 28 weeks are added, the estimates are only slightly higher. One study provides an estimate of 13 per cent beginning at 7 weeks and ending at 28 weeks (Pettersson 1968).

Some of the variability between these estimates could reside in different methods of computing life-table probabilities.[6] When the same computation is applied to each study, however, the variation is not much decreased. For this purpose, we selected five prospective studies for closer scrutiny (Table 4-4). On the Island of Kauai, the probability of loss before 28 weeks is 23 per cent (or better, about 21 per cent when ectopic pregnancies are excluded). Estimates from the other four studies are lower, and range from 10 to 15 per cent. Nearly all of the variation between studies occurs in the first trimester of pregnancy (see Figure 4-2).

Although each study included women from the fourth week after the last menstrual period, they all yield weak estimates of early pregnancy loss because the numbers of very early registrants were small. Thus, estimates for losses before 8 weeks draw on samples that are largely composed of women who entered in weeks 6 and 7. Before the eighth week of pregnancy, the rate of loss on the Island of Kauai is 11 per cent, three or more times that observed elsewhere. This difference accounts for the overall higher estimate of the probability of loss obtained on the Island of Kauai. For pregnancies that survive to 8 weeks and beyond, the probabilities of loss are far more comparable between studies, ranging from 8 to 12 per cent (see Table 4-4).

The higher estimate from Kauai is largely explained by the unique method of ascertaining pregnancies, which extended beyond those identified through medical facilities. All women in the community were encouraged to notify the study team if menstruation was delayed. Forty-five per cent of the 273 pregnancies that eventually ended in loss were first identified from direct reports to the study team. Among losses, 22 per cent were not recorded in medical records. Thus, the study captured pregnancies that were either never seen in a medical service or not seen until the time of loss.

On Kauai, the probability of loss in pregnancies identified through a medical facility (about 10 per cent)[7] is comparable to estimates from the

[6]For example, the 17 per cent estimate given by Erhardt (1963) was obtained by extrapolating observations backwards from gestations of 8 weeks and later to earlier gestations; further extrapolation to conception produced an estimate of 30 per cent.

Gestation-specific rates of loss were computed in 4-week intervals by French and Bierman (1962), in single weeks by Pettersson (1968), and in women-days by Taylor (1969) and Harlap et al. (1980a). The probability of loss decreases rapidly in the early stages of gestation whereas the number of pregnancies available to observation increases with gestation. For this reason, the use of 4-week gestational age intervals, rather than shorter intervals, tends to underestimate the probability of loss. This underestimate may be as much as 50 per cent, judging by two studies that estimated the gestation-specific probabilities of loss in relation to the number of women-days of observation (Taylor 1969; Harlap et al. 1980a). The underestimation is most marked in the gestational interval before 8 weeks.

[7]To estimate the probability of loss for pregnancies first registered at a medical facility on the Island of Kauai, we assumed that those ending in loss were identified in the same 4-week gestation interval as the loss.

Table 4–4 Life-table estimates of the probability of reproductive loss (%)[a] at various intervals of gestation (LMP)

Interval	French & Bierman 1962[b] Kauai, Hawaii, 1953–56	Erhardt 1963 New York City, 1960	Pettersson 1968[c] Uppsala County, 1963–64	Taylor 1969[c] Vicinity of San Francisco, 1959–66	Harlap et al. 1980a[c,d] Vicinity of San Francisco, 1974–77
to 8 weeks	10.8	3.2	1.4	2.9	1.6
to 28 weeks	22.7	14.8	12.8	11.8	9.5
to term	23.7	15.9	13.3	13.0	NC[e]
From 8–28 weeks	11.9	11.6	11.4	8.9	7.9
Total number of pregnancies	3083	2573	1258	16,170	32,167

[a]To facilitate comparison between studies, probabilities of loss have been recomputed for all studies using gestational intervals of 4 weeks and the equations of French and Bierman (1962). See Leridon (1977) for alternatives. Published data to compute intervals by days were insufficient.

The table includes the one subsample from the study by Erhardt (1963) for which data were judged most complete. The sample of Shapiro et al. (1971), defined by terminations and not prospectively by registration, was excluded.

[b]Includes 16 ectopic pregnancies. Excluding ectopics, the rate to term is about 21 per cent. It is unclear whether or not the other studies enumerated ectopic pregnancies.

[c]Gestational intervals of one day were used by Taylor (1969) and Harlap et al. (1980a) and intervals of one week by Pettersson (1968). Recomputation using 4-week intervals lowers the estimates of loss. The original (and probably better) estimates of loss to 28 weeks gestation are 14.6, 14.4, and 13.0 per cent, respectively.

[d]Losses include 66 born alive before 28 weeks (LMP).

[e]NC = Not computed; data insufficient.

four other studies, which relied solely on medical facilities to identify pregnancies. Thus, pregnancies not identified through a medical facility presumably account for the high probability of loss at less than 8 weeks gestation on Kauai.

It could be argued that on Kauai, in contrast to the four other series, losses were overstated because a large proportion of these putative losses were actually episodes of amenorrhea unassociated with pregnancy. This proposition cannot now be evaluated. On the other hand, it can be asserted that studies that rely only on ascertainment by medical services understate early losses.

Notwithstanding better ascertainment, it could also be that the probability of loss was truly higher on Kauai than in the other samples. Two possible sources of higher rates are the demographic characteristics of the population on Kauai, and selection for lower-risk women in studies that drew solely from medical facilities. The Kauai population was rural, with large proportions of Polynesian and Asian women. The 23 per cent probability of a pregnancy loss before 28 weeks might thus relate to special features of place or population.

In the remaining four studies that relied solely on pregnancies ascertained at a medical facility, the probabilities of loss are remarkably similar to those observed in the hCG studies described earlier, in spite of different methods of study. These data suggest a probability of clinically recognized loss, among women who seek prenatal care early in pregnancy, of about 12 to 14 per cent.

Another approach to estimating pregnancy loss depends on ultrasonography. Beginning with pregnancies visualized at 7 to 10 weeks (LMP), loss was estimated at only 10 per cent by 28 weeks. Eight per cent had been considered not viable on ultrasonography, leaving only 2 per cent of pregnancies considered viable that ended in loss (Gilmore and McNay 1985). In a similar study at 8 to 12 weeks gestation, rates were slightly lower, as might be expected with somewhat later pregnancies: 5 per cent were judged nonviable and 2 per cent were judged viable but were lost by 28 weeks (Cashner et al. 1987). The rates of loss estimated from these ultrasonography studies agree well with life-table estimates beginning at 8 weeks.

Retrospective and cross-sectional studies also provide estimates of the frequency of reproductive loss. In epidemiologic studies frequency is usually measured by the *fetal death rate,* which relates the numbers of losses to the number of pregnancies identified. (In statistics from vital records, the frequency measure tends to be the *fetal death ratio,* which relates the numbers of losses to the numbers of births.)

One problem, in populations without access to legal induced abortion, is that the frequency of clinically recognized loss may be inflated by the misclassification in the numerator of induced abortions as spontaneous. A majority of reported studies are beset by this problem. On the other hand, in populations with access to legal induced abortion, the denominator requires modification. The denominator pregnancies have typically included both losses and births. A pregnancy terminated by induced abortion precludes a spontaneous pregnancy loss at gestational ages beyond that event; their unmodified inclusion deflates rates of loss, and their exclusion does the opposite. An appropriate modification, derived from fetal life-table methods, is to add to the denominator an estimated number of pregnancies that were at risk of spontaneous loss before they were terminated by induced abortion (Susser 1983; Susser and Kline 1984).

Both retrospective and cross-sectional studies identify pregnancies—whether by report or observation—not on recognition but at termination. For this reason, estimates of the probability of reproductive loss might differ from those obtained in prospective studies. In retrospective studies the closeness of the rate of loss to the true probability of loss will vary with the accuracy of the reproductive histories obtained. In cross-sectional studies the closeness of the estimate to the true rate depends on the extent to which women use medical care for miscarriages, births and, in some populations, for induced abortion.

Rates of reproductive loss in retrospective and cross-sectional studies span a large but overlapping range. To facilitate comparison, Table 4-5 gives fetal death rates for losses (whenever data were given) before 20 weeks, from 20 to 27 weeks, and from 28 weeks on.

No systematic variation with study design is apparent. Some of the variations between studies could result from risk factors differently distributed between samples, and these are explored in later chapters. Another part of the variation could result from other differences in method, including the types of losses enumerated and the gestational range covered. These variations reflect some of the changes that have attended the definition of fetal death and of spontaneous abortion or miscarriage in particular (see Chapter 11).

In *1950,* the World Health Organization defined *fetal death* as "death prior to the complete expulsion from its mother of a product of conception, irrespective of the duration of pregnancy; . . . the foetus does not breathe or show any other evidence of life . . ." (WHO 1950). The Expert Committee recommended that fetal deaths be classified as *early* (<20 completed weeks of gestation LMP), *intermediate* (20 up to 28 weeks), *late* (28 completed weeks or more), or *not classifiable.* They recommended against the use of the terms "abortion" and "stillbirth," but considered the latter synonymous with late fetal death.

In *1970* the World Health Organization again grappled with definitions of pregnancy terminations. They defined *spontaneous abortion* as nondeliberate fetal death of an intrauterine pregnancy before 28 completed weeks of gestation, corresponding to a fetal weight of approximately 1000 grams. The traditional limit of 28 completed weeks was

Table 4–5 Fetal death rates per 100 pregnancies in retrospective and cross-sectional studies

Study	Design	Sample	Definition of fetal death	Fetal death rate
Yerushalmy et al. 1956	Retrospective	Obstetric histories from women born since 1900, Kauai sample, 1953	<20 weeks 20+ weeks	5.5 2.6
Stevenson et al. 1959	Cross-sectional	All pregnancies known to hospital or Medical Officer of Health, Belfast, 1957	<20 weeks 20–27 weeks	11.1 0.6
	Retrospective	Obstetric histories of 983 women experiencing miscarriage	<28 weeks	16.8
Warburton and Fraser 1964	Retrospective	Obstetric histories of families of children with birth defects counseled at Montreal Hospital, 1952–62	<6½ months	14.7
Pettersson 1968	Retrospective	Obstetric histories from medical records of women enrolled in a prospective study of pregnancy loss, Uppsala	<28 weeks	19.6
	Retrospective	Obstetric histories of women delivered at university clinic, Uppsala 1963–64	<28 weeks	15.3
	Retrospective	Obstetric histories of women hospitalized for abortion (both induced and spontaneous), in university clinic, Uppsala 1963–64	<28 weeks	16.4
Pettersson 1968	Retrospective	Obstetric histories of women applying for legal abortion, Uppsala 1963–64	<28 weeks	6.2
Jain 1969	Retrospective	Obstetric histories of women living with their husbands; Taichung City 1962	To term	7.6[a]
Shapiro et al. 1971	Cross-sectional	Pregnancies terminating in New York City Health Insurance Plan 1958–60	<20 weeks 20–27 weeks 28+ weeks	12.5 0.8 1.0
Naylor 1974	Retrospective	Most recent previous pregnancy of pregnant women enrolled in U.S. Collaborative Perinatal Project 1959–66	<20 weeks	12.6
Leridon 1976	Retrospective	Representative sample of females of childbearing age in Martinique 1968	No mention	12.1

Table 4–5 (Continued)

Study	Design	Sample	Definition of fetal death	Fetal death rate
Leridon 1976	Cross-sectional	Women attending obstetric clinic in a public hospital, Creteil 1974	No mention	~11.5
	Retrospective	Obstetric histories from this same group	No mention	15.3[a]

[a]For comparability with other studies, induced abortions are excluded from the denominator.

retained because it complemented the definition of stillbirth noted in the 1950 recommendations. However, the preference of the Scientific Committee was to limit spontaneous abortions to losses before 20 weeks gestation, following the common medical definition of abortion that denoted termination before the fetus attained viability.[8] (By 1970, a number of infants weighing 400 or 500 grams had survived.)

In *1977*, the World Health Organization recommended that *abortion* be defined to include embryos and fetuses weighing 500 grams or less (20 to 22 completed weeks of gestation) and "an otherwise product of gestation of any weight and specifically designated (e.g., hydatidiform mole) irrespective of gestational age and whether or not there is evidence of life . . . (WHO 1977)." This recommendation marks a departure from the 1970 definition in a variety of ways: by using birth weight as a criterion for losses containing an embryo or fetus; by not requiring death prior to expulsion (but assuming that fetuses of 500 grams or less are nonviable); by including losses beyond 28 weeks in which there is no recognizable embryo or fetus (presumably, for example, missed abortions); and by failing to exclude explicitly extrauterine pregnancies. *Stillbirth* is defined as the birth of a fetus weighing more than 500 grams when there is no evidence of life after birth. In the United States, requirements for reporting fetal deaths vary among jurisdictions, with most reporting deaths at or beyond 20 weeks (corresponding to 350 grams) (National Center for Health Statistics 1980).

The epidemiologic studies listed in Table 4-5 all include early fetal deaths (before 20 weeks gestation), and several extend to 28 weeks or term. Excepting three samples, fetal death rates range from 11 to 20 per

[8]The Committee favored the term "spontaneous abortion" over "miscarriage." They considered the use of miscarriage in a scientific context as obsolescent (WHO 1970). In this text, however, we use the term miscarriage to describe clinically recognized loss; for the epidemiologist the simpler term permits no ambiguity between spontaneous and induced abortion under the rubric of abortion. Further, with this everyday term we remind the reader that measures of pregnancy loss vary between studies both at the earlier and later bounds of gestation, earlier according to recognition and later according to the definition of viability.

cent. Differences in definition such as the inclusion or exclusion of ectopic pregnancies, of live births before 28 weeks, or of missed abortions occurring after the gestational age cutoff used all occur at low frequencies, and effects on rates should be minor.

Three samples—women on the Island of Kauai in 1953 (separate from the cohort study discussed previously), Swedish women seeking induced abortion, and married Taiwanese women—provide considerably lower fetal death rates, in the range of 5 to 8 per cent. It is unclear what part is played in these low rates by differences in method, on the one hand, and in risk factors between populations on the other. However, in both Kauai and Taiwan, at least part of the deficit appears to be due to underreporting of loss (Yerushalmy et al. 1956; Jain 1969).

One practice, the inclusion of losses that lack physical confirmation of a pregnancy, might produce differences that reflect the conditions and design of studies. Some episodes of this kind of unconfirmed loss were included in each of the studies listed. The proportion of such unconfirmed losses identified at a medical facility, however, is likely to be smaller than that in pregnancies reported retrospectively. Thus, in general, the cross-sectional studies undertaken in a medical facility probably provide more uniformity in diagnostic criteria than retrospective studies based on reproductive histories, but to an extent that remains to be measured.

EXPECTATIONS OF SURVIVAL AND LOSS THROUGHOUT GESTATION

For a given cycle in which a supposedly fecund couple engages in sexual intercourse around the time of ovulation, what is the probability of fertilization, implantation, and survival to birth? Answers to such questions, we have seen, must be tempered by the assumptions and guesses forced by scanty data and tenuous inferences. They must also be tempered by the fact that no study represents all pregnancies in a population, and many are biased in one way or another.

Our best estimates of the probabilities follow. It seems likely that when sperm and ova are present together, fertilization will take place 60 to 80 percent of the time or more. During the first 7 days after fertilization, it is certain that a loss of zygotes takes place. What is uncertain is the extent of the loss, though it is likely to be steep. Thereafter the probability of loss decreases, with the rate of decrease slowing as gestation lengthens. In Figure 4-3, we set out several estimates of the probability of loss from fertilization to term and the data sources for these estimates.

1. Beginning at fertilization, estimates of loss must depend on the single value of 50 per cent suggested by the descriptions of eight pre-implantation ova (Hertig et al. 1959).

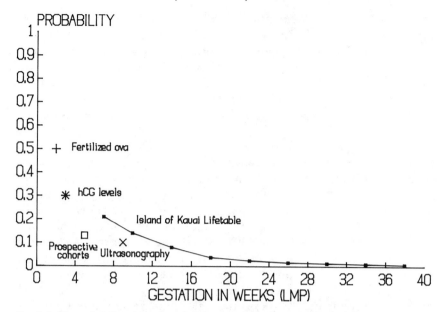

Fig. 4–3 The probability of loss (to term) given survival to various stages of gestation estimated from several sources. Fertilized ova: Hertig et al. 1959. hCG levels: Wilcox et al. 1988. Prospective cohorts: Miller et al. 1980; Edmonds et al. 1982; Whittaker et al. 1983; Wilcox et al. 1988. Ultrasonography series: Gilmore and McNay 1985; Cashner et al. 1987. Island of Kauai life-table: French and Bierman 1962

2. The probability of loss for conceptions that have survived to the early postimplantation stage (say, days 25–28, LMP) is around 30 per cent (Wilcox et al. 1988). This probability derives from a single study of pregnancies diagnosed early by the presence of hCG, and it is similar to the estimate obtained from studies of fertilized ova retrieved at hysterectomy in the postimplantation stage (Hertig et al. 1959). The hCG study sample was relatively homogeneous and comprised well-educated volunteers. Higher loss rates might apply to less advantaged women.

3. The probability of loss among intrauterine pregnancies that have survived to clinical recognition (around 5 to 7 weeks, LMP) ranges between 12 and 21 per cent. The lower estimates derive from hCG studies carried out in the 1980s in women who volunteered to be studied over the period during which they were trying to conceive, and also from life-table analyses of women seeking prenatal care. The highest estimate of 21 per cent derives from the community-based study of the Island of Kauai in the 1950s (modified from the reported 23 per cent by excluding ectopic pregnancies).

Beginning in week 8 (LMP), the probabilities of loss decrease with increasing gestational age. This observation derives from prospective studies analyzed with life-table methods. From this stage losses constitute about 10 per cent of surviving pregnancies. Of those pregnancies that appear viable on ultrasonography, however, only 2 to 3 per cent are lost. Prospective hCG studies that enrolled women before conception have not reported data on the natural pattern of attrition throughout gestation; in any event, the cohorts are probably too small to provide stable rates. When ultrasonography is used for cohort definition or description, the picture of attrition may also be incomplete because some pregnancies judged nonviable are medically terminated, thus disrupting the natural timing of loss.

The data summarized here leave uncertain the exact extent of reproductive loss beginning at conception: the single estimate of 50 per cent derives from morphologic descriptions of preimplantation conceptions. There is less uncertainty about the rate of loss after implantation: most likely it is on the order of 30 per cent. This estimate derives from a single prospective study. Despite the uncertainties that attend unreplicated observations, the estimate is bolstered by two other observations: the nearly identical estimate obtained from morphologic study of postimplantation conceptions, and the agreement in the rates of clinically recognized loss between this study and other prospective hCG studies. Approximately 70 per cent of postimplantation losses are biochemical. Among the remaining 30 per cent of losses, the majority (perhaps 80 per cent) are of a conceptus that did not reach the fetal stage of development. These observations suggest that, of 100 postimplantation losses, 70 are biochemical and 30 are clinically recognized; of these 30, 24 are prefetal and 6 reach the fetal stage.

The tabulation below draws on the sources summarized in Figure 4-3 to estimate the probabilities of loss at successive stages from fertilization to term. Because the estimate of the frequency of preimplantation loss is especially tenuous, we also provide estimates beginning with conceptions that survive to implantation.

	From fertilization			From implantation		
Stage	Number reaching stage	Number lost before next stage (%)	Cumulative loss %	Number reaching stage	Number lost before next stage (%)	Cumulative loss %
Conception	1000	272 (27)	—			
Implantation	728	160 (22)	27	1000	220 (22)	—
Clinically recognized pregnancy	568	54 (10)	43	780	74 (10)	22
Fetal stage	514	14 (3)	49	706	19 (3)	29
Live birth	500	—	50	687	—	31

5 Developmental Abnormalities: I. Measuring Frequencies

Intrauterine survival depends on the attributes of the conceptus, the attributes of the mother, and the biological interaction between the two. We have seen that perhaps half of all conceptions are lost before birth, so that infants born alive are the survivors of cohorts of conceptions that have experienced severe attrition. Among survivors at birth, most will be undamaged. A small minority—having been defective from the start or having sustained insults during gestation—will be damaged in a manner and to a degree that did not prevent a live birth. Others will not be born alive but result in stillbirths or miscarriages or subclinical losses. Among stillbirths or late fetal deaths, still only a small minority will have detectable damage. Among conceptions that fail to survive to birth, the majority will be abnormal; the remainder will appear to be normal to the extent that karyotype and gross anatomy establish normality.

Abnormalities of the conceptus arise in different ways and at different times. Some abnormalities, such as inherited defects and most chromosome aberrations, will have been present at or around the time of the formation of the zygote. Other abnormalities arise during gestation. Early in pregnancy, dysmorphic embryonic development and focal malformations arise; their origin could be in causes operating before conception as well as soon after. Later in pregnancy, abnormalities in growth can be recognized, and a number of deformations of joints, limbs, and trunk appear; many of these are likely to be owed to insults during pregnancy.

CHANGING PERSPECTIVES

At first, available techniques limited the description of embryonic abnormalities to morphology (Mall 1917; Streeter 1920; Mall and Meyer 1921; Hertig and Sheldon 1943). Even so, compelling evidence that the conceptus was often abnormal was provided by classic pathological studies of fertilized ova (Hertig et al. 1959; see Chapter 4). In the 1960s, the advent of cytogenetics changed the focus of embryonic research. Techniques for karyotyping cultured cells had caused the revision of the accepted human chromosome number from 48 to 46 (Tjio and Levan 1956), comprising a single pair of sex chromosomes and 22 pairs of autosomes.

Karyotyping led soon to the discovery of chromosomal aberrations in surviving individuals. In 1959, aberrations of the autosomes were first recognized, notably chromosome 21 in Down's syndrome (Lejeune et al. 1959), as well as aberrations of the sex chromosomes: XO with Turner's syndrome (Ford et al. 1959), XXY with Klinefelter's syndrome (Jacobs and Strong 1959; Ford et al. 1959), and XXX (Jacobs et al. 1959).

Systematic searches for aberrations followed, for instance, among institutionalized and patient populations and among the newborn (reviewed by Jacobs 1982). In institutions for mentally retarded persons, males and females with extra sex chromosomes (XXY and XXX) were found to be overrepresented (Maclean et al. 1962), and the XYY karyotype was linked with aggressive behavior in tall males (Jacobs et al. 1965). Among patients with primary amenorrhea, a high prevalence of XO and XO mosaics was found, and in some the typical stigmata of Turner's syndrome were present (Jacobs et al. 1961). Around the same time, karyotyping was applied to conceptuses culled from miscarriages (Delhanty et al. 1961; Penrose and Delhanty 1961).

After the discovery of the extra chromosome in Down's syndrome, the rising prevalence of the syndrome in older children and adults began to attract notice. Improved environment and medical care had increased survival in the hazardous early years of life (Carter 1958; Tizard 1964; Susser 1968; Stein and Susser 1971b; Fryers 1984). Rising prevalence provoked scientific as well as public health interest in the possibilities of prevention. Once cytogenetics made refined classification of Down's syndrome and other chromosomal syndromes possible, investigators began to look for the effects on the chromosomes of a range of environmental factors.

Most studies have used births to seek variations in the prevalence of defects; they are accessible to clinical observation and tend to be systematically recorded. Such studies must contend with the lack of statistical power contingent on the rarity of many specific defects. They are also incomplete because, by definition, they exclude anomalies that are incompatible with delivery at term. Even for those defects that do survive to term, however, studies of births could be misleading because of our ignorance of the pattern of losses between conception and birth. An association of a suspect factor with a birth defect need not reflect a simple increase in the incidence of the defect at conception or later. Such an association could be produced if the probability of intrauterine loss for defective conceptuses is decreased, or if the probability of intrauterine loss for conceptuses without the defect is increased. In studies of births alone, neither hypothesis can be ruled out.

The point is illustrated by one group of investigators who found, in areas in South Wales of high prevalence of neural tube defects, rates of reported miscarriage lower than in areas of low prevalence (Roberts and Lloyd 1973). To explain these geographic variations in prevalence, they postulated that variations in the *survival* of affected embryos, rather than variations in *incidence,* were reflected in miscarriage rates; with fewer miscarriages, more defective embryos survive to birth.[1]

Studies of developmental abnormalities at miscarriage have begun to alleviate our ignorance of the epidemiology of the prenatal phase. Such studies, although not devoid of problems, have advantages peculiar to themselves. At miscarriage, a wider range of developmental abnormalities can be observed: chromosome aberrations that are rarely or never seen at birth are brought within the reach of researchers. Also, abnormalities can be captured early in their course. Enumerations made early in gestation more closely reflect incidence than those made at birth. The shift back in developmental time toward the point of origin strengthens causal inferences about the association of a factor with observed abnormalities; opportunities are reduced for the conflation of factors that promote the survival of abnormal conceptions with factors that are actual determinants of the abnormalities.

The chromosome aberration trisomy 16 illustrates the disparities between incidence at conception and frequency at miscarriage and at birth. This trisomy far outnumbers all other trisomies among miscarriages, accounting for about 30 per cent of the total (Hassold et al. 1984b). Incidence at conception can be presumed to be of similar order. Yet this aberration has never been observed in births at or around term. With so lethal an abnormality, a cause that increases their incidence obviously could not be detected in studies of births. In one special class of cases— namely, genetic disorders that at birth exhibit frequencies in conformity with Mendelian models for single major gene defects—the correspondence between incidence rates at conception and prevalence rates at birth can be taken to be close. On theoretical grounds, a genetic disorder that exhibits a Mendelian conformation at birth is bound to have had a similar conformation at conception.

In studies of miscarriages, it soon became apparent that a striking proportion were chromosomally aberrant (Carr 1965; Dhadial et al. 1970; Boué and Boué 1970, 1973b; see Carr 1971 for a review of the early studies), with estimates ranging from 22 to 61 per cent. The recognition that so large a proportion of karyotypes could be aberrant crystallized a notion about the causes of miscarriage—one entertained as

[1]Further evidence favoring this hypothesis has not been forthcoming. A subsequent comparison of the rates of neural tube defects in chromosomally normal miscarriages in New York City and London does not support it. The hypothesis requires that rates of the defect at miscarriage and birth vary inversely. In New York City the rates of neural tube defects were low among both chromosomally normal miscarriages and births, whereas in London they were higher at both these endpoints (Byrne and Warburton 1986).

long ago as the eighteenth century by Morgagni (1762)—that the role of maternal factors and the role of factors inherent in the ovum or embryo were distinct. Before the advent of karyotyping, the abnormalities in the anatomic development of very early embryos had provided some foundation for the postulate (see, for instance, Hertig and Sheldon 1943). Cytogenetic studies gave the postulate fresh force; it became evident that, on average, more than 90 per cent of chromosomal aberrations were lethal in utero. There could be virtual certainty that the primary cause of the miscarriage of a chromosomally aberrant conceptus resided in the abnormality.

With the capacity to distinguish chromosomally normal and aberrant miscarriages, we also acquired the capacity to explore with greater precision the separate sources of reproductive loss in the women and the conceptus. An appropriate model could assign causal factors to their origin at three loci. One source is the intrinsic defects of the conceptus, as indicated for instance by chromosome aberrations. Another source is the environment of the conceptus (most immediately the uterus but, at one remove, the woman and her characteristics and environment). The third source is the interactions between the conceptus, the woman and the external environment. Although the role of intrinsic defects in miscarriages will be most apparent with chromosomal aberrations, the role of environment will be most apparent with the chromosomally normal. This is not to say that the chance of miscarrying an aberrant conceptus might not be influenced by maternal characteristics. It is to say that, because most chromosomal aberrations are lethal in utero, the added contribution of extrinsic factors to such miscarriages cannot be large, and the detection of their effects will be difficult. On the other hand, not all chromosomally normal miscarriages are the consequence of factors extrinsic to the conceptus. In chromosomally normal abortuses, disruptions in early morphologic development are rather frequent; among these, and perhaps also among apparently normal fetuses, undetected genetic effects such as homozygosity for harmful recessive genes could play a part.

MEASURES OF FREQUENCY

In studies of developmental defects at miscarriage and birth, problems in the measurement of frequencies and their interpretation require special attention. Studies of developmental defects draw on medically attended miscarriages and births. We noted that a majority of the one-half or so of all conceptions that do not survive to term are lost before they come to attention which, ordinarily, can be no sooner than the first missed menstrual period at about 2 weeks after fertilization. Most abnormalities also arise before this time, at conception or in the weeks immediately after conception. It follows that the majority of developmental defects seen in clinically recognized pregnancies must be those prevalent at the time of observation and not those incident at conception or soon after. Incidence refers to newly arising cases, and prevalence to existing cases. Thus, even at miscarriage, although abnormalities are culled at a time closer to the moment of inception than those at birth, the counts are still of prevalent and not of incident cases.

An *incidence rate* measures the frequency with which new cases of a disorder arise in a population over a given time period. In an open or dynamic population—one subject to recruitment and losses—the numerator of the incidence rate is the number of new occurrences of a disorder over the time period; the denominator is the sum of the durations of observation for all members of the population and can be measured in units of person-time (e.g., person years). This denominator is ordinarily estimated from the average number of persons present in the population over a defined time period. The traditional incidence rate for an open population has been termed *incidence density* (Miettinen 1976), or *period incidence* (Susser 1985). Incidence density is meant to convey the concept of "instantaneous" incidence, which is to say it measures the rate of new disease at any instant in time and also as it changes with time, much as a speedometer measures instantaneous velocity in an automobile. (The concept of incidence density is especially applicable in survival analysis, when it is called the hazard rate, which is the instantaneous rate of morbidity or mortality expressed in units of cases per person-year. An older term for the hazard rate is the force of morbidity or mortality.)

In a closed population it is also meaningful to measure the *cumulative incidence* over a defined time period. Such a closed population or cohort is defined by its point of entry (e.g., conception, or birth, or recognition of pregnancy, or hospital admission). The cumulative incidence rate equals the proportion of the fixed cohort that develops the disorder over a specified period of time. The time period of observation may relate either to calendar time or to a defined span of the life course (e.g., gestation). The cumulative incidence depends on the incidence density, much as the distance traveled in a day depends on the instantaneous velocity during the journey.

Cumulative incidence can also be usefully and equivalently expressed as the average *individual risk* of developing the disorder in a specified time period for a member of the cohort observed; this probability ranges from 0 to 1. In the ideal example, the cumulative incidence rate of developmental defects would relate to a cohort of pregnancies identified at conception and followed until termination. Since it is not yet possible to identify and describe very early pregnancy losses, practically speaking, only the cumulative incidence of those defects that are not lost before the time pregnancy is clinically recognized can be observed.

In cumulative incidence rates, calendar period and life course overlap and are confounded. Data from different calendar periods are needed to separate the effects of a particular stage in the life-course from those of the historical time period. An additional difficulty arises in cohorts in which entry is defined, not by a fixed stage in the life course, but by the time that observation begins—such as recognition of pregnancy or hospital admission. In such cases cumulative incidence can be estimated by life-table methods, which appropriately account for changes in the cohort that result from staggered entry at different stages in the life course.

Prevalence rates describe the proportion of a defined population that is affected by an existing disorder. For prevalence relating to *calendar time,* usually in an *open population,* the numerator of the rate comprises existing individuals who have the disorder at a particular point in time; the denominator comprises the population among which those with the disorder are found. For prevalence relating to the *life course,* usually in a *closed population,* numerator and denominator are enumerated at a point in the life course and not at a point in calendar time. For example, the number of congenital defects found at birth, as numerator, relates to total births as denominator; or the number of chromosomal aberrations found at miscarriage, as numerator, relates to the number of pregnancies extant at the same stage of gestation in the same population as denominator. At each stage of gestation from which any of these observations are drawn, conceptions with and without defects are the survivors of processes of genesis and attrition that began at conception. At birth, the numerator of the prevalence rate of a given defect is a function of its cumulative incidence from conception on, and of its probability of surviving until birth. The denominator of a prevalence rate at birth is a function of the total of all conceptions and their probabilities of surviving until birth.

We have formalized the relationship between the prevalence of a defect at birth and its incidence at conception in the model illustrated in Figure 5-1 (Stein et al. 1975c). The equation from this model allows us to interpret the ways in which changes in several factors can affect the prevalence of a given defect among births. After conception, abnormal conceptuses are lost either subclinically, in miscarriages or as stillbirths. Thus, each type of abnormality of the conceptus has its own probability of occurrence or cumulative incidence rate (in Figure 5-1, p_a denotes the probability of abnormality a) and its own probability of loss (r_a). Conceptuses without the specific abnormality can also undergo intrauterine loss before they become viable or, if they reach viability, can be born before term. These too have their own probability of loss (r_n in Figure 5-1).

The model is, like all models, a simplification. There are many abnormalities, each with its own developmental staging and its own probabilities of occurrence and of loss: different anomalies enter the cohort of

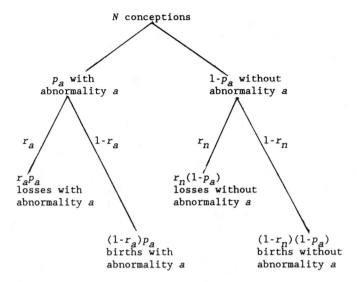

Prevalence of abnormality a at birth:

$$F_B = (1 - r_a)p_a/[(1 - r_a)p + (1 - r_n)(1 - p_a)]$$

$$p_a = \frac{\text{number of conceptions with abnormality } a}{\text{number of conceptions}}$$

$$r_a = \frac{\text{losses with abnormality } a}{\text{conceptions with abnormality } a}$$

$$r_n = \frac{\text{losses without abnormality } a}{\text{conceptions without abnormality } a}$$

Fig. 5–1 Model illustrating the relation between the prevalence of an abnormality at birth (F_B) and the rates of loss for conceptions with and without the abnormality.

pregnancies, and are lost from it, at different times in gestation. The time of occurrence can affect the choice of denominator. Only those pregnancies in progress at the time the abnormality arises are truly at risk of the defect. The incidence rates (p_a) for abnormalities that arise at conception have all conceptions as their true denominator. The incidence rates for abnormalities that arise during gestation, such as microcephaly, for some purposes could also be calculated with the same denominator. More restrictively, their exact denominator includes only those pregnancies that survive to the time during gestation when the abnormality arises.

The timing of loss can affect the numerator. For example, many chromosomal aberrations tend, as we shall see, to have a characteristic pattern of intrauterine survival. It follows that the probabilities of loss at different stages of gestation vary among aberrations. Chromosomal ab-

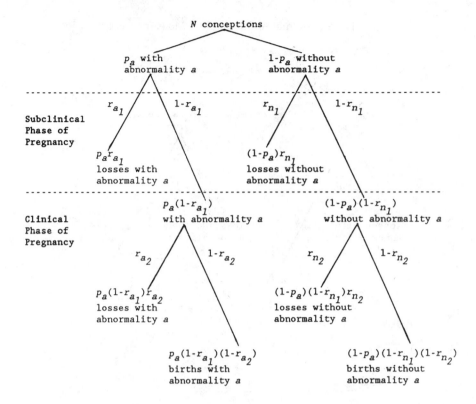

Prevalence of abnormality a at birth:

$$F_B = \frac{p_a(1 - r_{a_1})(1 - r_{a_2})}{p_a(1 - r_{a_1})(1 - r_{a_2}) + (1 - p_a)(1 - r_{n_1})(1 - r_{n_2})}$$

Prevalence of miscarriage with abnormality a:

$$F_M = \frac{p_a(1 - r_{a_1})r_{a_2}}{p_a(1 - r_{a_1}) + (1 - p_a)(1 - r_{n_1})}$$

Proportion with abnormality a among miscarriages:

$$P_M = \frac{p_a(1 - r_{a_1})r_{a_2}}{p_a(1 - r_{a_1})r_{a_2} + (1 - p_a)(1 - r_{n_1})r_{n_2}}$$

Fig. 5-2 Model illustrating the relation between the prevalence of an abnormality at miscarriage (F_M) and at birth (F_B), and the rates of loss for conceptions with and without the abnormality.

$$p_a = \frac{\text{number of conceptions with abnormality a}}{\text{number of conceptions}}$$

$$r_{a_1} = \frac{\text{number of subclinical losses with abnormality a}}{\text{number of conceptions with abnormality a}}$$

$$r_{a_2} = \frac{\text{number of miscarriages with abnormality a}}{\text{number of clinically recognized pregnancies with abnormality a}}$$

$$r_{n_1} = \frac{\text{number of subclinical losses without abnormality a}}{\text{number of conceptions without abnormality a}}$$

$$r_{n_2} = \frac{\text{number of miscarriages without abnormality a}}{\text{number of clinically recognized pregnancies without abnormality a}}$$

errations lost early in gestation are not present to be counted in the later stages. In contrast, abnormalities arising late in gestation, such as deformations, cannot be counted early on.

The model shown in Figure 5-1 ignores these complexities; it depicts only the incidence (p_a) and overall rates of loss (r_a) of a single abnormality that arises at conception, and the overall rate of loss of all other conceptions (r_n). Nonetheless, the model suffices to show that the prevalence of a defect at birth is a function not only of its incidence and its probability of survival, but also of the probabilities of survival for all other conceptions.

Figure 5-2 extends the model by dividing pregnancy into two stages—before clinical recognition and after. By definition, all conceptions that do not survive to be clinically recognized end in subclinical loss. Figure 5-2 incorporates the notion of such losses. It illustrates that, as with prevalence at birth, the frequency of anomalies that miscarry is also a prevalence rate. The numerator of this prevalence rate comprises clinically recognized losses with abnormality a; the denominator comprises all clinically recognized pregnancies, whether they end in miscarriage or birth. Both numerator and denominator exclude subclinical losses.

The most commonly used measure of the frequency of clinically recognized losses with abnormality a is the *proportion* with abnormality a among such losses. The interpretation of the proportion abnormal among clinically recognized losses raises difficulties beyond those of prevalence rates. The haze of a changing denominator may obscure the true variation in the rates of a particular abnormality. For example, the denominator of a proportion chromosomally aberrant comprises, besides the aberrant miscarriages of the numerator, chromosomally normal miscarriages that are themselves a result of the depletion of surviving pregnancies. The rate at which these chromosomally normal miscarriages occur differs with the stage of gestation, the age of the woman, and the environmental situation. Thus, when a denominator is confined to miscarriages, the proportion aberrant varies as variation in the rate of chromosomally normal miscarriages increases or reduces the denominator, irrespective of the rate of chromosomally aberrant miscarriages. Such changes in the denominator because of variation in chro-

---

Note: The most commonly used measure of the frequency of miscarriages with a given abnormality a is the proportion with abnormality a among miscarriages (P_M). The expression for this proportion allows for the effect of subclinical loss among conceptions with and without abnormality a. The numerator of the proportion with abnormality a among miscarriages includes a term for the numbers of conceptions with abnormality a that survive to clinical recognition ($1 - r_{a_1}$). It also includes a term for the probability of miscarriage among the survivors to clinical recognition (r_{a_2}). The denominator similarly allows for the diminution of the cohort of conceptions available to observation, both with and without abnormality a, through subclinical loss. This denominator is composed of miscarriages only. Since it excludes pregnancies from the same conception cohort that continued to term, the proportion with abnormality a among miscarriages is not a prevalence rate. The prevalence rate for miscarriages with abnormality a (F_M) excludes only subclinical losses from the denominator; the denominator includes miscarriages and births.

mosomally normal losses could either suppress variation in the chromosomally aberrant numerator, if both changes were in the same direction, or exaggerate it if they were in opposite directions.

These considerations make evident the propensity for an index of the proportions chromosomally aberrant or normal to veil the source of cytogenetic variation. As an example, one study found the proportion chromosomally aberrant to be higher among miscarriages that had been preceded by oral contraceptive use. The authors considered that this effect was, for various reasons, more likely a reflection of a lower frequency of chromosomally normal miscarriages than of a higher frequency of chromosomally aberrant miscarriages (Alberman et al. 1976). In general, when data are limited to proportions among miscarriages only, present-day knowledge about the effects of risk factors on chromosomally normal miscarriage is seldom enough to allow a choice between such alternative interpretations.

The ambiguities in this seemingly simple index (the proportion abnormal among miscarriages) emerge more clearly when we are reminded of the actual phenomena the index is intended to measure. The index describes an endpoint of a process with many facets. The processes include the recruitment of members of multiple cohorts of conceptions, the losses that occur at differing stages of gestation among those conceptions, and the conditions that govern their survival or loss throughout pregnancy. Moreover, the women among whom the particular endpoint of pregnancy is observed can be variously characterized; they are exposed to differing conditions, any one of which might influence the incidence of abnormality or survival patterns. Yet, by the nature of the data that can be brought to bear, we are obliged to infer the frequencies with which abnormalities arise merely from knowledge of the proportions that are abnormal at miscarriage.

ISSUES OF SAMPLING

To the difficulties of interpreting indices of frequency, one must add those of the selective sampling of karyotypes among recognized pregnancies. In general, miscarriages that can be successfully karyotyped underrepresent clinically recognized losses early in pregnancy. One reason for this is that in roughly 30 per cent of miscarriages no recognizable fetal tissue is found, and these are not randomly distributed but tend to be of earlier gestational ages (Creasy et al. 1976; Hassold et al. 1980a; Byrne et al. 1985).

A second reason is that no hospital-based population captures all early pregnancies ending in miscarriage, including those that can be clinically recognized. From the prospective study on Kauai (see pp. 60–62), in which special efforts were made to ascertain pregnancies as soon as possible after conception, it appears from life-table estimates that of recognized miscarriages (up to week 28 of gestation) 70 per cent occur before the twelfth week (French and Bierman 1962). In karyotype studies, the proportions of losses before the twelfth week do not approach these estimates (see Chapter 7). This kind of underrepresentation arises, in part, from the ways in which women perceive and act on the need for medical care. Among women in New York City who gave a history of miscarriages in their first pregnancy, 12 per cent who miscarried before 10 weeks of gestation had not sought medical care; only 2 percent who miscarried later had not sought care (unpublished data).

Variation in laboratory technique is another factor one must always guard against in comparing studies. Karyotyping is no exception and technique alone may produce variations in the proportion aberrant. Some investigators obtain a karyotype in about 9 out of 10 cultures, others in only 6 out of 10 (see Table 7-1). Success in karyotyping has been found to be influenced by gestational age, morphology, type of tissue cultured, maceration, and the time elapsing before the tissue culture is set up (Creasy et al. 1976; Hassold et al. 1980a; Kajii et al. 1980; Warburton et al. 1980b; Byrne et al. 1985).

Some aspects of sampling are within the control of the investigator. Both the study definition of miscarriage and the selection of particular tissues for cell culture may result in the exclusion of certain types of loss from study. When, for these reasons, inclusions and exclusions differ, estimates of the proportions chromosomally normal and aberrant can also be expected to differ. For instance, when the karyotyping of fragmentary specimens is not attempted (Creasy et al. 1976), the result is a deficiency of early miscarriages and of the aberrations that occur especially among them. As we shall see, specific chromosomal aberrations differ in the level of morphologic development they attain, and so are not equally distributed early and late in gestation.

The choice of an upper gestational age threshold for the definition of miscarriages (which has varied from 18 to 28 weeks in karyotype series) affects the numbers sampled in which the conceptus reaches the fetal stage and also, therefore, some of the proportions derived from the data. Since the frequencies of chromosomal aberrations are lowest in fetal specimens, differences in overall proportions follow.

In summary, direct and complete measures of true frequencies of the prenatal phenomena of our concern are an unattainable ideal. Much of the loss of incident chromosomal aberrations is inaccessible to observation. With very early loss of a pregnancy (e.g., when the only sign of pregnancy is a short-lived elevation of hCG), there can be no determination of the karyotype. Consequently, what can be observed are aberrations among clinically recognized pregnancies, for the most part at their termination. Even among these, not all losses can be karyotyped. Prevalent aberrations constitute, at any observable gestational interval and for any chromosomal aberration, only a residue. This residue provides the numerator for estimated frequency rates.

Because pregnancy losses go unrecognized or unrecorded, no studies of karyotyped miscarriages have been able to describe, even approximately, the universe of pregnancies that initially gave rise to the miscarriages. Indeed, up to the present no karyotype study has satisfactorily described those surviving to the point in the life course at which the miscarriages appeared: none could completely specify a defined population, either pregnant or nonpregnant, from which the observations were drawn. No study of karyotyped miscarriages has begun with a cohort of pregnancies; in all instances, observations describe miscarriages at termination. Hence, even for clinically recognized pregnancies taken alone, the base for a population denominator is lacking. Further, such knowledge as we have of the epidemiology of karyotyped miscarriages is founded entirely on the portion of miscarriages that are medically attended. The sole parameter against which to set the frequencies of a particular karyotype is thus the frequency of the remaining miscarriages from which other specific karyotypes are culled. This yields a ratio or proportion which, we have seen, is not the equivalent of a prevalence rate from a cohort of pregnancies. The reader should bear these deficiencies, perhaps even distortions, in mind as later chapters unfold.

6 Developmental Abnormalities: II. Frequencies Observed

Armed with an appreciation of the limitations of available measures, we proceed to consider the frequency of developmental abnormalities as they appear at the termination of pregnancy. Abnormal development is culled and concentrated in abnormal terminations. For the study of abnormalities, epidemiologists must seek out the circumstances in which they are concentrated, and for this reason miscarriages deserve particular attention. Developmentally normal pregnancies nearly always terminate in live births, although a small proportion end in stillbirths and miscarriages. Few developmentally abnormal pregnancies terminate in live births, a larger proportion end in stillbirths, and most end in miscarriages.

The developmental abnormalities we deal with fall into two classes: aberrations of the chromosomes and anomalies of morphology. In our review of reproductive loss owed to these abnormalities, we aim to clarify the separate and joint contributions of both the woman and the conceptus. From the observed frequencies of abnormalities among clinically recognized miscarriages, stillbirths and births, we can find a basis for weighing the role of fetal and maternal factors in attrition and survival throughout the stages of gestation. By the nature of the observations, however, all these data on terminations are of the cross-sectional kind, and in the first instance frequencies appear as proportions and not rates.

NAMING ABNORMALITIES

In the literature on developmental abnormalities, a number of terms occur that are often used regardless of initial definitions, usages or etymology. We ourselves have contributed to this confusion. Indeed, some terms have no single standard technical definition, and some categories of abnormality have no single standard technical term. In this text, we cleave to a terminology that has the virtue of internal consistency if not necessarily of universal consent.

Developmental abnormality is used as a nonspecific term to cover every kind of abnormality. These divide readily into a morphological class of anomalies and a chromosomal class of aberrations.

Morphologic anomaly, or simply anomaly, is the general term we use for all disorders of developmental form and morphology. These anomalies divide into a fetal class of malformations and a prefetal class of dysmorphisms.

Malformations are anatomical defects of organs or organ systems in well-formed organisms. They can be further characterized as *focal malformations,* which are localized to particular organs. Because organs and systems appear only as development proceeds, malformations tend to manifest and to be recognized in fetuses rather than in embryos. (Fetuses are distinguished from embryos by the completion of organogenesis; although the dividing line between embryos and fetuses is hazy, it is usually placed at the end of the eighth week after conception.)

Dysmorphism, in its general usage, describes any disorder of morphological development.

Gross dysmorphism, in our qualified usage, is confined to the prefetal stage, and describes general structural disorganization of the conceptus, for example, empty sacs or disorganized embryos.

Chromosomal aberration, in our usage, covers all departures from normality in the chromosomal constitution or *karyotype* of the cell. Normal karyotypes must be normal both in number and in structure of the chromosomes; an aberration may involve either number or structure or both.

Euploidy describes any balanced set of chromosome pairs, whether the normal diploid number (23×2) or multiples thereof, as with *tetraploidy* (23×4), *triploidy* (23×3), or *haploidy* (23×1). In humans tetraploidy and triploidy are unequivocally abnormal; haploidy is normal for some stages of cell development. Thus normal germ cells are haploid, having but one set of 23 chromosomes.

Aneuploidy unambiguously describes all departures in number from euploidy, for instance, the imbalance in *monosomy* (with an absent chromosome) or *trisomy* (with an added chromosome). (In this text, we avoid the broadening and loosening of the term to cover, along with imbalance in chromosome number, such aberrations of chromosome structure as rearrangements and deletions and so-called partial or segmental aneuploidies.) In the haploid state, too few chromosomes are designated by the term *hypohaploidy* and too many by the term *hyperhaploidy.*

Heteroploidy encompasses all departures from the normal number of chromosomes, whether or not the departure is an exact multiple of the normal number. Thus, along with the aneuploidies, it includes *polyploidies* such as triploidy and tetraploidy, as well as haploidy that is abnormal as in somatic cells. Heteroploidy, like aneuploidy, excludes aberrations solely of chromosome structure, for instance, rearrangements and deletions (Hook 1985; Rieger et al. 1976).

FREQUENCIES

Chromosomal Aberrations

Table 6-1[1] provides estimates of the frequencies of a number of chromosomal aberrations among miscarriages, stillbirths and live births. The frequency of such aberrations among miscarriages is about seven times higher than it is among stillbirths and about 70 times higher than among live births. About 40 per cent of miscarriages are chromosomally aberrant, about 6 per cent of stillbirths, and less than 1 per cent of live births.

Among karyotyped miscarriages, the variety as well as the number of chromosomal aberrations is many times greater than among births. All trisomies have been observed, although some rarely. At birth, trisomies 13, 18 and 21 and trisomies of the sex chromosomes predominate, although trisomies of other autosomes (8, 9, 20, 22) occur on occasion (Kunze 1980). Among miscarriages, triploidy and monosomy X each account for about 6 to 8 per cent; among births, triploidy has only occasionally been reported (Niebuhr 1974; Creasy 1977), and monosomy X occurs at a frequency of less than 1 per 10,000. Among miscarriages, tetraploidy occurs in about 2 per cent; at birth, most of the occasional cases are mosaics with a diploid cell line (Scarbrough et al. 1984).

Miscarriages clearly provide a rich source of lethal chromosomal aberrations. This concentration of many kinds of aberrations in miscarriage opens up the possibility of identifying the factors that might produce them and increase their incidence. A minority are of concern because they may be viable. All are of concern because we may learn from them about the nature of the disorders and even about the underlying order of the reproductive process.

The data shown in Table 6-1 derive from cross-sectional studies of pregnancies identified by particular kinds of terminations in different populations and at different times. On their own, data confined to live births, stillbirths, or miscarriages cannot yield prevalence rates of abnormality among all clinically recognized pregnancies. A rough estimate can be made by applying the frequencies of abnormalities observed at each kind of termination to estimates of the probabilities of loss from a cohort of pregnancies recruited as soon after conception as possible.

Among karyotyped miscarriages, some 90 per cent have endured in the uterus for at least 8 weeks. Pregnancies at 8 weeks after the last menstrual period thus provide a sufficient and convenient base population for making forward estimates from that time in pregnancy. Of all pregnancies that survive to 8 weeks, we estimate that roughly 13 per cent

[1]The table draws on three studies of miscarriages in which chromosomes were routinely banded, thus permitting counts of trisomies of individual chromosomes rather than of chromosome groups.

Table 6–1 Chromosomal aberrations in miscarriages, stillbirths, and live births: rates of selected aberrations and estimated per cent distribution among the three outcomes (N = number karyotyped)

Aberration	Rates per 1000			Distribution among outcomes (%)[d]		
	Miscarriage[a] (N = 3,353)	Stillbirth[b] (N = 452)	Live birth[c] (N = 31,521)	Miscarriage	Stillbirth	Live birth
Autosomal trisomies						
13	11.0	2.2	0.1	93	2	5
16	55.8	0.0	0.0	100	0	0
18	8.4	13.3	0.2	78	12	0
21	20.0	8.8	1.1	71	3	26
other	118.1	13.3	0.0	99	1	0
Trisomies of sex chromosomes	3.3	4.4	1.5	24	3	73
Monosomy X	83.5	0.0	0.1	99	0	<1
Triploidy	57.9	4.4	0.0	99	1	0
Tetraploidy	23.9	0.0	0.0	100	0	0
Total aberrant[e]	415.2	57.5	6.0	90	1	9

[a]Miscarriages: combined data from Denmark, N = 255 (Lauritsen 1976); Honolulu, N = 1000 (Hassold et al. 1980a); New York City, N = 2098 (Kline 1986).

[b]Stillbirths: combined data from London, N = 156 (Machin and Crolla 1974); Edinburgh, N = 195, and Adelaide, N = 18 (Sutherland et al. 1974); USSR N = 83 (Kuleshov 1976).

[c]Live births: combined data from studies of consecutive births in Aarhus County, Denmark, N = 11,148; London, Canada, N = 2081; New Haven, Connecticut, N = 4353; Winnepeg, Canada, N = 13,939 (Hook and Hammerton 1977).

[d]In computing the distribution among miscarriages and stillbirths, we estimate that among conceptions surviving to 8 weeks post-LMP, 12.9 per cent will end in miscarriage and 1.2 per cent in stillbirth (French and Bierman 1962 recomputed excluding ectopic pregnancies).

[e]Total aberrant includes all types of aberrations; selected aberrations are listed.

will miscarry by 28 weeks, and 1.2 per cent will result in a stillbirth. These frequencies derive from the life-table constructed from the prospective study of pregnancies on the Island of Kauai (French and Bierman 1962). At the time of writing, this study provided the only available data in which an attempt was made to represent all pregnancies in a total population and follow them to term. As we discussed earlier (in Chapter 4), beginning at 8 weeks gestation these frequencies are similar to those that have been observed in smaller prospective hCG studies of women enrolled before conception, as well as in life-table analyses of women seeking prenatal care.

At 8 weeks after LMP, it appears that about 6 per cent of surviving pregnancies are chromosomally aberrant. This estimate is derived by combining our estimates of frequencies of loss with the proportions chromosomally aberrant observed in cross-sectional studies at successive intervals of gestation. The estimate is consistent with observations from induced abortions carried out at 7 to 9 weeks gestation (Kajii et al. 1978; Yamamoto and Watanabe 1979; Ohama et al. 1986). From 8 weeks on, the proportion of chromosome aberrations lost by miscarriage exceeds 90 per cent for all but four types of chromosomal aberrations. The exceptions are trisomies 21, XXX, XXY and XYY.

Prevalence rates of chromosome aberrations estimated from pregnancies that survive to 8 weeks gestation provide limited insight into the incidence at conception of such aberrations (p_a). As pointed out in the previous chapter, in very early pregnancy attrition rates might differ among chromosomally aberrant and normal pregnancies. If they do differ, at later stages of pregnancy prevalence rates for aberrant and normal karyotypes will not reflect the balance that existed in the cohort at fertilization. Consequently, at conception incidence rates for aberrant karyotypes may be higher than, the same as, or lower than prevalence rates estimated from various observation points suggest.

Some kinds of evidence, but not all, point to higher incidence of chromosome aberrations at conception than is suggested by frequencies observed in clinically recognized pregnancies. Subclinical losses, which may well be substantial, are bound to include additional aberrations of the types rarely culled from miscarriages, and perhaps even autosomal monosomies that have only rarely been observed among losses. If rodents offer any guide, we can expect to find monosomies almost exclusively in the preimplantation stage (Gropp 1973). A Japanese study of karyotyped induced abortions also suggests that incidence at conception may be higher than frequencies at later stages suggest. The proportion chromosomally aberrant was highest among induced abortions carried out at 5 to 6 weeks gestation (9.3 per cent of 108; confidence limits 3.8, 14.7), and then roughly constant at 6 per cent from 7 to 12 weeks (Yamamoto and Watanabe 1979).

One circumstance in which the incidence of chromosomal aberration in human zygotes can be observed is after in vitro fertilization. Because the process does not reflect the natural experience, extrapolation could be treacherous. The unusual antecedent circumstances of the infertile couple, and the zygotes selected for karyotyping from the in vitro process, might influence the incidence of aberration. The zygotes karyotyped and not transplanted in the uterus may be predisposed to aberration: they are usually those judged least likely to yield a successful pregnancy, because they are either multinucleated (Rudak et al. 1984) or are dividing less well than other ova obtained from the same insemination (Angell et al. 1986). In at least one circumstance selection bias can be ruled out, namely, in those ova donated by women requesting sterilization that are fertilized and karyotyped solely for research purposes. The 15 such embryos so far available, 4 of which were chromosomally aberrant (Angell et al. 1986), are too few to guide us in estimating the possible bias in clinical series, or in estimating incidence in vivo.

The frequency and the types of chromosomal aberrations in human germ cells, as antecedents to the zygote, might also yield information bearing on the incidence of developmental aberrations. Studies of unfertilized and preovulatory oocytes and of sperm provide some evidence of this kind. In these studies, again, the numbers of individuals contributing samples are small and the procedures technically difficult. Estimates may change as data accumulate and techniques yield higher rates of retrieval.

Studies of oocytes all derive from samples of infertile women; they include preovulatory oocytes, "spare" oocytes retrieved for in vitro fertilization but not inseminated, and oocytes that were not successfully fertilized in vitro. Here we consider only the frequency of hyperhaploidy. We disregard hypohaploidy because artifacts of technique can produce aneuploidies in vitro, and these are thought to be more likely to deplete than to increase the number of chromosomes.

Rates of hyperhaploidy are variable, ranging from 2 per cent in "spare" oocytes (1/50; Martin et al. 1986), to 8 per cent in unfertilized oocytes (15/188; Pellestor and Sele 1988), to 9.1 per cent in preovulatory oocytes (2/22; Wrambsy et al. 1987). The rate of hyperhaploidy is likely to vary depending on whether the source of the infertility is in oocytes or in sperm. In the largest of these studies (Pellestor and Sele 1988), a high estimate of 10.1 per cent was obtained from the 129 oocytes in which the sperm were adequate and the more likely reason for failed fertilization resided in the oocytes. A low estimate of 3.4 per cent was obtained from the 59 oocytes obtained from attempted fertilizations in which the sperm appeared defective. Although the range and circumstances of these observations must leave doubt as to the incidence of hyperhaploidy in oocytes of fertile women, the low estimate would seem better to approximate frequencies in normal women.

Sperm can be visualized upon insemination of a preparation of nude hamster ova. These studies also give variable rates of hyperhaploidy and of structural aberrations as well. The frequency of hyperhaploidy has varied by a factor of about 3—from about 0.6 per cent (Brandriff et al. 1985; Kamiguchi and Mikamo 1986) to 1.8 per cent (Martin 1985). The frequency of structural aberrations, the most common type of aberration described in sperm, has also varied by a factor of 3, ranging from 4 to 13 per cent.

These various observations of chromosomal aberrations in germ cells permit a wide range of estimates of the incidence of aberrations at conception. Such estimates depend heavily on the frequencies of chromosomal aberrations in oocytes and sperm chosen for the calculation. They also require assumptions about those chromosomal aberrations, such as autosomal monosomies, that have rarely appeared in human conceptions. Thus, one assumption is that germ cells with hypohaploidy of autosomal chromosomes occur and are fertilized (producing monosomies) at the same frequency as germ cells with hyperhaploidy (producing trisomies), but virtually all such conceptions end in subclinical loss. With this assumption, a high estimate of the incidence rate of chromosome aberrations at conception (assuming hyperhaploidy in 8 per cent of oocytes and 1 per cent of sperm) is about 18 per cent; a low estimate (assuming hyperhaploidy in 3.4 per cent of oocytes and 1 per cent of sperm) is about 9 per cent.

The low estimate of the incidence of aberrations admits the possibility that the rate at conception is no higher than the frequency among clinically recognized pregnancies. The estimate is nearly the same as that reported at 5 to 6 weeks gestation in one study of induced abortions. The equivalence obtains even though the estimate allows for autosomal monosomies to be added at frequencies that balance those of trisomies (on the theory indicated earlier that each trisomy must have its complement in a monosomy). This similarity between the low estimate and observed frequencies raises the possibility, therefore, that conceptions with hypohaploid germ cells may not equal those with hyperhaploid germ cells. The low estimate might also be taken as compatible with another observation: before 8 weeks gestation, the proportion chromosomally aberrant among miscarriages is consistently lower than at 8 to 11 weeks (28 per cent versus 52 per cent; see Chapter 7).

The low estimate of incidence challenges the view that aberrations at conception, because of high attrition rates soon after, far exceed those observed in clinically recognized pregnancies both in number and in type. One should take note of the vulnerable assumptions built into the estimates of incidence based on germ cells, whether high or low. Despite the preceding arguments, the low proportion of aberrations observed before 8 weeks compared with later miscarriages might easily give a false impression of incidence rates. It is a reasonable anticipation that at conception chromosomally normal zygotes substantially outnumber aberrant zygotes. If so, a *rate* of early loss lower among chromosomally normal than among aberrant conceptions (as would be expected) is still compatible with a *proportion* of chromosomally aberrant conceptions that is lower among very early losses than among later ones. A rate of early loss among the chromosomally normal equal to or greater than that among the aberrant would certainly lead to the same result, that is, a lower proportion of chromosome aberrations in early losses than in late ones.

Later in gestation, rates of loss among the chromosomally normal and the aberrant do diverge in a way that changes the balance in their proportions observed at miscarriage. As we shall see, nearly all chromosomally aberrant conceptions miscarry in the first half of pregnancy; nearly all chromosomally normal conceptions survive beyond that time.

MORPHOLOGIC ANOMALIES

Miscarried products of conception take several forms: mere fragments of membrane, empty amniotic sacs either intact or ruptured, amniotic sacs with a blighted ovum, disorganized embryos, organized embryos, and organized fetuses. A fetus is distinguished from an embryo by the completion of organogenesis; all organs except the external genitalia are present in rudimentary form, and subsequent development involves growth and elaboration. In a normal pregnancy, embryos cross the threshold of fetal development toward the end of the eighth week after conception (or 10 weeks after the last menstrual period); hence the definition of 56 days from conception for the separation of fetuses from embryos (Moore 1988).

Some chromosomally normal miscarriages show an early failure of development. The abortus may consist of a severely disorganized embryo or only of a sac with or without a small blighted ovum. These disorders halt all development and, of course, have no counterpart in the fetus. More developed chromosomally normal miscarriages consist of an organized embryo or fetus. At these later developmental stages, focal malformations may be recognizably similar in type to those found among births. In embryos and in macerated specimens, however, the diagnosis may be clouded.

The true frequency of gross dysmorphism and focal malformation among chromosomally normal pregnancies is somewhat uncertain. The uncertainty stems from the problematic quality of the materials examined. In roughly 30 per cent of miscarriages, specimens are not set up for tissue culture and karyotyping at all because fetal tissue cannot be identified (Lauritsen 1976; Creasy et al. 1976; Takahara et al. 1977; Hassold et al. 1980a; Byrne et al. 1985). In many miscarriages that are karyotyped and known to be chromosomally normal, what is found are mere fragments of membrane, or apparently empty sacs, ruptured or intact. Such remnants preclude judgment about the stage and type of embryonic development or even about whether an embryo developed at all.

These various losses to observation, incurred for both natural and technical reasons, tend to occur early in development; they are therefore strongly selective and likely to seclude gross dysmorphisms from detection. Among chromosomally normal miscarriages, the proportions cultured from incomplete specimens have ranged widely, from 11 to 52 per cent (Creasy et al. 1976; Takahara et al. 1977; Byrne et al. 1985). The gross dysmorphisms or malformations discovered at observation, it is evident, bear no certain relationship to the true proportions among clinically recognized losses, especially early losses.

Among later losses, uncertainty is relieved about the relations of what is observed to what exists. Confidence in the diagnosis of malformations increases in the fetal stage, and frequencies in fetuses at miscarriage can reasonably be compared with frequencies at birth. Table 6-2 shows such a comparison. The malformations selected for inclusion in the table are those that are likely to have similar chances of being ascertained both at miscarriage and at birth. The result was unexpected. For most organ systems, the proportions malformed varied little at the two endpoints.[2] This constancy in fetuses and births implies that in the fetal stage the rates of loss of normal and malformed fetuses are equal. Since the organ system categories are broad and the malformations included are selective, the result does not mean that particular types of defects might not occur more frequently in fetuses at miscarriage. Neural tube defects in England in the 1960s and early 1970s, for example, were found frequently among stillbirths (about 10 per cent), less frequently among chromosomally normal embryos and fetuses (3 per cent), and far less frequently among live births (0.15 per cent) (Carter and Evans 1973; Creasy and Alberman 1976).

The limitations of these comparisons of miscarriages and births should not be ignored. The miscarriages came from a single study and produced a relatively small number of malformations, with rates that cannot be expected to be entirely stable even when grouped by organ

[2]A study of embryos and fetuses obtained from induced abortions in a Japanese sample reported higher rates of malformations than have been observed in studies of the newborn (Nishimura 1970). The interpretation was that the probability of loss was higher for malformed than for anatomically normal embryos and fetuses. Unfortunately, these data do not provide information about the frequency of malformations among embryos and fetuses that are chromosomally normal. Only some were karyotyped and, among those that were, data on chromosomal and morphologic characteristics were not presented together. Hence, the data do not allow any conclusion about the frequency of miscarriage of malformations that occur in chromosomally normal pregnancies.

Table 6–2 Malformations in chromosomally normal fetuses at miscarriage and in births: selected major malformations of different organ systems

Organ system[c,d]	Chromosomally normal fetuses[a]		Births[b]
	Number	Rate/1000	Rate/1000
Central nervous	2	5.0	5.3
Cardiac	3	1.1	0.8
Musculoskeletal	2	5.0	5.2
Respiratory	2	5.0	3.2
Gastrointestinal/abdominal	2	5.0	3.4
Genitourinary	2	5.0	2.8

[a]Data from 400 abortuses in the New York City series (Byrne et al. 1985). Cardiac defects from 277 chromosomally normal fetuses were examined anatomically and microsopically (Ursell et al. 1985).

[b]Data on 50,282 births in the National Collaborative Perinatal Project (NCPP), from Heinonen et al. (1977), limited to major malformations that might be diagnosed in a similar manner in births and miscarriages.

[c]Malformations in fetuses by organ system include the following:
Central nervous—microcephaly; hydrocephaly
Cardiac—tetralogy; VSD; VSD and ASD, 2nd degree
Musculoskeletal—limb reduction deformities
Respiratory—diaphragmatic hernia; partial cleft lip and palate
Gastrointestinal/abdominal—asplenia; omphalocele
Genitourinary—fused kidneys; L-shaped kidney (same fetus as with asplenia)

[d]Two major malformations—arthrogryphosis and micrognathia—are excluded because ascertainment is not comparable in births and miscarriages.

system. Further, among the selective exclusions made to enhance comparability of miscarriages with births[3] were all embryos, whether organized or not, as well as several types of diagnosable malformations.

FACTORS IN THE ATTRITION OF ABNORMAL AND NORMAL CONCEPTIONS

The viability of a pregnancy is determined by both fetal and maternal attributes, acting separately or jointly. We begin by considering characteristics intrinsic to the conceptus. We then move to consider factors

[3]Most stillbirths in the United States Collaborative Perinatal Project that provided the data were examined for external and internal malformations. For surviving births, malformations were discovered either at the newborn examination or during follow-up to 4 years of age. The malformations selected were those visible on inspection or associated with perinatal death or morbidity in infancy. Malformations detectable at autopsy but unlikely to produce perinatal death or postnatal morbidity (e.g., Mullerian malfusion, malrotation of gut, accessory spleen) were excluded as were those in which a diagnosis in the fetus might be difficult (e.g., arthrogryphosis, micrognathia, clubfoot).

extrinsic to the conceptus, and in particular the attributes and experiences of the woman.

The Contribution of the Conceptus

Plausible propositions about the role of the conceptus in miscarriage include the following: (1) the risk of intrauterine loss is generally higher for abnormal conceptions (r_a) than for conceptions that are normal chromosomally and morphologically, that is, $r_a > r_n^*$, where r_n^*, denotes the probability of loss for a conceptus that is chromosomally *and* morphologically normal; (2) particular abnormalities are characterized by modal patterns of survival; and (3) attributes of the conceptus other than abnormality influence the risk and pattern of intrauterine loss.

The data that support these propositions draw largely on clinically recognized pregnancies. The hiatus in observation produced by subclinical losses limits and, as always, could easily confound interpretation. To keep a clear distinction between postulated frequencies at conception and observed frequencies, we use the notation r_{a_2} and r_{n_2} to refer to the rates of clinically recognized loss for pregnancies with and without abnormality *a*, respectively (see Figure 5-2, in Chapter 5).

Proposition 1: Losses of Abnormal versus Normal Conceptuses. $r_a > r_n^*$. Chromosomally aberrant pregnancies have a risk of clinically recognized loss (r_{a_2}) certainly higher than that in all chromosomally normal pregnancies (r_{n_2}); the subgroup that is chromosomally normal and also morphologically normal (r_n^*) has the lowest risk. For chromosomally aberrant pregnancies, estimates of clinically recognized loss depend on the aberration, and range from 25 to 100 per cent (see Table 6-1). For chromosomally normal pregnancies, estimates of loss are more tentative but much lower: for chromosomally normal pregnancies as a whole the rate of clinically recognized loss is about 8 per cent, and for the chromosomally and morphologically normal subgroup it is probably no more than 2 to 3 per cent.[4]

Most trisomies are incompatible with survival to birth; irrespective of the extent of subclinical loss, r_a is 100 per cent. Chromosomal aberrations compatible with live births all have rates of intrauterine survival substantially lower than chromosomally normal pregnancies (with the possible exception of the 47XXY Klinefelter karyotype), although the rates vary markedly. Less than 1 per cent (0.05 per 1000) of monosomy

---

[4]We obtained the estimate of 8 per cent by combining evidence on the probability of miscarriage at 8 weeks gestation or later from a single prospective study of loss (French and Bierman 1962) with estimates of the proportion chromosomally normal within 4 week gestational age intervals from four large karyotype series (Table 7-4). The estimate of 2 to 3 per cent derives from studies that followed pregnancies judged normal by ultrasound in the first trimester (Gilmore and McNay 1985; Cashner et al. 1987; Simpson et al. 1987).

X conceptuses survive to birth; as many as 25 per cent of recognized trisomy 21 conceptions do so. [We note in passing that monosomy X births and miscarriages differ in that the frequency of mosaicism, usually with a normal cell line, occurs in the majority of births and the minority of miscarriages (Hassold et al. 1988).]

With chromosomally normal fetuses, we have seen that the presence of focal malformations may not systematically increase the rate of clinically recognized loss. If they do not, r_{a_2} must be roughly equal to r_n^*. This result goes against the intuitive biological assumption that the damage from a major organ malformation is bound to raise the risk of miscarriage.

With r_{a_2} equal to r_n^*, one explanation could be misclassification: a proportion of chromosomally and morphologically normal fetuses have hidden abnormalities that render them vulnerable to miscarriage, for instance, homozygosity for a recessive gene. Another explanation could be that loss of chromosomally normal fetuses with focal malformations is influenced primarily by maternal as opposed to fetal factors. Cardiac anomalies, for example, may not interfere with intrauterine survival. Thus, the proportion and types of defects observed in a detailed systematic anatomical and microscopic study of fetal hearts in New York City were similar to those reported for live births (Ursell et al. 1985). That the cardiac anomaly itself causes no intrauterine problem during a phase when its primary function is in abeyance is perhaps not surprising. Even so, as we saw with neural tube defects, for particular malformations the chance of prenatal survival may be lower than for normal organisms.

Proposition 2. Modal Patterns of Survival. Specific chromosomal aberrations are associated with different degrees of intrauterine viability that set the schedule for survival. In karyotyped miscarriages, several chromosomal aberrations exhibit a modal configuration of survival. This phenomenon was first described in a study in Paris (Boué and Boué 1973b; Boué et al. 1975, 1976) of karyotyped miscarriages classified by developmental (but not by gestational) age (see Figure 6-1). Tetraploidies and trisomies of groups C and E (chromosomes 6–12 and 16–18,[5] respectively) ceased development early; in each the modal developmental age was 3 weeks. Trisomies of groups D and G (chromosomes 13–15 and 21–22, respectively) and monosomy X continued to develop somewhat longer, and had a modal developmental age of 6

---

[5]The majority of trisomies in group E, we have since learned from banding techniques, are trisomy 16.

$\longrightarrow$

Fig. 6–1 Distribution of various chromosomal aberrations by developmental age at miscarriage: (a) monosomy X (=45); triploidy (=69); tetraploidy (=92); (b) trisomies 6–12 (=C); trisomies 13–15 (=D); trisomies 16–18 (=E); trisomies 21–22 (=G). (From Boué et al. 1976)

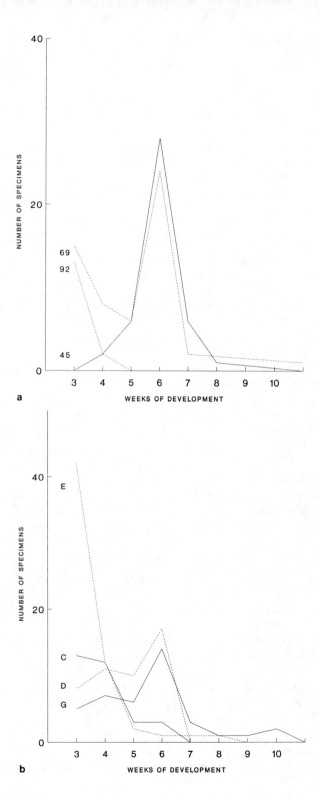

a

WEEKS OF DEVELOPMENT

b

WEEKS OF DEVELOPMENT

weeks. Triploidies had a bimodal pattern, with peaks at both 3 and 6 weeks (see also Chapter 7).

In the Parisian study, the distribution of developmental ages was truncated by the restriction of cases to less than 12 weeks of development. Developmental age was estimated from the stage of embryogenesis or, when no embryo was present, from placental histology (Philippe and Boué 1970). Although the sample must underrepresent miscarriages in which the conceptus reached the later stages of fetal development, the patterns observed for chromosomal aberrations generally conform with series that selected cases by gestational age (Kline and Stein 1987). Trisomies and also monosomy X each manifest a modal gestational age, and triploidies do not. We infer that these patterns of survival and loss reflect an intrinsic limit on development: different chromosomal aberrations are capable of sustaining different degrees of morphologic development. The most viable of the autosomal trisomies is that of chromosome 21, most of which reach the embryonic stage. Trisomy 16 is not viable, and embryonic development is rare (Kline and Stein 1987).

With focal malformations, modal patterns of survival are less well-studied than with chromosomal aberrations. By the nature of the phenomenon, we have noted, malformations can be ascertained only in conceptions that reach a stage of development in which the defect has become manifest. On the whole, this is the fetal stage. We can deduce that most fetuses with focal malformations must survive to 28 weeks gestation: as noted, the proportions malformed appear to be similar among fetuses miscarried before 28 weeks and births after 28 weeks, and the absolute frequency of births is about 50 times that of miscarriages of chromosomally normal fetuses.

Data on malformations in stillbirths are generally too sparse to add much to our understanding of the viability of specific malformations. Under good conditions, stillbirths constitute 1 to 2 per cent of all births. Thus, the majority of malformed fetuses will be liveborn, excepting malformations that are about 50 to 100 times more frequent among stillbirths than among live births. This was the case with neural tube defects reported from London (Carter and Evans 1973; Creasy and Alberman 1976).

Proposition 3: Attributes of the Conceptus   With certain anomalies, attributes of the conceptus other than the anomaly may moderate loss. For that majority of chromosomal aberrations in which r_a is close to 100 per cent, little room is left for other attributes to influence the rate of loss. This does not rule out other influences that might affect the course of development before it ceases. Triploidy provides a possible example.

Nearly all triploidies are nonviable. This anomaly carries an extra set of chromosomes that may be either paternal or maternal in origin. In a Honolulu study of karyotyped miscarriages (Jacobs et al. 1982), the results suggest that with triploidy the parental origin of the extra complement of chromosomes sets some of the conditions for the course of development. The extra chromosome complement was paternal in 54 triploidies; every one of these was found in a hydatidiform mole. Of the 54 moles, 53 were partial and only 1 was complete.[6] The extra chromosome complement was maternal in 15 triploidies; only 3 of these were found in moles: 2 of these 3 moles were partial and 1 was complete. Paternally derived triploidies (and hence partial moles) miscarried at later gestational ages than maternally derived triploidies (most of which did not occur in moles).

Sex is another condition that affects the probability of loss. Among live births, the male : female ratio (number of males : number of females) is greater than 1, and generally ranges from 1.04 to 1.07 (Visaria 1967). Among perinatal deaths, the male : female ratio is exaggerated, with some 20 per cent added to the male excess in births. By our computation, the male : female ratio for all perinatal deaths in the British Perinatal Survey of 1958 (Gruenwald 1969a,b) is 1.24: the ratios respective to antepartum and intrapartum stillbirths were 1.23 and 1.10, and the ratio for early neonatal deaths was 1.41. In this British Perinatal sample, males outnumbered females for most causes of death, as with immaturity, prematurity, Rh isoimmunization and trauma. For neural tube defects on the other hand, as expected from other surveys, there was an excess of females (Gruenwald 1969b).

Among karyotyped perinatal deaths, the findings are consistent with those for all deaths regardless of karyotype: the male : female ratios among chromosomally normal deaths have ranged from 1.15 to 1.62 (Machin and Crolla 1974; Sutherland et al. 1978). Among chromosomally normal miscarriages, the true male : female ratio is probably in the same direction as for perinatal deaths. Although in several series (reviewed by Hassold et al. 1983) the male : female ratios appeared at first to be reversed (less than unity), some miscarriages are liable to be misclassified as females. One study provides an estimate of the extent of such misclassification: in a substantial number of cases (6 to 20 per cent depending on the criterion), cells of maternal rather than fetal origin had been inadvertently karyotyped. The male : female ratio adjusted for misclassification was estimated at 1.32 (Hassold et al. 1983).

Operations to induce abortions are carried out at roughly the same time in gestation as miscarriages are likely to occur. Among chromosomally normal induced abortions, the male : female ratios in several studies disperse around unity, varying from 0.92 to 1.07 (Sasaki et al. 1971; Hahnemann 1973; Yamamoto et al. 1977; Kajii et al. 1978;

[6]In a complete hydatidiform mole, there is generalized hyperplasia of villi in classic grape-like form and no embryo or fetus. In a partial mole, only some of the villi are swollen and an embryo or fetus is present. The diagnosis of the two complete moles in this series was tentative because of the small amount of tissue available.

Hassold et al. 1983; Ohama et al. 1986). It seems likely that, as with miscarried products, some males have been misclassified and thus the true ratio exceeds unity.

Insofar as the male : female ratio among induced abortions is in fact similar to that among births, and the ratio among chromosomally normal miscarriages is higher, then the rate of attrition during gestation must be higher for males than for females. A simple hypothesis postulates a male excess at conception that is steadily depleted by the preferential attrition of males in the course of gestation and through the first week of life. The hypothesis must remain insecure as long as we remain ignorant of the male : female ratio of a high proportion of conceptions.

The Maternal Contribution

A woman provides a buffer that protects the "perfect parasite" in her womb against the severities and hazards of the external environment. At the same time, the buffer is not perfect; the woman also provides the sole access to the growing organism for those agents and infections that can breech the placental barrier once she has inhaled, ingested, introjected or absorbed them.

A maternal attribute or exposure might influence the risk of intrauterine loss through several mechanisms. Interference with the development of the conception might produce an abnormality that is ultimately lethal and followed by loss. In the production of chromosomal aberrations, if the factor has not acted on the germ cells of one of the parents, it must act no later than at the time the zygote is formed. Other types of damage occur after conception; as we discussed earlier, the forms they take depend on their timing. Damage to the placenta and the supply system of the developing organism, rather than direct damage, might also produce disorders of growth or development. In all these instances, intrauterine loss would be consequent on the impairment of the conceptus. With a normally developing organism that fails to survive to term, some other mechanisms might come into play. An adverse factor might prove rapidly lethal in utero without causing abnormality. Alternatively, an adverse exposure or unfavorable uterine environment might precipitate the premature expulsion of a normal conceptus before it had acquired the potential for autonomous existence.

In practice, knowledge of both the maternal state and the reproductive outcome is often too incomplete to allow us to distinguish between pathogenetic mechanisms. For example, fever during pregnancy has been associated with chromosomally normal miscarriage, and the data are compatible with several mechanisms (Kline et al. 1985). The fever alone, or the infection of which it was a symptom, might have produced an abnormality in the conceptus that made it vulnerable to subsequent loss; the fever or infection might have been lethal for the developing organism without producing abnormality; finally, the fever or the infection could have impaired the placenta, the uterus, or the endocrine system and thus caused the expulsion of a normal but not yet viable organism.

Maternal characteristics and experiences may influence the probability of pregnancy loss, or the time during gestation that the loss occurs, or both. Factors extrinsic to the developing organism that influence losses are most readily detected among chromosomally normal pregnancies. Even here, the conceptus may be the determinant of the miscarriage. In most cases, development has ceased before the fetal stage and many are grossly dysmorphic. For abnormalities incompatible with survival to birth, there can be no increment in losses; the only effect on survival that could be observed is a shift of the intrauterine loss to earlier or perhaps later gestational ages. On the other hand, with trisomy 21, one-quarter of which do survive to birth, maternal factors could influence rates of survival and loss.

Extrinsic factors might act at any time in gestation to affect intrauterine survival. We noted previously (see Chapter 4) that in the first trimester 5 to 8 per cent of pregnancies were judged not viable on ultrasonography, and another 2 to 3 per cent thought to be viable later miscarried (Gilmore and McNay 1985; Cashner et al. 1987). Assuming that (as in miscarriages overall) about half of the nonviable pregnancies were chromosomally normal, it follows that in a majority of chromosomally normal miscarriages the factors leading to the loss have acted before the end of the embryonal phase.

The list of potential maternal influences on reproductive loss is long. It includes characteristics of the woman such as age, obstetric history and medical and gynecologic conditions; exposures such as smoking, alcohol drinking, medications and contraceptives; and disorders such as infection, diabetes and epilepsy. These characteristics and exposures are considered in relation to the risk of miscarriage in later chapters. Factors extrinsic to the conceptus, one should bear in mind, might also reduce the probability of miscarriage. This could hold not only for conceptions that are normal in karyotype and morphology but, against intuition, for conceptions with abnormalities that do not prevent survival to birth.

Joint Action of Maternal and Fetal Factors

The most complex source of variation in rates of miscarriage might reside in the joint action of maternal with embryonic or fetal factors. We use joint action here in the biological sense of the enhancement of separate effects by synergy, or their suppression by antagonism. Enhancement or suppression by *biological interaction* results in effects larger or smaller than the simple combination of the effects of the participating factors, and produces one form of statistical interaction (Susser 1973).

That the pregnant woman and fetus jointly contribute to reproductive outcome is the common knowledge, not always expressed, of obstetricians. Incompatibilities of the Rh and ABO blood groups between the pregnant woman and fetus provide notable examples. For instance, 15 per cent of Caucasians[7] are Rh negative. With random mating (among Caucasians), an Rh negative woman might be fertilized by a man carrying either two genes with the incompatible factor (39 per cent of the population) or one such gene (48 per cent of the population). This means that in Rh negative women about 60 per cent of conceptions can be expected to have incompatible Rh blood types. When fetal blood cells gain access to the maternal bloodstream, as they commonly do in the course of labor, the pregnant woman develops antibodies against Rh positive blood and remains sensitized thereafter. With each subsequent Rh positive fetus, the mother's antibodies become increasingly sensitized and tend to cause increasing degrees of fetal damage in successive pregnancies; the range runs from hemolytic disorder of the newborn, through kernicterus and hydrops fetalis, to perinatal death. Thus, the chance of sensitizing a fetus is influenced not only by the concordance of its Rh type with that of the mother but also by the effects of previous conceptions on her immune state.

Another example of possible interaction between maternal and fetal factors is seen with the recurrence of neural tube defects at birth. Women with one affected pregnancy are at increased risk of having an affected offspring subsequently, and risk is even higher after two affected pregnancies (reviewed in Elwood and Elwood 1980; Seller 1981). This increasing recurrence risk may be due jointly to genetic factors and to environmental factors. On the environmental side, deficiency of specific nutrients is a candidate under hot pursuit as a causal factor.[8] An early randomized trial of folic acid supplementation before conception (Laurence et al. 1981) was too small to permit a conclusion; recurrences occurred in 2 of 60 supplement-treated pregnancies (both to women who had not adhered to the regimen) and in 4 of 51 placebo-treated pregnancies.

A larger but nonrandomized trial carried out in England and Northern Ireland suggests that the risk of recurrence might be reduced by a maternal supplement, before conception, of a mix of vitamins. Vitamins A, B complex, C, and D, folic acid, and iron were all given together. In this trial one cannot be discriminated from another and the hypothesis of a specific folic acid deficiency could not be tested. The favorable result held in two series of women, although not in a third. In the first

[7]Ethnic variation is marked with the Rh blood groups. Only 5 per cent of blacks in the United States are Rh negative.

[8]Several randomized clinical trials (Wald and Polani 1984; Elwood 1983; Czeizel and Rode 1984; reviewed in Rhoads and Mills 1986) are now underway to test whether various vitamin supplements lower the risk of neural tube defects.

two series, the rates of recurrence among fully supplemented women were reduced to 0.7 per cent (3 out of 429), compared to 4.7 per cent (24 out of 510) among unsupplemented women (Smithells et al. 1981, 1983, 1985; Wild et al. 1986). In the third series, of smaller sample size, the rates were similar between fully supplemented and unsupplemented women (4 out of 157 or 2.5 per cent versus 2 out of 135 or 1.5 per cent) (Seller and Nevin 1984).

If the overall beneficial effect suggested by the combined data is upheld in randomized trials, two etiological interpretations might apply. It is possible that persisting nutritional deficiencies alone increase the likelihood of neural tube defects in each pregnancy. Alternatively, the nutritional state of the woman may be a condition that interacts with the genetic constitution of the conceptus. In other words, the embryonic predisposition to developmental error may be modified by the nutrients supplied by the woman. The latter hypothesis is consistent with animal experiments in the curly-tailed field mouse, a species genetically susceptible to neural tube defects. Vitamin A either increases or decreases the frequency of the defect depending on the timing of the treatment and the sex and genotype of the progeny (Seller 1982).

Few instances of the joint action of maternal and fetal factors have been analyzed quantitatively in terms of *statistical interaction*. When present, biological interaction is bound to give rise to statistical interaction, although the reverse does not hold (Susser 1973). Interaction implies that, if we give primacy to the woman, fetal outcome varies with the presence or absence or the degree of maternal attributes or conditions. If we give primacy to the conceptus, analogous differences among conceptions would result in maternal responses conditional on those differences and produce outcomes that vary likewise.

In theory, interaction between maternal and fetal factors in miscarriage implies that the joint effect of these factors on the probability of loss is greater or less than the sum of their effects taken separately. In practice, differences between women that relate to reproductive loss are poorly understood and seldom quantified. Hence, conditional relations between the woman and the conceptus can often be discussed only on the presumption rather than the fact of interaction.

The extremely high frequency of abnormalities found at miscarriage initially prompted the notion of maternal–fetal interaction in miscarriages. Miscarriages, we proposed, might be seen as a maternal screening device for the rejection of abnormal conceptuses and thus for the maintenance of effective reproduction in the face of a high rate of biological error at fertilization (Stein et al. 1975c). The unknown mechanisms by which an abnormal conceptus is miscarried, we supposed, involve a maternal response to a signal from the conceptus. Whether or not the abnormality is lethal in utero, activation of the uterus must precede the expulsion of the conceptus. When the abnormality is of a potentially viable type—for instance trisomy 21, trisomies of the sex chromosomes and focal malformations—maternal factors extrinsic to the conceptus might influence the probability of loss. When the abnormality is not viable and loss is inevitable, maternal factors might yet influence the time of loss.

The theory of screening for the early detection of disease provides a conceptual framework in which to consider maternal-fetal interactions in the relations between r_a and r_n^* (Stein et al. 1975c). *Sensitivity* can be defined as the ability of a screening test to recognize abnormality, and *specificity* as the ability to recognize normality. An analogy for reproduction equates the probability of loss for abnormal conceptions (r_a) with sensitivity, and the probability of survival for normal conceptions ($1 - r_n^*$) with specificity.

In screening for disease by means of a particular screening test, these two properties are inversely related. When the test criterion used to define likely cases of disorder is lowered, the resulting increase in sensitivity is accompanied by a decrease in specificity, and vice versa. If the analogy with a particular screening test were exact, with a decline in sensitivity one might expect that fewer abnormal conceptions would be lost; at the same time specificity, if not 100 per cent to start with, would improve reciprocally, and more normal conceptions would survive.

In the maternal screening hypothesis, however, the presumption is that a woman with an efficient maternal screening mechanism would cause the rejection of all abnormal conceptions including potentially viable ones (high sensitivity) and allow all normal ones to survive (high specificity). A more appropriate analogy is therefore with the comparison of two tests, one of which is more accurate than the other. In this instance one could expect a change across the board in maternal capacity to discriminate between normal and abnormal conceptions. In other words, if the postulated maternal screening mechanism exists, a decline in accuracy is likely to depress both sensitivity and specificity; respectively, fewer abnormal conceptions might be lost (r_a) and fewer normal conceptions might survive ($1 - r_n^*$).

We have seen that with miscarriages, the opportunity to test the operation of a postulated screening mechanism must be largely limited to that minority of chromosomal aberrations that are potentially viable and to malformations. Maternal aging provides a circumstance in which the efficiency of a screening mechanism might be expected to decline. Among recognized pregnancies, the effect of maternal age on the frequency of miscarriages of both chromosomally normal and trisomic conceptions seems to be in the same direction (Stein et al. 1980). The frequency of chromosomally normal miscarriage increases in women beginning in their late thirties (Chapter 16), and this increase is accompanied by a decrease in the survival time of the conceptus indicated by mean gestational age (Warburton et al. 1986). Effects of maternal age on gestational age are also seen with aberrations that are potentially viable such as trisomies 13, 18 and 21, but not with the lethal aberration trisomy 16 (Warburton et al. 1986). With trisomy 21, the proportion miscarried appears to rise in women in their forties.

Thus, at least among clinically recognized losses, the best fitting postulate appears not to support a screening model: rather, maternal age seems to increase the general liability to miscarriage, rather than the capacity to discriminate between normal and abnormal conceptions. As we shall discuss in Chapter 17, some of us have suggested that this conclusion cannot simply be extended to subclinical loss, when attrition may be substantial (Stein et al. 1986). In the subclinical phase, a screening model cannot yet be rejected.

CONCLUSION

Miscarriages are not a homogeneous class of events. Cytogenetic studies display an astounding range of types and frequencies of aberrations. We shall see, too, that morphologic studies reveal heterogeneity in the development of both chromosomally aberrant and normal miscarriages. For chromosomally normal losses such studies reveal both early disruptions in development and losses of apparently normal embryos and fetuses. In later chapters we consider in greater detail the patterns of intrauterine survival for the various types of miscarriage and the factors that might determine these patterns.

7 Karyotypes at Miscarriage: Variations and Regularities

Traditional wisdom for epidemiologists facing a new problem and searching for leads is summed up in a few cogent questions: what? who? when? where? The answer to "what?" requires that the investigators define, in ways serviceable for data collection, the "cases" that are the object of attention; or, if the object of attention is a potential hazard of some sort, that they characterize and provide measures of "exposure." Answers to the questions of who, when, and where demand quantitative knowledge of the occurrence of cases in populations, times and places. Which kinds of people are affected and at risk and what are their attributes? What changes are observed through time in chronologies that may be secular, seasonal, diurnal, or pointedly epidemic? Which places—town or country, slum or suburb, tropic or temperate—are burdened and which untouched? In epidemiology these variations and regularities are the foundation for the inference by induction from which plausible hypotheses about causes can be derived and tested.

Available knowledge about the occurrence and frequency of aberrant karyotypes allows us to answer only a few of the questions posed. We begin our exploration of chromosomally aberrant and normal miscarriages by considering variations in frequencies between studies. All studies use cross-sectional samples of medically attended miscarriages. As guideposts, we offer several propositions at the outset. A previous analysis of existing data (Kline and Stein 1987) provides the groundwork for these propositions; naturally, we expect them to be modified as fresh data accumulate.

Chromosomally Aberrant Miscarriages

1.1. The frequencies of specific types of chromosomal aberrations at miscarriage exhibit a high degree of constancy in different peoples and at different times and places (provided only that maternal age at childbearing is similar among them). These constancies are a feature of chromosomal aberrations at all reproductive endpoints—induced abortions, amniocenteses, stillbirths and live births.

1.2. Specific chromosomal aberrations exhibit typical and idiosyncratic patterns of development and viability.

1.3. The constancy underlying the observed patterns of development and loss of chromosomal aberrations is best explained by the primacy of the aberrations themselves in determining the patterns typical for each.

1.4. The constancy of patterns of frequency, development and loss of chromosomal aberrations leaves a limited role for environmental factors in both incidence and survival rates, but it does not exclude them.

1.5. The factors that determine incidence are particular to each type of chromosomal aberration. Whatever these factors might be, their action is most likely to occur early, that is, before or at conception. The hiatus that exists in observations of development and attrition during the subclinical phase of pregnancy needs to be weighed in interpretations of incidence.

Chromosomally Normal Miscarriages

2.1. The proportions of chromosomally normal miscarriages vary. This variability is a feature mainly of the second trimester, when in some part it reflects true variations in incidence.

2.2. The variability in the proportions of chromosomally normal miscarriages at late stages in gestation is best explained by the effect of maternal and other environmental factors on the viability and survival of the fetus.

2.3. The consistency of the proportions of chromosomally normal miscarriages at earlier stages in gestation leaves a limited role for maternal and other environmental factors in incidence but (as in 1.4 under Chromosomally Aberrant Miscarriages) does not exclude them.

2.4. The majority of chromosomally normal miscarriages have not reached the fetal stage. Thus, most factors that influence incidence must act early, that is, before conception, at conception, or in the subclinical phase. At the maximum they must act by 8 weeks after conception.

OVERALL VARIATION IN CHROMOSOME ABERRATIONS

Table 7-1 summarizes the nine largest series of karyotyped miscarriages now available. Three continents, three decades and many ethnic groups are encompassed by these studies. The overall proportions that are chromosomally aberrant range widely, from 22 to 61 per cent.

Table 7-2 shows the specific chromosomal aberrations found in the five largest series of the nine shown in Table 7-1; all include more than 500 karyotyped miscarriages. Despite the twofold variation across studies in the overall proportion of chromosomal aberration, the proportions of specific aberrations among all aberrations are remarkably similar. Trisomies occur in roughly 50 per cent of all chromosomally

Table 7-1 Selected studies of karyotyped miscarriages: study setting, definition of miscarriage, sample sizes, karyotype rate; among those karyotyped, proportions chromosomally aberrant, less than 12 weeks gestation, 20 weeks gestation or more, and fetuses

| Study | Definition[a] | Number of miscarriages | | Karyotyped[c] (%) | Chromosomally aberrant | Karyotyped specimens (%) | | |
		Identified[b]	Karyotyped			<12 weeks	≥20 weeks	Fetuses
Boué et al., 1975, Paris	<12 weeks DA postconception	NR	1498	70	61	NA	NA	NR
Kajii et al., 1980, Geneva	Crown-rump length < 100 mm	806 s	402	71	54	NA	NA	NR
Lauritsen 1976, Aarhus County, Denmark	≤18 weeks GA	460 w	255	89	55	<64[d]	0	NR
Takahara et al. 1977 Ohama[e] Hiroshima	<20 weeks GA	NR	505	~65	47	44	1	~5
Carr 1967, London, Ontario	<22 weeks GA and <500 g	400 s	227	57	22	NR	NR	NR
Dhadial et al. 1970, London, England	≤24 weeks GA	1000 s	423	63	24	<34[d]	NR	NR
Hassold et al. 1980a[e], Honolulu	<500 g	NR	1639	~89	49	44	5	NR
Creasy et al. 1976, London, England	<28 weeks GA	2620 s	941 singletons	57	30	14	26	45
Warburton et al. 1986, New York City	<28 weeks GA	6342 w	2314	62	38	36	18	32

[a]DA = developmental age; GA = gestational age (LMP).

[b]NR = not reported; NA = not applicable, cases selected by developmental age; s = number of specimens identified; w = number of women identified.

[c]Per cent karyotyped among specimens set up in tissue culture.

[d]Per cent first trimester; per cent <12 weeks not reported.

[e]Personal communication.

Table 7–2 Chromosomal aberrations at miscarriage: per cent distributions by type in selected studies

	Paris[a]	Hiroshima[b]	Honolulu[c]	London[d]	New York City[e]
Chromosomally aberrant: % (N)	61.5 (921)	46.9 (237)	49.2 (807)	30.5 (287)	37.6 (789)
Among chromosomally aberrant (%)					
Autosomal trisomies	53.7	57.0	50.1	49.8	49.3
Monosomy X	15.2	16.9	20.4	23.7	16.4
Triploidy	19.9	20.3	14.5	12.9	14.6
Tetraploidy	6.2	2.5	6.7	4.2	5.2
Rearrangements	3.8	1.3	5.3	3.1	3.4
Other[f]	1.2	2.1	3.0	6.3	11.2

[a]Paris: Boué et al. 1975.
[b]Hiroshima: Ohama, personal communication.
[c]Honolulu: Hassold, personal communication.
[d]London: Creasy et al. 1976.
[e]New York City: Kline and Stein 1987.
[f]Includes mosaics, hypertriploidies, others
(N) = number aberrant.
Source: Adapted from Kline and Stein 1987.

aberrant miscarriages, monosomy X in 15 to 25 per cent, and triploidy in 12 to 20 per cent. Combined, these three classes account for about 85 per cent of all chromosomally aberrant miscarriages.

The small differences between studies in the proportions of these three largest specific classes of chromosomal aberrations cannot explain the large differences in the overall proportions aberrant. For instance, the overall proportion aberrant is 60 per cent higher in Honolulu than in London. Trisomy, monosomy X and triploidy, on the other hand, comprise proportions of all aberrations that are nearly identical. Variations in proportions, we have taken care to explain, might be produced by changes in either the numerator or the denominator. The similarity of the distributions of specific aberrations across series argues for a source of the variations in the denominator, particularly in the chromosomally normal component (see Propositions 1.1 and 2.1).

Artifactual Differences between Studies

Much of the variation between studies in the overall proportion chromosomally aberrant results merely from disparate sampling. The proportions chromosomally aberrant are quite different in early and in late developmental stages. It follows that differences in the distributions of developmental stages sampled will lead to differences in the overall proportions aberrant and normal. As discussed before, with early miscarriages selective sampling arises especially from ascertainment practices and from selection of materials for laboratory study. With late miscarriages, it arises especially from differences between studies in the cutoff points for length of gestation from which the eligibility of a pregnancy termination as a case is decided.

Two studies, in London and in New York City, karyotyped all miscarriages through the second trimester (under 28 completed weeks of gestation). This period covers a majority of fetal losses; the data can thus be used to illustrate the sharp differences in proportions chromosomally aberrant between the organisms that survive into the fetal stage and those that do not (Table 7-3). In prefetal miscarriages, whether or not an organized embryo is present, the proportion chromosomally aberrant is around 50 per cent; in fetal miscarriages it is about 5 per cent.

The effect of unrepresentative sampling of early and late miscarriages is again seen in comparing London and New York City studies with the Hiroshima study. Both in London and in New York City, fetal miscarriages are overrepresented in the karyotyped sample, although for different reasons.[1] In Hiroshima, fetal miscarriages must be underrepre-

---

[1] In London, because fragments were not routinely cultured, the proportion of prefetal miscarriages was reduced; in New York City, karyotyping was more often successful with fetal than with prefetal miscarriages, which raised the proportion of karyotyped fetal miscarriages.

Table 7-3 Per cent (rounded) chromosomally aberrant within each morphological class at miscarriage (numbers karyotyped in parentheses)

Morphology	London		New York City	
	%	(N)	%	(N)
Fragments	29	(17)	45	(248)
Empty and ruptured sacs	52	(297)	58	(301)
Organized and complete embryos	54	(105)	57	(120)
Organized and complete fetuses	4	(421)	6	(430)
Total[a]	30	(941)	40	(1356)

[a]Disorganized embryos, specimens with a cord stump only, and incomplete embryo/fetus are included in total, but not in the proportions above because the classification system for the two former categories differed between studies.

Source: Data from New York City (Byrne et al. 1985) taken from an earlier phase of the study than those included in Tables 7-1 and 7-2. Data for London come from Creasy et al. 1976.

sented simply because of the virtual exclusion of losses after 20 weeks gestational age. In London, with 45 per cent of karyotypes from fetuses, the overall proportion chromosomally aberrant is 30 per cent. In New York City, with 32 per cent of karyotypes from fetuses, the proportion chromosomally aberrant is 40 per cent. In Hiroshima, with only about 5 per cent of karyotypes from fetuses, the proportion chromosomally aberrant is 47 per cent.

In Honolulu, descriptions of morphology were not recorded. Hence, whether or not a lowered frequency of fetal miscarriages accounts for the combination of relative deficiency of late karyotyped miscarriages with the higher proportion chromosomally aberrant is a question that cannot be answered. The criterion for inclusion in the series was a fetal weight of less than 500 grams. Judging by the New York City data, this criterion should have encompassed all but 1 per cent of losses up to 28 weeks gestation. Yet the impression of the Honolulu investigators (Hassold, personal communication) is that large fetuses of the type frequently encountered in New York City were uncommon. Ascertainment of miscarriages was not in the hospital wards but through the hospital laboratory designated to receive products of conception and fetuses less than 500 grams. One possible explanation for the apparent dearth of larger fetuses was that these had been routed to a second hospital laboratory. This possibility, checked partway through the study, was thought not to be the case.

Artifacts still less easily interpreted are created by the use of different indicators to select and classify the abortuses, that is, by a lack of uniformity in the definition of a case. Studies that assign a "developmental age" inferred from the stage and type of organization of the conceptus or placenta, and those that assign a chronological age inferred from length of gestation or "gestational age," will not agree. All fetuses, having by definition completed the developmental stage of the eighth week postconception, by the same definition miscarry later than the tenth week (LMP). On the other hand, embryos—all of which have by definition ceased developing before the eleventh week (LMP)—often miscarry later than that. In the New York City study, about 30 per cent of prefetal conceptions miscarried after the first trimester defined as 12 completed weeks (LMP).

Early Miscarriages: Prefetal Forms

The marked divergence among miscarriages between early and late stages of development in the frequency of chromosomal aberration indicates that the population of surviving organisms at each stage is sufficiently different to require separate treatment. In a consideration of early miscarriages, we at once meet an impediment in comparing karyotype studies. The two selection criteria—developmental age and gestational age—have been used exclusively in different studies, but they relate differently to the stage of morphologic development.

If, as was suggested by the Parisian investigators (Boué and Boué 1973b), expulsion of the abortus indeed occurs an average of 5 to 7 weeks after its development has ceased, then the sample selected and classified by the index of developmental age will depart markedly from one for which the index is gestational age. Most karyotype studies have used gestational age—length of gestation at the termination of pregnancy—to select miscarriages (see Table 7-1). Besides the difficulties of obtaining precise dates of fertilization, if after development has ceased expulsion is delayed for several weeks, the gestational age index will obviously be a flawed indicator of the time when development becomes abnormal or ceases.

Developmental age therefore contends with gestational age as the better index of development. In practice, published data based on developmental age are too few to permit comparisons between studies. Data based on gestational age are more plentiful. To examine variations in the patterns of attrition for chromosomally normal miscarriages, therefore we rely solely on a recasting of available data based on gestational age (Table 7-4). Inconsistencies between samples with a divergent range of gestational ages can be dealt with by making comparisons within the same limited gestational age intervals. Inconsistencies between studies in the proportions of chromosomally aberrant or chromosomally normal miscarriage might then reflect true disparities, and consistency might reflect true similarities.

In fact, the data for first-trimester miscarriages are persuasive of similarity between populations. Consistency is evident between different

Table 7–4 Per cent (rounded) chromosomally aberrant within gestational age intervals at miscarriage (numbers karyotyped in parentheses)

Gestation (4 week intervals)	Hiroshima[a]		Honolulu[b]		London[c]		New York City[d]	
	%	(N)	%	(N)	%	(N)	%	(N)
≤7	14	(44)	37	(82)	———	(0)	26	(91)
8–11	41	(167)	54	(641)	50	(121)	53	(594)
12–15	56	(210)	50	(620)	44	(376)	46	(632)
16–19	69	(51)	40	(209)	21	(168)	24	(266)
20–23	———		44	(55)	10	(145)	12	(248)
24–27	———		46	(28)	0	(83)	14	(91)
Total	48	(472)	49	(1635)	31	(893)	38	(1922)
Unknown	25	(28)	50	(4)	19	(48)	28	(176)

[a]Hiroshima: Ohama, personal communication. Although miscarriages of 20 weeks were not systematically obtained, the investigators also report 5 losses at 20 to 23 weeks, 2 of which were aberrant.

[b]Honolulu: Hassold, personal communication.

[c]London: Creasy et al. 1976.

[d]New York City: Kline and Stein 1987.

Source: Adapted from Kline and Stein 1987.

ethnic groups and across far-flung locations. Four of the five largest karyotype studies exhibit consistent proportions of chromosomally aberrant and chromosomally normal throughout the first trimester (Table 7-4 and Figure 7-1). In each, the proportion aberrant rises to a peak between 10 and 12 weeks gestation (LMP) and then declines slightly. Three of the four studies included miscarriages that occurred before 8 weeks (LMP). As noted in Chapter 5, the proportion chromosomally aberrant is lower in the earliest period than in the immediately subsequent period (Kline and Stein 1987). The proportion chromosomally normal is, of course, complementary: highest before 8 weeks and lower in the remainder of the first trimester.

The general consistency of these results is compatible with biological explanations (see Chapter 5). Here we need to draw attention to the Paris study (Boué and Boué 1973b), which classified abortuses by developmental age; the proportions of chromosomal aberrations obtained thereby challenge the consistency of the other studies, which classified by gestational age. In the Paris series, the specimens in which development was presumed to have been arrested very early were more frequently chromosomally aberrant than normal. At the very earliest stage of 2 weeks developmental age, the proportion chromosomally aberrant was highest (78 per cent of 23 specimens); at the stage of 3 to 6 weeks the proportion was lower (62 to 70 per cent of 1018 specimens); and at later stages of developmental age the proportion declined further.

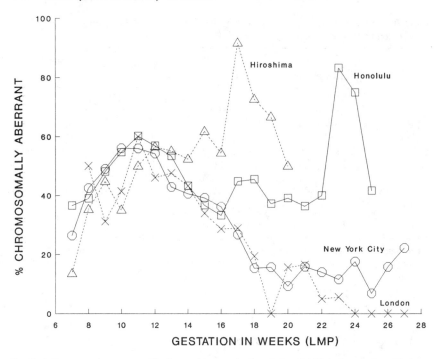

Fig. 7–1 Per cent chromosomally aberrant by week of gestation (LMP) in four series of karyo-typed miscarriages. (From Kline and Stein 1985b)

Taken at face value, these observations permit an alternative explanation for the finding, among karyotyped series classified by gestational age, of a dearth of aberrant relative to normal karyotypes in the earliest stage, that is, before the gestational age of 8 weeks. It might be that chromosomally aberrant conceptuses in which development ceased at 2 to 3 weeks after fertilization may miscarry later in gestation than chromosomally normal conceptions of the same developmental age. The lower proportion aberrant before 8 weeks gestational age might then reflect a difference, not in development, but in the time a conceptus with aberrant or normal karyotype is retained in the uterus after development has ceased.

In the main, we face an issue of interpretation because of differences in the operational definitions of age. This difficulty does not detract from one significant issue of fact, which is the consistency in those studies that have used the same definition of age for the conceptus.

Fetuses and Later Miscarriages

The consistency between studies in the proportions chromosomally aberrant and normal in the first trimester is not sustained later in gestation. In the second trimester, the patterns of East and West diverge (see Table 7-4 and Figure 7-1). On the one side, in London and New York City the proportion chromosomally aberrant declines steadily, from a peak at 11 weeks gestation until the end of the second trimester, which was the cutoff point for miscarriage in both studies. On the other side, in Hiroshima (where losses at 20 weeks and later were not systematically collected) the proportion chromosomally aberrant does not decline, and in Honolulu the decline continues only up to 16 weeks of gestation and is more modest and less regular than in the East. The proportions chromosomally normal are necessarily complementary. In London and New York City, where the proportions chromosomally normal rise as the length of gestation increases, the proportions at 20 weeks and later are 85 per cent or more. In Honolulu, with an irregular and much less marked rise in the proportions chromosomally normal as gestation increases, the proportion at 20 weeks and later is 55 per cent.

The disparity between East and West most likely arises from variations in the chromosomally normal component of miscarriages (Proposition 2.1). Chromosomally normal miscarriages, unlike the chromosomally aberrant, vary markedly in their distributions across gestational age (Figure 7-2). The proportions of all chromosomally normal miscarriages that occurred at 20 weeks gestational age and later are roughly 35 per cent in London, 25 per cent in New York City, and only 6 per cent in Honolulu.

The differences between these several locations in the gestational age distributions of chromosomally normal miscarriages contrast with the similarities seen for trisomies, monosomy X and triploidies (Figure 7-2). The low proportion of chromosomally normal miscarriages late in gestation in Honolulu might reflect a low incidence of such later losses in the population sampled. The low proportion might also reflect unrepresentative ascertainment and sampling after 16 weeks of gestation, when the proportion chromosomally normal clearly begins to diverge from those in London and in New York City. Differences in methods of ascertainment between these studies exist, but they may not explain the whole of the divergence between East and West.

An argument against selective bias in ascertainment is provided by the dissimilarity of the results for Honolulu and London notwithstanding similar ascertainment procedures and, conversely, by the similarity of the results for London and New York City notwithstanding different procedures. In Honolulu and London, where the proportions chromosomally normal later in gestation are low and high, respectively, the samples were defined in terms of miscarriage specimens identified through hospital laboratories. In New York City, with karyotype distributions similar to London, the sample was defined in terms of women. All women seeking care for miscarriage at any location in three medical centers were identified by a review of admission records, medical charts,

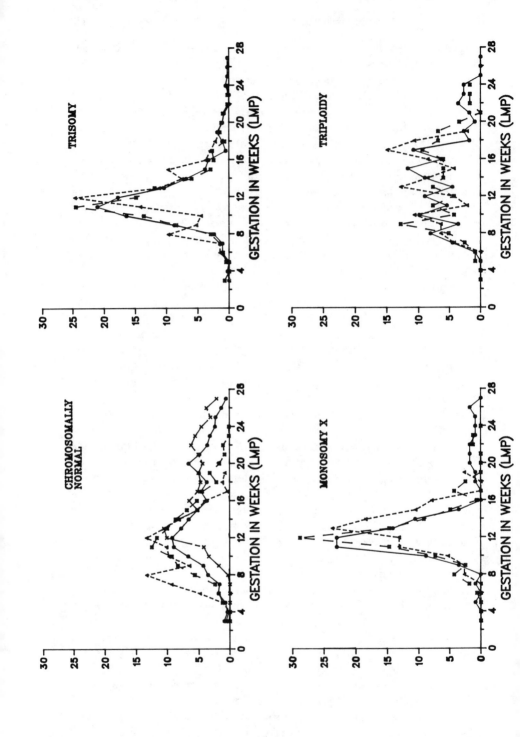

operating room schedules, pathology logs, and the collection of miscarried products of conception.

Ascertainment is thus unlikely to explain the low proportion chromosomally normal in later miscarriages in Honolulu compared with New York City and London. Nor do the different success rates of centers in culturing tissue for karyotyping seem likely to explain these disparities late in gestation, since they produce no evident disparities early in gestation.

A reasonable interpretation of the relative dearth of late chromosomally normal miscarriages in Honolulu is simply that fewer were collected than in New York City and London: large fetuses, and losses of 20 weeks gestation and later were far less frequent in Honolulu. Selective sampling, from what can be discovered, seems not to have occurred. If this bias is ruled out, the best remaining explanation is that true geographic or ethnic differences in the rate of loss of chromosomally normal fetuses underlie differences between the Eastern and Western sites.

SPECIFIC CHROMOSOMAL ABERRATIONS: PATTERNS OF VIABILITY

Survival and continuing development are two facets of the viability of an organism. It follows that departures from normality in capacity for survival, and in the stage of development attained by an organism, are often aspects of the same underlying defect in viability. In accordance with this proposition a number of chromosomal aberrations, at miscarriage as at birth, manifest both characteristic phenotypes and characteristic survival patterns (Proposition 1.2).

Morphologic Development

Critical descriptors of miscarriages that bear on the viability of chromosomally aberrant forms are the stage and type of morphologic development. These descriptors support the idea that the type of chromosomal aberration determines the patterns of development and loss. At birth, several aberrations manifest typical phenotypes: Down's syndrome characterizes trisomy 21, Turner's syndrome characterizes monosomy X, Edward's syndrome characterizes trisomy 18, and cri-du-chat syndrome characterizes a deletion of the short arm of chromosome 5. By backward extrapolation from such observations at birth, chro-

Fig. 7–2 Per cent distribution by week of gestation (LMP) for chromosomally normal, trisomy, monosomy X, and triploidy miscarriages from four series of karyotyped miscarriages: ▲ Hiroshima; ■ Honolulu; ● New York City; X London. (From Kline and Stein 1987)

mosomal aberrations seen at miscarriage might also be expected to display typical phenotypes in their morphological development. This proposition is difficult to evaluate. To consider the difficulties, we need to digress somewhat before moving to conclusions.

A first and mundane difficulty inheres in the process of ascertainment through medical facilities. By the time a woman has sought medical attention, the products of conception often cannot be obtained intact and hence described. The products might be lost either in the normal process of expulsion or in the process of treatment by dilatation and curettage or other surgical procedures. In some specimens that are retrieved, even the previous existence of an embryo cannot be assumed with certainty: mere fragments of membrane and ruptured embryonal sacs without a cord can comprise from 20 per cent to as many as 45 per cent of all karyotyped specimens (Creasy et al. 1976; Takahara et al. 1977; Byrne et al. 1985). In other specimens, such as a ruptured sac with only a portion of umbilical cord, the existence of an embryo can be assumed but no embryo is on hand.

A second and remediable difficulty that obscures the connection between karyotype and phenotype again arises from a lack of uniformity in methods. Both the techniques used to study specimens and the schemes used to classify the observations affect comparisons. The Paris study (Boué and Boué 1973b) used both embryo and placenta to classify the abortus. Phenotypes and developmental age were judged from gross anatomy and from the histology of placentas. Other studies have described the miscarried products macroscopically in variable detail (Singh and Carr 1967; Lauritsen 1976; Creasy et al. 1976; Takahara et al. 1977; Kajii et al. 1980; Byrne et al. 1985). The definitions of most morphological classes in all these studies are comparable, but the methods of examination and thus of categorization may vary.

Even with these difficulties of comparison, it is clear that morphologic development as well as viability may be determined by the karyotype. To illustrate, we describe three aberrations—monosomy X, trisomy 16, and trisomy 21—that display characteristic phenotypes and also differ in their likelihood of survival to birth (Kline and Stein 1987).

> **Monosomy X** is compatible with survival to birth. Of recognized conceptions, about 5 per 1000 are born alive. At miscarriage, monosomy X tends to be associated with an intact amniotic sac. Most often, the remains of an embryo are found at the end of a well-defined cord (Boué et al. 1976; Byrne et al. 1985). In about one-third, an organized embryo or fetus is found. Although embryos generally have appeared normal, fetuses have manifested defects, such as bronchial swelling, that are typical of Turner's syndrome at birth (Singh and Carr 1967; Boué et al. 1976; Creasy et al. 1976).
>
> **Trisomy 16,** always lethal in utero, seems to be incompatible with development beyond an early stage. The predominant phenotype is a sac, either empty or containing a small blighted ovum (Boué et al. 1976).

Trisomy 21 is compatible with survival to birth in about 25 per cent of recognized pregnancies. At miscarriage, the majority have formed an embryo or fetus (Boué et al. 1976). Major malformations among miscarried trisomy 21 fetuses have been infrequently detected. In New York City, one of seven trisomy 21 fetuses was found to have a heart defect on dissection (Byrne et al. 1985). In the same study, smaller fetuses with the trisomy 21 aberration were characterized by short limbs and a dysmorphic appearance.

Other trisomies may also exhibit characteristic morphologic development at miscarriage, as the Paris study suggests (Boué et al. 1976, 1985).[2] Certainly, the proportions with organized embryos or fetuses seem to vary with the type of trisomy (Table 7-5).

To conclude on the relation of chromosomal aberration to phenotype, the intrinsic character of the chromosomally aberrant conceptus, it seems clear, imposes narrow limits on variations in phenotype and viability.

Length of Gestation

Another index of the capacity for survival of a chromosomally aberrant conception is provided by the duration of gestation the conceptus can sustain. For this purpose, we examine the distribution of gestational age at miscarriage for specific classes of chromosomal aberration. In this exploration, we give heed especially to the consistency between studies.

The necessary data are available from three studies conducted in Hiroshima, Honolulu and New York City (see Figure 7-2). The three largest classes of aberration—autosomal trisomies, monosomy X, and triploidies—each manifests a distinctive pattern of gestational age at miscarriage that holds across the three studies. Trisomies and monosomy X both evince a modal distribution: for trisomies, the mode is at 11 to 12 weeks; for monosomies, the mode is at 11 to 13 weeks. Triploidies tend to miscarry evenly throughout the gestational interval, stretching from 7 to 18 weeks.

In summary, the data on survival patterns point up sharp contrasts between organisms of aberrant and normal karyotype. With the chromosomally aberrant, the modal distributions by length of gestation displayed by the three largest classes are so similar between studies, in the face of the potential for artifactual fluctuations emphasized earlier, that they must be counted striking. Consistency in the face of heterogeneous geography, culture and ethnicity argues for patterns of intrauterine

[2]In Paris, miscarriages of less than 12 weeks developmental age were studied. In theory, the exclusion of miscarriages at later stages in development might have biased observations relating specific aberrations to morphologic development. In practice, the potential for this bias is not large; it can affect only the few aberrations (trisomies 13, 18, 21, XXY, monosomy X, and triploidy) that are compatible with the formation of a fetus.

Table 7–5 Morphologic development in trisomic miscarriages: per cent (rounded) embryos and fetuses by type of trisomy[a]

Type of trisomy	Per cent with organized embryos or fetus	Total number of specimens examined
2	0	25
4	9	11
5	0	1
7	18	17
8	0	14
9	0	14
10	0	9
13	23	26
14	20	15
15	26	38
16	3	136
17	0	2
18	46	26
20	25	8
21	52	40
22	31	32

[a]Combined miscarriage data from Aarhus County (Lauritsen 1976), London (Creasy et al. 1976), and New York City (Byrne et al. 1985); all used a gestational age criterion for eligibility. The numbers of banded autosomal trisomies studied were 60, 89 and 265, respectively.

survival peculiar to each kind of aberration, regardless of the population source. Modal survival, it appears, is mainly determined by the anomalous character of the conceptus itself, and not by extrinsic factors.

CONCLUSION

To conclude, consistency between settings points to the karyotype as the commanding determinant of the state of morphologic development attained before miscarriage, and of patterns of survival into successive stages of gestation (Proposition 1.3). Thus, typical patterns in relation to karyotype could be recognized at miscarriage: specific chromosomal aberrations exhibit modes for stage of development (inferred from morphological form); and classes of aberration, except for triploidy, exhibit modes for survivability (inferred from gestational age attained by the organism). These regularities appear despite indices of frequency and form that are far from ideal. They appear across studies that have used different criteria to select miscarriages for study. And they appear despite diversity of peoples and environments. When manifest variation is so limited, we can expect the usually difficult search for environmental determinants to be even more difficult (see Proposition 1.4).

The different classes of chromosomal aberration differ in underlying genetic mechanisms. Some, such as trisomies, arise most of the time from errors in the parental germ cells; others, such as triploidies, arise most of the time at conception. In all, however, factors that influence incidence must act before or at conception. Since different genetic mechanisms give rise to the different aberrations, such factors may be specific to each type (see Proposition 1.5).

Even the earliest observable chromosomal aberrations, we repeat, are prevalent and not incident cases. It follows that observable frequencies can relate not only to factors affecting incidence, but also to factors that influence subclinical loss.

If the type of chromosomal aberration is the primary determinant of development, we might suppose that, at least for some aberrations, the modes seen at terminations in clinically recognized miscarriage could reflect the true norms of their capacity for survival. Animal experiments provide some support for this proposal. Aberrations produced by the breeding of hybrid mice have exhibited specific unimodal patterns of survival: where chromosomal material was deficient, the conceptions were rarely observed beyond the preimplantation stage; where chromosomal material was excessive, conceptions could be observed beyond the early postimplantation phase, although not at birth (Gropp 1973; Ford and Evans 1973).

The supposition that modes of survival observed at miscarriage are true norms for survival requires that there is only one mode. In that case, the numbers of each specific aberration observed at miscarriage might be close to the numbers at conception; further, such factors as are found to relate to such aberrations might be unconfounded by selective attrition in the subclinical phase of pregnancy. This is only one among several possible interpretations. Earlier modes for losses in the subclinical phase of pregnancy cannot be ruled out. Subclinical losses in human beings are probably substantial; biochemical losses alone might be twice as common as clinically recognized losses. Since subclinical losses are inaccessible to karyotyping and exact counts (Chapter 4), the possibility of bimodal distributions of survival for chromosomal aberrations remains.

With chromosomally normal miscarriages, distributions by length of gestation are dissimilar across studies. The differences are centered in the second trimester. In part, these divergencies may reside in method, but they could also stem from true variations in the rate of late chromosomally normal miscarriages (see Proposition 2.1). Causes may lie in the geographic, socioeconomic, ethnic, and cultural factors that distinguish these three locations (see Proposition 2.2).

8 Environmental Factors, Miscarriage and Karyotypes

In this chapter we consider environmental factors, as they might be manifest both in karyotypic aberrations, and in miscarriage as an adverse outcome in its own right regardless of karyotype. Environmental factors, in our broad definition, are all factors extrinsic to the conceptus that influence its development or its survival to birth. The environment provided for the developing organism by the pregnant woman goes beyond her own physiological and anatomical attributes. All external influences that impinge on her, and that through her may impinge on the developing organism, are part of this environment.

Although the scope of environmental factors is vast, we are quick to admit that the limits of our scientific knowledge are narrow. To understand environmental effects, we need to comprehend the meaning of variation in the chromosomally aberrant and normal conceptuses observed at different stages of pregnancy. For several chromosomal aberrations, the pointers to the processes of genesis and survival come from studies of miscarriages alone. For a few only, notably trisomy 21, evidence from studies of births is also substantial. Recently prenatal diagnosis has added to the evidence.

Maternal factors can act at the genesis of abnormal conceptions to alter incidence, and so may affect prevalence observed at subsequent stages of pregnancy in a primary way. Maternal factors can also act to the same effect in a secondary way, by altering the balance between attrition and survival for the conceptus, whether chromosomally aberrant or normal. Survival up to any point, we have emphasized, determines prevalence at that point. Paternal factors have less scope than maternal factors, both before and after fertilization, to affect outcome.

We have already noted that chromosomal aberrations may arise either in the germ cells of one parent or at the time of fertilization. Knowledge about the possible mechanisms gives some clue to the timing of an active factor and its maternal or paternal source. Regarding chromosomal aberrations, the evolution of germ cells takes different courses in females and in males. In the course of this evolution, the germ cells might be especially vulnerable to the disruption of the chromosomal structure during the rearrangements of normal meiosis. Far less time is needed to complete the process of meiosis in the germ cells of males than of females. In females, the first stage of meiosis begins in the oocyte while the woman-to-be is still a fetus in her mother's womb. After this beginning, a long stretch of preconceptional environmental experience must intervene before an ovum ultimately comes to be fertilized in a woman of mature reproductive development. Consequently, ova at fertilization could carry in their chromosomes and cytoplasm the imprint of maternal exposures impressed on them at any point in that long stretch. In males, meiosis in spermatocytes is a process that begins around the time of puberty. New spermatozoa, produced continuously, survive about 10 weeks. Exposures that could affect the zygote by disrupting the meiosis in spermatocytes are likely to be limited to the brief span of development that precedes fertilization.

Intrinsic defects in the conceptus produced before or at conception may be either maternal or paternal in origin. In defects produced around the time of conception, it seems possible that paternal pathways for environmental factors may involve not only the spermatozoa but also the semen. Studies in rats have yielded some provocative results. Cyclophosphamide fed to males has been found in a sequence of stages that indicate absorption of the substance by the dam and subsequent transmission to the conceptus: the substance has been detected in the ejaculate; in the mated female, to its detriment; and it has also resulted in cytopathological effects in the conceptus and preimplantation loss (Trasler et al. 1985; Hales et al. 1986). Even if the origin of the aberration can be fixed at fertilization, however, questions about parental source and about the exact time of initiation in relation to the fertilization process sometimes remain open. Triploidies provide an example. The mechanism that gives rise to most triploidies is the fertilization of a single ovum by two spermatozoa (Jacobs et al. 1978). Double entry by spermatozoa is normally averted by the response of the vestments of the ovum to the entry of a first spermatozoon; the electrical "acrosome reaction" repels penetration by subsequent sperm (Gould and Stefano 1987). In theory, with regard to parental source, this response might fail because of a defect in either ovum or spermatozoon. With regard to timing, the arrival of the two sperm might not be consecutive but simultaneous; by their coincidental arrival and penetration, they might jointly evade the acrosome blockade.

Once the zygote is formed, maternal factors are obviously more salient than are paternal factors, and they are more salient for the survival of normal than aberrant karyotypes. With aberrant karyotypes, we have seen that survival must be in the main a function intrinsic to the conceptus. With normal karyotypes, on the other hand, although survival may also be a function of the conceptus and its capacity for normal development, there is more leeway for maternal factors. Paternal influence in intrauterine loss can be ruled out because of the inaccessibility of the conceptus to the male parent except in very special circumstances. For example, it is not impossible that a pregnant woman might be exposed to compounds such as lead or vinyl chloride carried on the person and the clothes of her male partner, or to his tobacco smoke.

MISCARRIAGE AS THE FOCUS OF STUDY

Clinically recognized pregnancies, we have noted, miscarry in the range of 12 to 21 per cent (see Chapter 4). We have noted further that most severe developmental anomalies that can survive to recognized pregnancy are lost, so that miscarriages concentrate chromosomal aberrations and gross disruptions in morphologic development. They thus provide a source in which to seek environmental determinants of developmental anomalies (always keeping in mind that the factor might alter their probability of survival to clinically recognized pregnancy instead of their incidence). Miscarriages are currently the sole source from which to seek environmental determinants of losses of apparently normal conceptions.

We once suggested that changes in the *overall* rate of miscarriage might signal not only the involvement of maternal factors in losses of apparently normal conceptions, but also changes in the incidence of developmental anomalies (Stein et al. 1975c). We have since come to understand that, in reality, a very large change must occur in the incidence of any particular anomaly, say a single chromosomal aberration, to produce even a modest change in the overall miscarriage rate. For example, trisomy—the most common of the chromosomal aberrations among miscarriages—would need to increase in prevalence nearly six-fold to produce a doubling in the overall rate of miscarriage (Kline 1986). Doubling of the overall miscarriage rate could more easily be produced by chromosomally normal miscarriages, since their frequency is far higher than that of any single chromosomal aberration or class of aberrations. At the same time, one must recognize that the anticipated accretion of statistical power in studies of chromosomally normal losses might be reduced by heterogeneity among them, especially in the morphological form of the conceptus. If an environmental effect were to be specific to each abnormal form, increases in the overall rate of loss might not be readily detectable.

The advantages of studying miscarriages go beyond their relatively high frequency. Miscarriages reflect a diversity of abnormal processes in pregnancy, and specimens accessible to examination in a variety of ways can provide information about the mechanism of the loss. The products of conception can be karyotyped, classified by morphology, and examined histologically, biochemically and immunologically. In epidemiology karyotyping, and to some extent morphology and histology, have so far been most used. Other techniques await further testing and development for large-scale application.

The chromosomal aberrations found in about 50 per cent of miscarriages can be divided into types according to structure—for instance, trisomy, monosomy X, triploidy and tetraploidy—or according to the postulated mechanism that gives rise to the anomalies, which may or may not coincide with structure. Trisomy is usually but not only the result of meiotic nondisjunction in the female germ cell; monosomy X is most likely the result of the loss of a chromosome in a very early mitotic division; triploidy often results from fertilization by two sperm; and tetraploidy results from the failure of the first mitotic division in the zygote. It is unlikely, if not impossible, that one agent will produce all these types of chromosomal aberration. When such associations are found, therefore, one looks for other explanations than a change in incidence that affects all types of aberration at once. Instead, attention is turned to a maternal effect that changes survival patterns either before or after clinical recognition of pregnancy, or to possible bias in the study design, for instance, in the maternal histories taken after the loss.

Against the advantages of studies of miscarriage in the search for the causes of chromosomal aberrations must be set the disadvantages. We have taken pains to show that interpreting observations is difficult when the proportions of aberrant and normal karyotypes among miscarriages are the measure of outcome. This has been the case in most studies of chromosomal aberrations; chromosomally normal losses drawn from the same sample have served as an internal comparison group by which to estimate the expected frequencies of exposure (Carr 1970; Dhadial et al. 1970; Lazar et al. 1973; Boué and Boué 1973b; Boué et al. 1975; Lauritsen 1975; Alberman et al. 1976).

In these cross-sectional data, in essence, the chromosomally aberrant and chromosomally normal are compared in regard to the proportions exposed and unexposed. Although the limitations of such internal comparisons are not disposed of, such data may sometimes yield to interpretation. When only one type of chromosomal aberration among many is associated with a risk factor, the plausible explanation is that incidence at conception has been altered. When only chromosomally normal karyotypes are associated with a risk factor, the most plausible explanation is an increase in the frequency of reproductive loss. The subclinical phase of pregnancy might be entertained as the source of an effect when data for the different observable phases of the reproductive process cannot be reconciled with each other. For example, incoherence between the parental age associations of trisomies and their parental origins led to the hypothesis that the incoherence relates to survival in the subclinical phase of pregnancy (Stein et al. 1986).

In other situations, interpretations are elusive. For instance, when an exposure occurs in excess among all types of chromosomal aberration, an interpretation of changed incidence is placed in doubt. Perhaps, contrary to biologic expectations, a single factor has increased the incidence of many chromosomal aberrations. Alternatively, the factor might have allowed aberrant conceptions to survive long enough to appear among miscarriages because of a maternal deficiency in rejecting such aberrations in the subclinical phase. Or the factor might have acted on chromosomally normal conceptions to improve their survival and not at all on the chromosomally aberrant. Such effects on intrauterine survival could lead to the spurious inference that the risk of chromosomal aberration had increased (Stein and Susser 1978). Even the seemingly straightforward case, in which exposure appears to relate neither to aberrant nor to normal karyotype at miscarriage, could be misleading. Because both karyotype forms at miscarriage could be adverse outcomes of an environmental exposure, two interpretations are possible. Either exposure is without effect—on either chromosomal aberrations or chromosomally normal loss—or it has affected both. In such an instance, to discover the existence of an effect requires knowledge of the baseline miscarriage rate and the changes that have ensued in relation to exposure.

Knowledge about the effects of risk factors on miscarriage is seldom firm enough to allow a choice between several alternative explanations to be made merely from cross-sectional observations relating exposure to karyotypes among miscarriages. For both chromosomally aberrant and chromosomally normal miscarriages, comparisons with pregnancies that do not miscarry are sounder. An early partial use of this strategy was made in a study of the effect of maternal irradiation on chromosomally aberrant miscarriages. Exposure to irradiation among chromosomally aberrant miscarriages was compared with exposure both among chromosomally normal miscarriages and among births (Alberman et al. 1972b). The New York City miscarriage study took this design strategy to its logical conclusion. All miscarriages seen in a hospital setting served as cases; pregnancies that did not miscarry, as shown by survival to at least 28 weeks gestation, served as the reference group for all miscarriages whether chromosomally aberrant or normal.

Factors implicated in miscarriages undifferentiatied by karyotype are many (see reviews by Leridon 1977; Lauritsen 1977; Strobino et al. 1978; Kline and Stein 1984). For most environmental factors, evidence is scant. Still, the list of determinants that must be given serious consideration remains too long to treat in full (Table 8-1). We focus on the few factors that have been examined in relation to karyotyped miscarriages in particular. Such studies refine the outcome and sharpen biological understanding. For trisomy 21 we also turn to studies of births and of prenatal diagnostic specimens.

First, we consider variation in the broad environmental context of

Table 8–1 Postulated environmental factors in miscarriage

Parental age
Previous or recurrent miscarriage (including immunological
    factors)
Induced abortion and/or dilatation and curettage
Maternal infections and/or fever
Maternal smoking
Maternal alcohol drinking
Oral contraceptives, conception with intrauterine device in
    place, use of spermicidal agents
Gynecologic conditions
Chronic maternal diseases: diabetes, epilepsy
Irradiation
Maternal medication and drug use
Socioeconomic characteristics
Stress
Nutrition, including consumption of specific substances
    such as caffeine-containing foods and beverages, sac-
    charin
Hormonal factors

social class and ethnicity. Then we turn to specific exposures that have been sufficiently studied to provide at least a modicum of evidence about their effects on prenatal development that become manifest in either reproductive loss or karyotype. The ordering of these specific factors in the text begins with those over which a woman can exercise individual control, namely, smoking, drinking, contraception, and induced abortion. Factors over which she usually has no direct control follow, namely, irradiation, fever and infection, and the workplace.

SOCIAL CLASS AND ETHNICITY

The influence of socioeconomic and ethnic factors on miscarriages overall, and on their karyotypes in particular, has not been the subject of thorough study. For the few data that do exist, interpretation is difficult. All such data derive from medically attended pregnancies. Entry to medical care is affected not only by necessity but by social and psychological factors. In general, women of higher social class have been more likely to obtain medical care than those of lower class (Susser et al. 1985b); patterns vary locally and over time with the manner of service provision, access, and availability as well as culture.

These variations can be expected to have had a powerful effect on the selection of first-trimester miscarriages seen in medical facilities. In some women an early miscarriage may cause little reaction: it may be seen as an event too insignificant to justify the time and expense of medical attention; or it may be passed off as merely an episode of irregular menstrual bleeding and go unnoticed. In the reported data on miscarriage, the ways in which selective factors act in reality remain obscure.

Associations with social class or ethnicity that are not owed to selection must reflect antecedent or intervening factors related to those statuses. As yet, even such known risk factors as maternal age have been little explored in relation to the social class configurations of miscarriage. The socioeconomic and genetic factors that are conflated with ethnicity also remain largely unexamined. For instance, a disadvantage for blacks can be discovered from a patchwork of data, but systematic study is lacking. In a prepaid health plan in New York City in 1958–60, the rate of miscarriage among nonwhites was double that among whites (Shapiro et al. 1971). In a California prepaid health plan the risk for blacks was also higher than that for whites. In the California study, maternal education, which serves as one index of social status, showed no association with miscarriage (Harlap et al. 1979b; 1980a). Aside from this, little is known of the underlying factors.

With karyotyped miscarriages, a London study found the proportion chromosomally aberrant to be greater in the higher social classes, a result that remained stable with adjustments for the effects of maternal age, oral contraceptive use, parity and smoking (Alberman et al. 1976). One explanation, which remains untested, is that higher-class women had fewer chromosomally normal miscarriages. Another is that higher-class women obtained medical care for miscarriages early in gestation more often than lower class women. Since, in the London sample, the chromosomally aberrant tended to miscarry earlier in gestation than the chromosomally normal, aberrant karyotypes would appear in larger proportions in prompt and assiduous users of medical care. In accord with this explanation, women of the higher social classes were overrepresented among all hospitalized miscarriages compared to what was expected from births (Creasy 1977).

In Hawaii, social class might underlie some of the ethnic differences observed in karyotypes at miscarriage (Hassold et al. 1980a). As elsewhere, ethnicity in Hawaii is to some degree a surrogate for social class: the four most numerous groups in the study—Caucasians, Orientals, Filipinos and Hawaians—can be placed in descending order on a social class scale. Hawaians, at the bottom of the scale, had a larger proportion of chromosomally normal miscarriages and a smaller proportion of trisomies than all other groups. This finding for Hawaians could relate to reproductive behavior connected with social position; the authors attributed it to a lowered risk of trisomy because of the younger maternal ages of Hawaiian women.

Caucasians, at the top of the scale, appeared in excess among hospitalized miscarriages compared with the expectation from live births.

This excess was present in both the study hospitals and the vital records for Hawaii. Environmental factors connected with ethnicity or class might explain such a difference. The Caucasian excess in hospitalized miscarriages was not accompanied by any change in the distribution of karyotypes, however, which was similar to that in Orientals and Filipinos. In the face of this Caucasian excess, the similarity of karyotype distributions for the three ethnic groups points away from an effect specific to the genesis or survival of particular karyotypes and favors an explanation such as selective use of medical care after miscarriage.

In the New York City study of miscarriages of 1974–81, however, an environmental or ethnic explanation seems more plausible than variable use of medical care. Social class selection for medical care at miscarriage, judged by comparisons of private and public patients, was not evident in the past histories of cases and controls. Whether private or public, patients reported using medical care equally often for previous miscarriages (Kline et al. 1982). On the other hand, in the index miscarriage, the proportion chromosomally normal was higher overall among public than among private patients (64 per cent and 57 per cent, respectively), and remained consistently so within 4-week gestational intervals (Warburton et al. 1986). Differences in ready use of medical care do not easily explain a difference in outcome that persists at all stages of gestation.

Ethnic differences nonetheless pervade these comparisons and could confound them. Private patients were predominantly white; public patients were black and Hispanic in roughly equal proportions. The proportion of chromosomally normal miscarriages was in excess in blacks but not in Hispanics. The results are compatible with the black/white differences in the earlier New York City study of miscarriage mentioned above. In that study, with medical care for all groups provided by the same prepaid health plan, the rate of miscarriage was higher among blacks.

The specific factors involved in the excess proportion of chromosomally normal losses with social disadvantage remain to be explained. Social class differences might reside in one or many of several factors besides ethnicity and race. In the New York City karyotype study, the two classes of patients differed demographically and with respect to various habits (Kline et al. 1986): private patients were better educated and older, on average, than public patients, and they were less likely to smoke and more likely to drink alcohol. Although this does not by any means complete the list of potentially relevant factors, cigarette smoking and alcohol drinking are widespread. They serve to illustrate how broad factors such as class and ethnicity may govern the distribution and hence the scale of the population effects attributable to more specific factors. The social distribution of habits like smoking and drinking has implications for analysis as well. Thus, in studies of the effects of these exposures in different populations and at different times, we can anticipate confounding from other habits and exposures as well as the use of medical care associated with class, ethnicity, or time period. As will become clear in what follows, the possibility of such confounding is a major problem.

Miscarriages undifferentiated by karyotype have been associated, separately, with both cigarette and alcohol consumption in some studies. Miscarriages differentiated by karyotype can be expected, by virtue of refinement in the dependent variable, to improve specificity-in-the-effect. Karyotype studies subject hypotheses to sharper tests of causality and, if they withstand the tests, might also shed light on pathogenesis. This idea has been followed particularly in our own work, but some of the results prove perplexing; neither causal nor methodological explanations are always compelling. In one aspect, the review of the effects of smoking and drinking that follows demonstrates the difficulties of interpretation often encountered in the absence of large, consistent or specific associations.

CIGARETTE SMOKING

Cigarette smoking has been adopted successively by different social groups, and to the extent that it has receded it has followed much the same order. Factors that enter into the distribution of smoking in society are many. Social desirability and social constraints, fashion, and the economics of production and marketing as well as individual psychology and needs are all involved. As value-laden customary and social activities, smoking and drinking pervade some social groups more than others, and both activities are often indulged in by the same individuals. For the same reasons, these indulgences are socially mobile.

Thus in developed countries, smoking was adopted first by men of the upper social classes and then those of the lower. Subsequently women, first of the upper and later of the lower social classes, came to indulge in growing numbers (Susser et al. 1985b). Pregnant women have not been excepted. Upper-class and more educated women have now begun to desist (Kleinman and Kopstein 1987). The awareness among women and their doctors that their pregnancies might be put at risk has undoubtedly induced a degree of caution.

Miscarriage undifferentiated by karyotype has been linked with smoking during pregnancy in several studies (Kullander and Kallen 1971; Kline et al. 1977b; Himmelberger et al. 1978; Harlap and Shiono 1980; Axelsson and Rylander 1982; Hemminki et al. 1983b). In all, the associations are modest. In some (Himmelberger et al. 1978; Harlap and Shiono 1980; Hemminki et al. 1983b) the risk ratios of about 1.2 to 1.3 are compatible with an absence of risk reported in others (Selevan et al. 1985; Axelsson et al. 1984). In three studies, on the other hand, a dose-related effect, growing larger with the amount smoked, supported the inference that a risk does exist (Kline et al. 1981b; Axelsson and Rylander 1982; Hemminki et al. 1983b).

In two studies, however, the initial observations indeed appear to have been confounded. The associations did not persist with statistical control, in one for alcohol use (Harlap and Shiono 1980), and in the other for unwanted pregnancy (Kullander and Kallen 1971). Yet adjustment for confounding does not resolve and sometimes adds to the conflict among studies. In two other studies, the association did persist with statistical control (Kline et al. 1977b; Himmelberger et al. 1978).

Refinement of the independent or exposure variable adds something to plausibility: in the New York City study, for example, miscarriage related to smoking, but only during pregnancy and not before (Stein et al. 1981b). The chief refinement of the dependent or outcome variable is by karyotype. Whether smoking impairs the capacity of a woman to sustain a pregnancy or the capacity of the conceptus to survive, effects should best be detected in chromosomally normal pregnancies.

Many more chromosomally normal than chromosomally aberrant conceptions are candidates for miscarriage upon exposure to an adverse factor. These candidates for miscarriage are confined to pregnancies that can be expected, under usual circumstances, to persist in utero until they are viable. Chromosomally normal conceptions constitute about 95 per cent of all clinically recognized pregnancies. Of these 95 per cent, as many as 8 per cent might subsequently be lost. Only about one-third of these losses (2 to 3 per cent of the total with normal karyotypes) are potentially viable, in that they reach the fetal stage. Slightly more than 90 per cent of all clinically recognizable pregnancies, therefore, might be karyotypically normal and potentially viable. All of these are available candidates that could add to the tally of miscarriage upon exposure to an adverse factor before the pregnancy reaches the stage of viability. Among the 5 per cent or so of all clinically recognized pregnancies that are chromosomally aberrant, almost the opposite obtains: more than 90 per cent are lethal, leaving fewer than 10 per cent that might reach the stage of viability, and that could add to the tally for miscarriage upon exposure to an adverse factor before they reach that stage.[1] With chromosomally aberrant pregnancies, some additional effect of a factor inimical to the survival of pregnancy might be found to shorten survival and hence shorten gestation, but this cannot add to the total tally of miscarriage.

Two early studies of smoking in karyotyped miscarriages relied, with inconsistent results, on comparisons of chromosomally aberrant and chromosomally normal losses. In a study in Paris, younger but not older

[1] It follows, when the appropriate calculations are applied to these frequencies, that chromosomal aberrations could add to the total tally of miscarriage in the ratio of 1 for about 220 chromosomally normal.

inhaling smokers had an increased proportion that were chromosomally normal (Boué et al. 1975); in a study in London, however, after adjustment for several other factors, smokers showed no such increase (Alberman et al. 1976).

The New York City case-control study took births as its reference group: exposures among women with miscarriages defined by karyotype (cases) were compared with those among pregnant women registering for prenatal care before 22 weeks, and not delivered before 28 completed weeks (controls). As regards smoking, this large study is the most closely analyzed so far available. All of the analyses reported here controlled statistically for age, ethnic group and education, and also simultaneously for the effects of alcohol drinking (Kline et al. in preparation).

The results in public patients point to a modest dose-related effect of smoking during pregnancy on chromosomally normal miscarriage: an odds ratio of 1.3 (95 per cent confidence intervals 1.1, 1.6) with 1 to 13 cigarettes per day rose to 1.6 (95 per cent confidence intervals 1.2, 2.0) with 14 or more per day. The results appear to be, as anticipated, specific to chromosomally normal miscarriage. For chromosomally aberrant miscarriage, with 1 to 13 cigarettes per day the odds ratio was 1.0; with 14 or more cigarettes per day, the odds ratio was 1.2 (95 per cent confidence intervals 0.9, 1.7).

The specificity of these results is perhaps clouded a little by the slightly raised odds ratio relating ex-smoking to chromosomally normal loss (1.2 with a lower confidence limit of less than 1); if real, this could imply a possible effect persisting from before pregnancy. Some previous results of the study, in relation to trisomy, have also seemed to cloud specificity. In the first phase of this study, smoking seemed to relate to trisomies in complex ways; in younger women the results pointed to reduced frequency of trisomies, in older women to possibly increased incidence (Kline et al. 1983). Fortunately, complicated interpretations can be dispensed with. The complete data set of the New York City study, which drew on two further phases of observation, indicates no such associations. In addition, an attempt to confirm, in older women, an effect of smoking on trisomies discovered at prenatal diagnosis refutes the earlier result. The lower rates of Down's syndrome at birth among smokers is most plausibly attributed to the depletion of trisomic pregnancies in the latter half of gestation (Kline et al. 1980c; Hook and Cross 1985, 1988; Shiono et al. 1986a; Christianson and Torfs 1988).

These variations between and within studies are not of a kind that dislodge the results of the a priori test of the hypothesis that smoking is a cause of miscarriage among public patients of the large-scale and focused New York City miscarriage study. The results among private patients, however, do give us pause in asserting what the nature of the relationship among public patients might be. Among private patients, no significant association was seen. Even disregarding statistical significance, the pattern of results does not resemble that for public patients. The odds ratio for smoking with chromosomally normal miscarriages was 1.2 (95 per cent confidence interval 0.8, 1.8) for 1 to 13 cigarettes per day and 0.8 (95 per cent confidence interval 0.5, 1.2) for 14 or more cigarettes per day.

A straightforward interpretation of these results is that smoking has a modest and conditional causal effect on miscarriage. That is to say, where there is social disadvantage, as in public patients, smoking has an effect on chromosomally normal loss; where there is no social disadvantage, as in private patients, any possible adverse effort is buffered. A plausible buffer would be, for instance, a more robust state of health. As always with modest associations in case-control studies, unidentified confounders and selection bias cannot be entirely ruled out, although every effort has been made to do so.

Alcohol Drinking

The drinking of alcohol shares with smoking all those characteristics that attach to a social phenomenon. As an indulgence much older than smoking, it is even more deeply encrusted with values and rituals of behavior. The forms of drinking, too, differ sharply between social groups and exhibit social mobility among them. Briefly, women in the past have used alcohol much less than men. In recent decades the gap between the sexes has been closing, and higher-class women were the first to become customary drinkers. As to drinking during pregnancy, the recognition of the possible danger has begun to affect women's behavior in that regard. It will become evident that the social factors involved in drinking lead to the same issues of the distribution of risk and difficulties of analysis encountered with smoking.

Miscarriage, undifferentiated by karyotype, has been connected with the drinking of alcohol during pregnancy in one cohort study and one case-control study.

In a California cohort (Harlap and Shiono 1980), women who drank had an increased risk of miscarriage in the second trimester. One or two drinks a day carried a twofold risk, and three or more drinks a 3.5-fold risk. In the first trimester, however, the relative risk from one or more drinks a day was only 1.2. In the New York City study, an early report— which did not differentiate between karyotypes—found drinking associated with miscarriage in both first and second trimester. In the miscarried pregnancies of public patients, drinking twice a week or more was more than twice as common (odds ratio 2.6) as in pregnancies terminating in births (Kline et al. 1980a). Women in poorer social circumstances were most affected; in those educated beyond high school, many of whom received private care, little or no association was detected (Kline et al. 1981b). The appearance of coherence in these results was later reinforced by the finding of a dose-related association with drinking during pregnancy but not before.

Any simple notions of causality entertained to explain the results are at once dispelled in the analysis by karyotype of the complete data from the three phases of the study. Two types of findings—conditional relationships and nonspecificity—place difficulties in the way of a causal interpretation.

First, the positive associations of miscarriage with drinking during pregnancy were again conditional on the adverse circumstances of social disadvantage. As with smoking, they were confined to the public patient stratum; the private patient stratum revealed no such associations.

Second, in the instance of alcohol, the associations were not specific to chromosomally normal miscarriages. Among public patients, drinking during pregnancy had a strong and consistent dose-related association with chromosomally normal miscarriage. At the same time, however, an equally strong and consistent dose-related association with chromosomally aberrant miscarriage thoroughly refutes the expectation of specificity-in-the-effect by karyotype. No ready explanation presents itself for the absence of specificity. Results could not be attributed, for example, to chromosomal aberration produced by drinking around the time of conception or before: drinking during this time period should be adequately described by reports of usual drinking, and usual drinking levels were similar among women with miscarriages that were chromosomally aberrant, women with miscarriages that were chromosomally normal, and controls.

In the interpretation of case-control studies, a first response in the face of confusing, inconvenient or unwelcome results is to question the comparability of cases and controls. In this study as in all others, grounds for question exist. In New York City, women who enter a particular medical center for an acute episode such as miscarriage may not represent the same universe as the prenatal clinic patients who serve as controls. Hence, in the absence of a causal relationship, drinking might be more prevalent a priori among women rushed into hospital as emergencies than among women who voluntarily embark on the sober path of preventive care for their pregnancies. In fact, there is evidence that cases and controls do derive from the same population: the reported levels of *usual* alcohol drinking, outside of pregnancy, are virtually identical in cases and controls. Numerous other sources of incomparability were explored without resolving the dilemma. None clarified the nature of effects that did not discriminate by karyotype.

We therefore turn from methodological to other kinds of explanation for the nonspecificity in this result. In matters involving early pregnancy and chromosomal aberration, one refuge is the uncharted periconceptional phase. In this instance, there is no avail in the possible action of alcohol either at conception or in the subclinical phase; as noted, any such action demands an association with usual drinking at least as strong as with drinking during pregnancy, since women who change their drinking habits tend to do so not before conception but after pregnancy is recognized.

A remaining speculation invokes an explanation that, though biological, is not causal. In this study, women tended to reduce their drinking with the advent of pregnancy. The association among public patients of both karyotype classes of miscarriage with drinking during pregnancy but not before depends on the fact that women who served as controls reduced their drinking more than women who had miscarriages. Thus, the connection of drinking during pregnancy with miscarriage regardless of karyotype may not be a reflection of the usual drinking habits of the women who miscarry; instead, one might look to reasons that induce women who have successful pregnancies to change their habits. For instance, the many women who stop or reduce the use of alcohol soon after conception might respond to signals (say, nausea, which portends a good prognosis) from sound and viable pregnancies, while those who continue drinking as usual might have an impaired conceptus that sends no signals and is already on the path toward miscarrying.

Finally, attention must be paid to the differences in results for public and private patients. In the absence of associations specific to normal karyotypes, environment is unlikely to account directly for the divergence in outcome. Instead, attention turns to issues of design, misclassification and confounding. A design problem, for public patients only, relates to the possibility of selective use of services (between emergency admissions for miscarriage cases and prenatal registration for controls). Differential misclassification of exposure, whether in public or private patients or both, might have occurred if retrospective reporting among cases were to have been biased by the event of miscarriage. Confounding could account for the differences between public and private patients if undiscovered maternal characteristics relate both to drinking habits and to pregnancy outcome but only among either the public or the private group. Hence consistency across social strata, while bolstering a causal inference when present, may or may not undermine it when absent.

CONTRACEPTION

The introduction of efficient barrier contraceptives facilitated a revolution in family size and spacing and in all aspects of human reproduction. In the course of the past century, family limitation by contraception has come to be almost universally practised in the developed world: as a result of economic development, the diffusion of modern techniques, and the efforts of international agencies concerned with population, contraception is also being increasingly practised in the less developed world.

Spermicides

Spermicides have been widely used as contraceptives either alone or in conjunction with an obstructive method such as a diaphragm. Risks of miscarriage attached to spermicide use, whether before conception or around the time of conception, are inconsistent across studies (Harlap et al. 1980b; Jick et al. 1982; Huggins et al. 1982; Scholl et al. 1983). The New York City miscarriage study does not support the idea that spermicides carry a risk of miscarriage: use either before or around contraception did not differ between women with chromosomally normal miscarriages and women with term births. In this large sample the odds ratios, adjusted for an array of potentially confounding factors, exclude even modest increases in risk (Strobino et al. 1986b).

Associations of spermicide use specifically with trisomy have been sought in several studies including one of miscarriages, one of prenatal diagnostic karyotyping, and at least nine of live births (Table 8-2). The types of trisomies available for study at these three stages of pregnancy are not the same. Miscarriages draw on a large proportion of nonviable trisomies; chorionic villus sampling (usually at 8 or 9 weeks) and amniocentesis (usually at about 16 to 18 weeks) draw mainly on the potentially viable trisomies 13, 18 and 21; births tap predominantly trisomy 21. In the matter of exposures, the majority of studies of live births have focused on spermicide use around the time of conception, excluding from their purview the long preceding period during which exposures could also be influential.

Among live births, all studies but one have failed to detect statistically significant associations with trisomy (reviewed in Kline and Stein 1985b). At the same time, only one study of births (Louik et al. 1987) has had sufficient statistical power to exclude a doubling or even trebling in risk. The one positive report defined exposure on the basis of prescription records (Jick et al. 1981). Subsequently, it appeared that at least two of the three cases initially considered "exposed" were unlikely to have been using spermicides at the time of conception (Watkins 1986). Two studies of births provide information on spermicide use previous to conception (Polednak et al. 1982; Louik et al. 1987). Neither study detected an association with Down's syndrome (Table 8-2). A truly raised risk for births seems unlikely, even improbable (Louik et al. 1987).

With miscarriages, in contrast, preconception spermicide use spanning periods longer than one year was, in the New York City study,

Table 8-2 Spermicide use and chromosomal aberrations (summary of epidemiologic studies)

Study	Time of exposure to spermicide	Outcome	Risk Ratio (95% CI)
Miscarriages			
Strobino et al. (1986b) New York City	Within 1 year before LMP	All trisomies	0.9 (0.5, 1.6)[b]
	Duration of most recent use 1 year or more		1.9 (1.2, 3.0)[b]
Prenatal diagnosis			
Warburton et al. (1987b) United States and Canada	1 month before to 1 month after LMP	Trisomies 13, 18, and 21	0.9 (0.5, 1.7)[b]
	Within 1 year before LMP		1.1 (0.7, 1.8)[b]
	Duration of most recent use:		
	1-4 years		1.0 (0.6, 1.7)[b]
	5+ years		1.1 (0.6, 1.9)[b]
Live births			
Jick et al. (1981) Seattle	Prescription within 600 days of delivery	Trisomy	15.3 (1.6, 147)
Rothman (1982)[a] Massachusetts	At the LMP	Down's syndrome with congenital heart disease	2.0 (0.6, 6.2)[c]
Shapiro et al. (1982) National Collaborative Perinatal Project	First 4 lunar months of pregnancy	Down's syndrome	1.8 (0.1, 9.9)[d]
Huggins et al. (1982) Oxford Family Planning	Ever used diaphragm	Down's syndrome	2.2 (0.4, 22.5)
Polednak et al. (1982) New York State	Within 1 year before LMP	Down's syndrome	1.2 (ns)[c]
	After LMP		0.7 (ns)[c]
Mills et al. (1982) Northern California	Within 1 year before LMP	Chromosomally aberrant	1.0 (0.2, 3.5)
	After LMP		0.6 (0.1, 2.9)
Bracken and Vita (1983) New Haven	At conception	Chromosomally aberrant	0.8 (0.1, 5.6)[c]
Cordero and Layde (1983) Atlanta	Perifertilization period	Down's syndrome	1.2 (0.4, 3.6)[c]
Louik et al. (1987) United States	1 month before to 1 month after LMP	Down's syndrome	1.2 (0.8, 1.8)[b]
	Lifetime duration of use:		
	<1 year		1.1 (0.8, 1.6)[b]
	1-3 years		1.3 (0.9, 2.0)[b]
	>3 years		1.0 (0.7, 1.6)[b]

[a]Defining diaphragm users as exposed.

[b]Adjusted or matched sample odds ratio.

[c]Odds ratio.

[d]Adjusted relative risk. All other risk ratios are relative risks.

Source: Updated from Kline and Stein 1985b. Samples of births, when trisomic or chromosomally aberrant, include mostly Down's syndrome.

nearly doubled in frequency among trisomy cases compared with controls (Strobino et al. 1986b). Once trisomies were sorted into potentially viable and nonviable classes, however, the association held only for nonviable trisomies. The absence of an association with the potentially viable trisomies is consistent with the absence of associations with trisomy at birth. Hence these results suggest that spermicides lead to an excess of nonviable trisomies but have no effect on viable trisomies. Because of small numbers and lack of statistical power, interpretations of this kind must remain inconclusive.

The New York City investigators also undertook a study of spermicides and trisomies that could test possible effects under different conditions (Warburton et al. 1987b). Data were collected on prenatal diagnostic karyotypes at 17 medical centers in the United States and Canada. Spermicide use was compared among trisomies and among chromosomally normal karyotypes at the same stage in gestation. All data on spermicide use were collected before the prenatal diagnosis was made, so that there was no potential for recall bias. Trisomy could not be linked with spermicide use. The study was sufficiently large to exclude risk ratios of 2 or more with confidence (Table 8-2). The finding held whether use was of short or long duration and irrespective of whether it covered the year before conception or, more narrowly, impinged only on the period around fertilization. This null result held for trisomies 13, 18 and 21 combined, and separately for the nearly two-thirds of all cases with trisomy 21.

An additional association with spermicide use around the time of conception was discovered by the New York City miscarriage study in its first phase. Two rare aberrations were involved, namely, tetraploidy and hypertriploidy. These arise from mitotic errors after conception. Since the spermicide exposure coincided in time with the pathogenesis underlying these aberrations, the finding seemed persuasive on biological grounds. It proved less persuasive on epidemiological grounds in that it did not persist over time into the later phases of the study (Strobino et al. 1986b).

In summary, the weight of the evidence indicates that the potentially viable trisomies, and in particular trisomy 21, are unrelated to spermicide use, whether around the time of conception, within the year before conception, or over periods of longer duration. The finding that trisomies not potentially viable are associated with spermicide use is not rejected but is less secure, since it rests on a single study.

Oral Contraceptives

Like barrier contraceptives, oral contraceptives have facilitated, and may have triggered, a revolution in the sexual behavior of women. For epidemiologists, the widespread use of oral contraceptives sparked a surprised consciousness of a new population hazard in medication and medical care generally (Susser 1971). Not long after the dissemination of oral hormonal contraceptives in the 1960s, investigators began to recognize unanticipated effects. Hypertension, cervical cancer, phlebothrombosis, coronary thrombosis, and breast disease both nonmalignant and malignant, all came under suspicion. Many if not all of the associations of oral contraceptives with disease have since proved inconsistent or benign.

Oral contraceptives have also been examined for possible effects on miscarriage and chromosomal aberrations. The overall rate of miscarriage among users of oral contraceptives is no higher than that among nonusers and perhaps lower (Royal College of General Practitioners 1976; Vessey et al. 1979; Harlap et al. 1980b).

The results of studies of karyotyped miscarriages, which began as early as the late 1960s, are less straightforward. In 1970, among women with karyotyped miscarriages who used oral contraceptives, a sixfold increase in the proportion of polyploidies was reported (Carr 1970). Subsequent studies did not confirm a specific association with polyploidies (Dhadial et al. 1970; Boué et al. 1975; Lauritsen 1975; Alberman et al. 1976). A slightly raised proportion of all aberrations was found, without specificity in type. This result could as well reflect a reduced risk of chromosomally normal miscarriages, and the contraceptive hormones might be seen as protecting pregnancies from miscarrying (Alberman et al. 1976). As always, however, nonspecific effects raise the possibility that unidentified confounders might be responsible. The fact that the effect did not vary with the interval between stopping contraceptive use and conception arouses suspicion. One might reasonably anticipate a decline in biological effects as the abstention from use grew longer.

Oral contraceptives are also largely absolved as a cause of trisomies among births. No association with use before contraception has been found (Petersen 1969; Janerich et al. 1976; Royal College of General Practitioners 1976; Rothman and Louik 1978), although in one instance an association with use in the periconception period was reported (Harlap et al. 1979a).

Intrauterine Devices

Among all types of contraception, an unequivocal reproductive risk attaches only to intrauterine devices. The risk of miscarriage is raised two- or threefold if an intrauterine device is in place when conception occurs (Vessey et al. 1974, 1979; Harlap et al. 1980b). The increase in risk persists even if the device is removed early in gestation (Harlap et al. 1980b). Two karyotype studies of miscarriage strengthen the finding. Both demonstrated an excess of chromosomally normal losses among women conceiving with an intrauterine device in place (Kline 1977; Creasy 1977). No increased risk of miscarriages has been found for conceptions that occur after the device is removed (Vessey et al. 1979; Harlap et al. 1980b). Hence the mechanism might relate to imperfect implantation.

INDUCED ABORTION

The 1960s and 1970s were marked by the success of movements to legalize abortion in several Western countries. In the wake of success, a question that has long been charged by ethical dilemmas has been super-charged by moral and political polemic. Among the thrusts exchanged between the antagonists were allegations, made the more easily in the absence of evidence, that the procedures of induced abortion either were or were not harmful to women.

One kind of objective evidence that epidemiologists have provided relates to the likelihood of miscarriage subsequent to induced abortions. That a single induced abortion does not raise the risk of a subsequent first-trimester miscarriage is the consensus of several studies (Daling and Emanuel 1977; Kline et al. 1978b; Harlap et al. 1979b; Levin et al. 1980; Madore et al. 1981; Chung et al. 1982); with two or more induced abortions, the case is not as firm (Hogue et al. 1982; Kline and Stein 1984).

Induced abortion might increase the risk of miscarriage in a subsequent pregnancy through damage to the cervix or uterus. Several mechanisms have been suspected of causing such damage. These include instrumental dilatation followed by curettage, wide dilatation, operative intervention early in pregnancy, and the inferior surgical techniques current before induced abortion was legalized (Alberman et al. 1973; Johnstone et al. 1976; Harlap et al. 1979b; Grimes and Cates 1979; Chung et al. 1982; Hogue et al. 1982). Still another possible mechanism is that curettage or infection could result in uterine adhesions which impede implantation or irritate the uterus.

If induced abortion were to increase the risk of subsequent miscarriage by damage to the cervix or uterus, the effect can be presumed to act during pregnancy. There is no biological basis for thinking that localized damage could increase the risk of chromosomal aberration at conception. Thus, the predominant association of induced abortion with subsequent miscarriage should be with chromosomally normal miscarriage. In the New York City study of karyotyped miscarriages, neither single nor multiple induced abortions were in general associated with chromosomally normal (or with chromosomally aberrant) miscarriage. Among public patients, odds ratios as low as 1.3 for multiple abortions can be excluded with confidence.

It appears, however, that while presentday techniques do not have sequelae, some earlier ones did (Kline et al. 1986). Among private patients in New York City, a history of multiple induced abortions beginning before 1973 was three times more common among chromosomally normal miscarriages than among term births; among public patients a similar association was observed in women who had had at least two abortions before 1973.

IRRADIATION

Irradiation produced the first hidden casualties of a major twentieth-century advance in medical technique. An excess of leukemias was first documented in radiologists exposed in the 1920s (March 1950; Seltser and Sartwell 1965) and later in a cohort irradiated for ankylosing spondylitis (Court-Brown and Doll 1957). In the late 1950s, medical irradiation during pregnancy was shown to produce an excess of leukemias in offspring (Stewart et al. 1958; MacMahon 1962), an effect that may not have persisted with change over time in the doses now encountered. Subsequently, other postnatal effects of prenatal irradiation were demonstrated; the surviving offspring of pregnant women exposed to the atomic bombing of Hiroshima and Nagasaki suffered an excess of microcephaly and mental retardation or, less drastically, had smaller head sizes and depressed mental performance (Wood et al. 1967a, 1967b; Miller and Blot 1972; Miller and Mulvihill 1976; Otake and Schull 1984). Similar effects on head size and mental performance were attributed to the practice in earlier decades of irradiating the heads of children to treat persistent ring worm (Albert et al. 1973; Modan et al. 1979).

In a long tradition, experimental geneticists have used radiation to alter the nuclear materials of flies, rodents, and other animals and to produce genetic mutations. With the advent of human karyotyping in the late 1950s, attention naturally turned to parental irradiation exposure as a factor in chromosomal aberrations in progeny. Twelve or more studies have focused on maternal exposures. A majority have studied chromosome aberrations in births, and hence have restricted the outcome to Down's syndrome (Table 8-3) (reviewed in Cohen et al. 1977; Schull and Bailey 1984; Kline and Stein 1985b). Three studies—two of miscarriages and one of induced abortions—are free of this restriction.

In studies of Down's syndrome at birth, both diagnostic and therapeutic irradiation have been implicated. Three studies suggest effects more marked in older than in younger women (Uchida and Curtis 1961; Uchida et al. 1968; Alberman al. 1972a). The interpretation that age sets the conditions for an effect is not straightforward. With irradiation—as with any recurring or persisting exposure—it is difficult to separate the effects of exposures accumulating as time passes from the intrinsic effects of age itself.

Taking the whole array of studies of irradiation and trisomy together,

Table 8–3 Irradiation and chromosomal aberrations: summary of epidemiologic studies

	Comparison groups	Exposure	Risk ratio (95% CI)
Lunn (1959), Glasgow	117 Down's syndrome 117 controls	"High gonad dose procedures"	1.1 (0.6, 2.0)
Carter et al. (1961), London	51 Down's syndrome 51 malformed controls	<4 abdominal x-ray ≥4 abdominal x-ray	0.8 (0.3, 2.3) 0.8 (0.2, 2.8)
Schull and Neel (1962), Hiroshima and Nagasaki	5582 exposed to atom bomb 9452 not exposed		Down's syndrome[a] 0.4 (0.1, 1.5)

Uchida and Curtis (1961), Winnipeg	81 Down's syndrome
	81 cleft lip/palate
	71 neighbors
		Versus cleft lip/palate:
		  <4 abdominal x-ray
		  ≥4 abdominal x-ray
		Versus neighbors:
		  <4 abdominal
		  ≥4 abdominal
			1.9 (0.8, 4.5)
			11.8 (3.3, 41.6)
			
			0.9 (0.4, 2.0)
			2.4 (1.0, 5.5)

Sigler et al. (1965a) Cohen and Lilienfeld (1970), Baltimore	216 Down's syndrome 216 controls	Diagnostic x-ray Diagnostic, fluoroscopic and thera-peutic x-ray	1.1 (0.7, 1.7) 2.4 (1.4, 4.0)
Uchida et al. (1968), Winnipeg	972 offspring of women previously exposed 972 offspring of women previously exposed	Born after abdominal x-ray Born before abdominal x-ray	Trisomy births 10.0 (1.3, 78.0) Down's syndrome 8.0 (1.0, 63.8)
Marmol et al. (1969), United States National Collaborative Perinatal Project	61 Down's syndrome 224 controls	Any abdominal/pelvic x-ray	1.1 (0.6, 2.0)

Study	Sample	Exposure	Relative risk / Odds ratio
Stevenson et al. (1970), Oxford	1052 offspring to 630 exposed women. Expectations based on maternal age	Salpingograms	Down's syndrome 1.4[a]
Alberman et al. (1972a), London	465 Down's syndrome 465 malformed controls	Estimated gonadal dose (mr) 0.1–1999 2000+	1.4 (0.9, 2.0) 3.1 (0.8, 12.6)
Alberman et al. (1972b), London	303 chromosomally normal miscarriages 103 chromosomally aberrant miscarriages 845 live births (controls)	Estimated gonadal dose (mr) 0.1–1999 2000+ 0.1–1999 2000+	Normal/control 0.9 (0.6, 1.6) 0.5 (0.1, 2.8) Aberrant/control 1.6 (0.6, 4.3) 5.4 (1.1, 25.8)
Boué et al. (1975), Paris	Miscarriages: 307 trisomies 92 monosomies X 156 polyploidy 323 chromosomally normal	Diagnostic and therapeutic x-ray Occupational (medicine, atomic industry)	"No associations" Trisomy/normal 1.1 (0.6, 2.3) Monosomy/normal 2.1 (0.9, 4.9) Polyploidy/normal 0.9 (0.4, 2.2)
Cohen et al. (1977), Baltimore	128 Down's syndrome 128 controls	Diagnostic only Diagnostic, fluoroscopic and therapeutic	1.0 (0.5, 1.9) 0.9 (0.4, 1.8)
Watanabe (1979), Niigata City	Induced abortions: 180 chromosomally aberrant 1170 chromosomally normal	Periconceptional x-ray Chest Abdominal	Aberrant/normal[a] 1.2 (0.4, 3.5) 2.4 (0.7, 8.9)

[a] Relative risk. All other risk ratios are odds ratios.

Source: Adapted from Kline and Stein 1985b.

those associations that appear are not consistent, and the inconsistencies seem not to be explained by such known variable factors as dose. Comparison across studies is complicated not only by differences in design but by problems in ascertaining and specifying exposure. Several of the case-control studies are liable to recall bias: parental reports of exposure could differ between cases with abnormal offspring and controls with normal ones. The level of exposure can often be no more refined than the dichotomy that exposure, say to x-irradiation in some diagnostic procedures, did or did not occur; unknown variations in dose may then contribute to inconsistencies. Untoward radiation doses—as in atomic bombings and nuclear accidents—have often been imprecisely estimated.

The problem of dosage is well illustrated by recent contention about the accuracy and the forms of radiation produced by the atomic bombings of 1945 in Japan. Revised estimates, both of the types of radiation and of total dosage from the bombs, have led to sharp upward revisions in the estimates of cancer risks at given levels of exposure to radiation. Notably, the risk of childhood leukemia has been multiplied by as much as ten (Roberts 1987; Radiation Effects Res. Found. 1987). Nonetheless, a positive association of prenatal irradiation with trisomy is most placed in doubt by the absence of detectable effects in the cohorts exposed to the atomic bombings in Hiroshima and Nagasaki.

This negative evidence from the atomic bomb exposures, it might be argued in counterpoint, could be a function of high levels of exposure. High-dose irradiation sufficient to cause radiation sickness has been associated with pregnancy loss (Yamazaki et al. 1954) and might prevent the emergence of an excess of trisomies in a depleted birth cohort (Wald et al. 1970). After the atomic bombings in Japan, we noted earlier, the birth cohort assumed to have been exposed in the 3 weeks after conception appeared to be somewhat depleted in numbers compared to cohorts exposed later in gestation (Miller and Blot 1972).

Collateral evidence does not give much help in resolving the issue. In mice, a variety of effects have been produced (Yamamoto et al. 1973; Russell 1981; Dobson 1983). One suggestion, therefore, is that human beings are less sensitive to irradiation than the animal species often used in experiment (Neel 1985). In human beings, when all the evidence is summed, the most we can say is that the effects of prenatal irradiation on chromosomes remain indeterminate.

FEVER AND INFECTION DURING PREGNANCY

Clinical lore has long held fever or the underlying infection to be a hazard to pregnancy and a putative cause of miscarriage. The literature on the subject is notably deficient of rigorous demonstrations of this link, perhaps because the effects were believed not to be in contention. The experimental literature hardly addresses the question directly. In experiments with guinea pigs, hamsters and rats, hyperthermia induced by placing pregnant dams in incubators (Edwards 1967, 1968, 1969a, 1969b; Kilham and Ferm 1976; Edwards 1981; Germain et al. 1985) has caused both resorption of embryos and malformations in surviving offspring. Various effects have also been observed in the bonnet monkey, the marmoset and the lamb (Poswillo et al. 1974; Hartley et al. 1974; Hendrickx and Stone 1976). Numerous reports on the effects of maternal hyperthermia during pregnancy followed. These focused on malformations in the offspring, particularly defects and deficits of the central nervous system (reviewed by Kline et al. 1985; Warkany 1986).

Effects on the maintenance of the pregnancy were sought less often. In human beings it is difficult to isolate the effects of fever from those of the disorder (usually an infection) of which it is the symptom. In the case of miscarriage in particular, it is also difficult to separate fever as a cause of miscarriage from fever as a consequence of the miscarriage itself turned septic. Among the few available reports on fever and miscarriage, some are not very informative because the data derive mainly from the second trimester, a period of low risk for miscarriage (McDonald 1961; Clarren et al. 1979).

The New York City case-control study of karyotyped miscarriages was able to deal with some of these problems (Kline et al. 1985). The frequencies and timing during pregnancy of fevers of 100°F or more among women who miscarried and control births were compared. Two hypotheses were posed. If fever were to be merely a symptom of the miscarriage itself, an association with miscarriage could be expected regardless of karyotype. If fever were to be a cause of miscarriage or a symptom of an illness causally related to miscarriage, an association could be expected with chromosomally normal but not with chromosomally aberrant miscarriage.

The latter proved to be the case. The odds of a history of fever during pregnancy were three times greater among women who had had a chromosomally normal miscarriage than among controls. The odds among women who had had a chromosomally aberrant miscarriage were not raised. Furthermore, the more recent the experience of fever, the stronger was the association with chromosomally normal miscarriage; for instance, the odds of a history of fever within the same calendar month as the miscarriage were six times those of a fever in controls during the calendar month of interview.

Fever might produce a direct effect through at least two processes: the fever might be lethal to the conceptus, resulting in its eventual expulsion; or the fever might cause uterine contractions, with expulsion of a nonviable conceptus occurring shortly after. Experimental studies provide some support for the hypothesis that fever can be lethal. Several mechanisms have been proposed, including cell death, disruption of mitosis or cellular migration or, for conceptions exposed during organogenesis, alteration in the patterns of protein synthesis necessary to the process (German 1984). In the human data, the induction of malformation by hyperpyrexia is not an intervening mechanism in miscarriages at the fetal stage; external morphologic characteristics of the abortus yield no suggestion of abnormality. Dysmorphism in the prefetal stage, however, was not examined in relation to fever and cannot be strictly ruled out as an intervening mechanism. It remains possible, also, that infection is the common underlying cause of both the fever and the miscarriage. The fact that the medical histories of fever reported by the women did not discriminate between types or sites of infection might weigh against specific infections and for fever itself as the underlying cause; not unexpectedly, however, these data were neither complete nor exact.

EXPOSURES IN THE WORKPLACE

A woman and the fetus in her womb, though separable entities, are locked in a biological and social union indissoluble except by delivery. Through the ages, hazards to women have by that fact alone been taken to be hazards to the conceptus. Even so, ethical, legal and political conflicts divide the interests of the dyad of woman and conceptus (Bertin 1986; Brandt-Rauf and Brandt-Rauf 1986). Until recently, concern about the effects of occupational exposures on reproduction focused largely on women, to the exclusion of men. This selective focus was further narrowed from the woman herself to her capacity to reproduce (Brandeis and Goldmack 1908; Baker-Faulkner 1925; Kessler-Harris 1984).

Exposure to lead is an outstanding example. The toxicity of lead was known in Roman times, and learned afresh in modern times when George Baker traced the Devonshire colic to lead-lined cider vats in the eighteenth century (Baker 1785; Wedeen 1984). The protection finally won at the insistence of organized workers was for men and not for women. Eventually, at the turn of the century in Germany, France and Britain, attention at last turned to women. The aim of this attention was not so much to protect women from toxic effects at work but to reduce the threat to reproduction by removing women from such dangerous workplaces as potteries and printing shops. Occupational hazards for women themselves gained attention as they entered the work force in numbers and joined unions that articulated their demands (Hamilton 1943; Hunt et al. 1979; Kessler-Harris 1984). Occupational effects on male reproduction aroused strong concern only in the late 1970s, when men exposed to dibromochloropropane (DBCP) discovered their shared infertility (Whorton et al. 1977).

Effects of the workplace on reproduction have been sought in many settings (see reviews by Chavkin 1984; Stein and Hatch 1986; Kline 1986). Our by now familiar refrain emphasizes once more the problems of method that beset these studies, as they do all studies of the external environment. The theoretical advantages of defined target populations involved in controlled manufacturing processes are offset by practical disadvantages of limited access, limited numbers and confounding. These difficulties color the interpretations of studies done thus far, and no doubt contribute to inconsistencies between them. Many problems can be averted when investigators are careful to elicit informed participation of the workers at every phase of the study (Rudolph 1986).

To begin with, employers may be reluctant to provide detailed information about the work environment. Cohorts of workers assembled in one setting may in any case be small, thus limiting statistical power. Occupation-related health effects can also be suppressed by comparisons of workers with nonworkers. This "healthy worker effect" is double-edged. Women in the workforce may be selected for better health than those whose work is to maintain their own homes; in addition, homes are by no means innocent of environmental hazards (Rosenberg 1984). Any one work setting may use multiple chemicals, making discovery of the salient exposure difficult. Moreover, evidence of the type and dose of maternal exposure is often obtained from the workers themselves or from records; consequently it is indirect, with job title or work location standing in as indicators. Reproductive and work histories obtained by questioning workers invite unintended bias, both through recall and through the effects of pregnancy outcome and work status on response rates: whether the outcome of pregnancy was favorable or adverse, and whether the work is suspected of being dangerous or not, may influence in a systematic way both readiness to respond and the response itself.

Work that entails exposure to anesthetics is the most often studied employment suspected of posing a danger to reproduction. Twelve studies of the effects of maternal exposure on miscarriage (reviewed by Kline 1986) have so far followed the initial report (Vaisman 1967). Estimates of the risk ratios linking miscarriage to anesthesia range widely (from 1.1 to 3.7). Five studies show low relative risks (around 1.2); in some instances these were taken to support an association (Askrog and Harvald 1970; Knill-Jones et al. 1972; American Society of Anesthesiologists 1974), whereas in others they were not (Pharoah et al. 1977; Hemminki et al. 1985). Five other studies show higher risk ratios of 2.0 or above (Cohen et al. 1971; Rosenberg and Kirves 1973; American Society of Anesthesiologists, 1974; Tomlin 1979); one of these, on chairside dental assistants, was taken to implicate nitrous oxide in particular (Cohen et al. 1980). In most of these studies response rates are low enough to make confounding by response bias a possible source of the association. Several studies also failed to seek out and adjust for the effects of potentially confounding factors for miscarriage.

A study of Finnish nurses (Rosenberg and Kirves 1973) imputed the effects found to stress rather than to anesthesia. Nurses exposed to anesthesia in the operating room had a rate of miscarriage similar to that of nurses who worked in intensive care units and were not so exposed. At the same time, the operating room nurses had rates greater than casualty (or emergency room) nurses unexposed to anesthesia but judged to be under less stress. In the one study in which biases in response rates and in recall can be excluded—a case-control study of Finnish nurses (Hemminki et al. 1985)—no statistically significant association between anesthesia and miscarriage was detected. As estimated from this study, if exposure to anesthesia during pregnancy does involve risk, the risk ratio is slight, on the order of 1.2.

Other industries, occupations, and workplaces have each been studied on one or at most a few occasions (reviewed by Kline 1986). Industries include metal, chemicals, and rubber and leather; workplaces include laboratories, hospitals, and offices. The suspect exposures include organic solvents, solder with resin, viruses, carbon disulfide, cytostatic drugs, ethylene oxide, video display terminals, and others. The sparse observations thus far preclude firm estimates of the risks for reproduction carried by these various exposures.

In the New York City study, employment histories were related to karyotype at miscarriage (Silverman et al. 1985). No evidence of adverse effects was found. Hospital workers and factory workers were similarly represented among chromosomally normal miscarriages and among controls. The data were insufficient, however, to test the effects of specific agents in the workplace.

CONCLUSION

Few environmental factors have been consistently associated with miscarriage. Detectable effects on miscarriage overall are most likely to occur with changes in chromosomally normal losses, the largest karyotypic component. On the whole associations still await testing by replication, since studies seeking links between exposure and karyotype at miscarriage are few.

With regard to cigarette smoking, although the link to miscarriage overall is inconsistent, the best available evidence indicates a risk for chromosomally normal loss among women at a social disadvantage that is modestly increased (with an odds ratio of about 1.6 with 14 cigarettes or more per day). Even with chromosomally normal miscarriages, however, the case may not yet be closed. Moderate risks, as well as inconsistencies between social strata, can always provoke doubt about a causal connection.

The use of alcohol during pregnancy also appears to give rise to a dose-related risk of chromosomally normal miscarriage, again only among women at a social disadvantage. The inference of a direct causal association cannot easily be sustained, however, in the face of the equal associations of alcohol use with chromosomal aberrations. Therefore a number of alternative hypotheses have been presented.

An intrauterine device in place of the time of conception is a risk factor for which a causal connection with chromosomally normal miscarriage seems certain. A causal connection of fever (or the illness of which it is a symptom) with chromosomally normal miscarriage is compelling on biologic and epidemiologic grounds. Nonetheless, the data derive from a single study, and it remains to test the association for replicability.

With respect to chromosomal aberrations, no environmental exposure has shown strong and consistent associations with any one aberration. This leaves us uncertain and often without coherent theory. Also, such theories as might be advanced may prove impervious to testing with available techniques. Since specific chromosomal aberrations differ in time of origin, mechanism, and parental source, they probably differ also in their determinants. When this heterogeneity is taken into account, samples are often rendered small and their statistical power low, making a convincing test of associations with specific aberrations difficult to mount.

Even so, the demonstrated impact of both maternal and paternal environmental exposures on the karyotype of conceptions might be judged meager. Possibly the human genome, or at least that part of it seen in aberrant forms in miscarriage, is not sensitive to the wider environment. Then again, the relevant exposures may not have been specified, or they may act within a sharply limited time—for instance, the few hours around the moment of fertilization—or on a small number of susceptible women. Poor measurement and misclassification can substantially reduce the apparent size of the risks detected or altogether frustrate their detection.

9 The Recurrence of Miscarriage and Chromosomal Aberrations

Universally, reproduction has been a repeated event in the life cycle of most women and most men. The repetition of events at once raises questions about the existence of patterns of events. Are some women or some couples favored by healthy outcomes or liable to repeatedly unfavorable outcomes? If patterns of favorable or unfavorable outcomes exist, can they be identified? Once patterns can be recognized, one may hope to predict the course of reproduction and discover the causes that underlie the recurrence of good or poor reproductive performance.

The recurrence of reproductive events can be followed in two ways: through the experience of individual women or couples, and through the experience of genetically related individuals. These dual approaches help both to improve predictability and to narrow the range of causes that could be at work. When patterns of recurrence are known, prognostications can be made about repetition in future pregnancies; at the same time, the nature of the possible causes is limited to those with the potential to produce recurrence. The causal factors that could operate in this manner cover a broad front. They include genetic factors, permanent or enduring attributes of the woman or her partner, and persisting environmental exposures. A systematic approach will devise strategies governed by the nature of the potential causes.

Patterns of recurrence, it is at once apparent, must be assessed quantitatively as matters of probability. A particular adverse reproductive outcome may be repeated in the successive pregnancies of the same woman (or the same couple). Some repetitions of such outcomes occur no more often than expected by chance; others occur in excess of expectation. A first concern is to distinguish between chance and excess. To address this concern, we begin by assigning to recurrence a meaning separate from mere repetition: *recurrence* is defined as the repetition, beyond chance expectation, of an outcome in a sequence of pregnancies. Thus, where recurrence exists, a first episode marks out the group of affected women (or couples) who in a later pregnancy are at raised risk of the same outcome.

A genetic factor underlies the recurrence of conditions inherited in a Mendelian manner, and also the recurrence of some conditions owed to structural rearrangements of chromosomes. Obviously, the recurrence of genetic conditions that result in births gives rise to a higher frequency among siblings. This type of recurrence manifests as *familial aggregation:* the given disorder occurs in the relatives of affected individuals at a frequency greater than that in the general population. The genes involved are transmitted by either parent or, with recessive traits, by both. Maternal conditions that are not genetic might also produce more than one affected pregnancy in an individual sequence. Cervical incompetence is such a postulated physical cause of recurrent miscarriage and prematurity.

Attributes of the couple rather than the woman alone are possibly involved, as they are with recessive heterozygous traits and immunological mechanisms. If inheritance is involved at all in immunological mechanisms, it is not in a direct way but through biological interaction. The mechanisms are presumed to become activated by the immunological conjunction of at least two of the three engaged parties—the male and female partner and the conceptus they produce. The immunological make-up of a woman and that of the conceptus she carries differ genetically in varying degree. The resulting effects first came to be understood with blood group incompatibilities; later and quite different formulations have been based on the generalization of allograft–host reactions. For instance, one theory postulates that in order to preserve a pregnancy within her own body, the woman's immune system must first recognize the conceptus as foreign, and then react in a manner that would not dislodge it as if it were an alien graft.

Environmental factors that endure may also produce recurrences. These may be factors in the physical environment, such as polychlorbiphenyls stored in a mother's body fat long after her initial exposure (Rogan et al. 1988). Recurrences could also occur when the first episode itself increases the risk of a repetition. For instance, one hypothesis postulated such a risk following a first miscarriage treated by dilatation and curettage (Alberman 1973). The hypothesis has not been supported by later studies of induced abortions in which the procedure was frequently used.

To establish that recurrence is present is a first step in focusing the search for causes. The assessment of recurrence has been approached in various ways. One way is to examine whether the number of women experiencing one, two, or more repetitions of the outcome is in excess of that expected were the risk constant for all women in all pregnancies. Another way is to examine whether the risk of the outcome is higher in women who have already experienced an episode than in those who have not. The most refined probabilities refer not to women but to couples, since male partners might also contribute to the recurrent outcome. The data necessary for such analyses, even if they happen to be available, are seldom considered.

The repetition of certain outcomes can readily give the false appearance of recurrence, especially when the outcome is common, as it is with miscarriage. One reason is the difficulty of disentangling recurrence from the changes that accompany aging with the passing of time, and from increasing gravidity as pregnancies succeed each other. Characteristics such as age or gravidity, as we shall show in detail in later chapters, are tied to the risk for some outcomes. These two characteristics necessarily change for each woman as her reproductive history unfolds through time. Thus the risks for the pregnancies that succeed each other may not be the same. When the risks for an adverse outcome increase with increasing age or gravidity, the repetition of the outcome may reflect no more than that fact, without any existing predisposition for the outcome to recur. To demonstrate a true risk of recurrence requires associations over and above those with age or gravidity; the risk must be estimated and judged against the baseline rates of the outcome as they change with age and gravidity.

Spurious associations of age or gravidity with a particular pregnancy outcome may also result from typical forms of reproductive behavior. Two elements that commonly affect such behavior—the response of couples to adverse outcomes and desired family size—can lead to bias. Some couples desist from childbearing because of an unhappy outcome such as a serious malformation; others persist in compensatory childbearing after a loss in order to reach a desired family size. Such self-imposed selection produces a bias in the reproductive histories of the women who advance from one pregnancy order to the next. As a result, the likelihood that women with an adverse outcome at one pregnancy order will be found among the ranks of those at the next pregnancy order is not the same as for women who have had normal pregnancies. Analyses that disregard phenomena of this type have led to sometimes egregious error, as others have shown (Mantel 1979; Golding et al. 1983). This problem is worked out in detail in Chapter 19.

To establish that women who experience one adverse outcome are at raised risk of another does not imply an equivalent risk for all in the group, nor that the recurrences of the particular outcome are the product of a single cause. The search for causes of recurrence, single or heterogeneous, may move along various paths.

One path is to refine description and classification of adverse outcomes, which may direct the search to certain types of causes. With miscarriage, for example, we can differentiate between karyotypes of the conceptus. The recurrence of structural rearrangements points to genetic factors in either parent. Recurrence of chromosomally normal miscarriages points first to the woman; attention might turn then to maternal immunologic factors, environmental exposures, nutritional deficiencies, gynecologic conditions and chronic disease.

Another path is to compare women who have repeated adverse outcomes with women who do not, in order to discover whether they differ in genetic, environmental and constitutional characteristics. Comparisons with women with a single episode among a number of pregnancies may sharpen distinctions between factors that raise risks for sporadic occurrences and those that raise the risk of recurrences. Once potential causes have been discovered, trials of treatments can help test causal hypotheses.

In this chapter we weigh the evidence, first, for the recurrence of miscarriage, and second, for the recurrence of trisomic conceptions. Maternal age must be dealt with in this discussion as a potentially confounding factor, since it affects both chromosomally normal miscarriage and trisomy. Full discussion of age as a risk factor for these outcomes is deferred to Chapters 17 and 18. We also defer to Chapter 15 the question of the recurrence and the aggregation of two other outcomes, namely, prematurity and low birthweight.

RECURRENT MISCARRIAGE

There is no doubt that women who miscarry give a history of miscarriage in previous pregnancies more often than women who go to term (Stevenson et al. 1959; Shapiro et al. 1971; Alberman et al. 1975; Kline et al. 1978a). They also sustain a higher risk of subsequent miscarriage (Warburton and Fraser 1964; Leridon 1976; Poland et al. 1977; Harlap et al. 1980a). After a first miscarriage, the chance of a second is about 60 per cent greater than after a pregnancy not preceded by miscarriage. Beyond the first miscarriage, however, elevations in risk with increasing numbers of miscarriages are slight (Warburton and Fraser 1964; Leridon 1976; Poland et al. 1977; Kline 1977; Harlap et al. 1980a; Harger et al. 1983).

The recurrence of miscarriage is most readily seen as an expression of the varying susceptibilities of individual women (Harris and Gunstad 1936); that is, a special risk besets some women. A history of one or more miscarriages is thus an indicator by which to assemble women at risk. Much the less likely alternative is that one miscarriage could be a direct cause of a subsequent miscarriage.

Recurrences in miscarriage could be the result of lethal abnormalities in the conceptus (whether genetic or not) or of maternal factors leading to the loss of a normal conceptus. Recurrences of lethal abnormalities at conception might be chromosomally aberrant or chromosomally normal. If conceptions with a lethal abnormality were typical or common in repeated miscarriage, we would look to the cause of the abnormality for an explanation. Thus, a small proportion of recurrent miscarriages results when one parent, who carries a balanced rearrangement of a chromosome, transmits it in unbalanced form at conception. The frequency of balanced rearrangements among couples with recurrent losses is about 4 per cent—10 times that in the newborn (reviewed in Warburton and Strobino 1987). This marks an upper limit for the proportion of recurrent losses attributable to inherited unbalanced chromosomal rearrangements.

In fact, the bulk of recurrences involve chromosomally normal miscarriages. Although undetected gene defects underlying such recurrences cannot at once be ruled out, with normal karyotypes mechanisms operating after conception become a focus of attention. The risk of subsequent miscarriages is greater after a first miscarriage if the karyotype is normal than if it is aberrant. In two studies, miscarriage in a later pregnancy was 50 to 100 per cent more likely when the previous miscarriage was chromosomally normal (Boué et al. 1975; Lauritsen 1976). Moreover, the subsequent miscarriage tends to be concordant with the first for chromosomal normality. The New York City and Honolulu studies assembled a sample of women who had experienced at least two miscarriages that had been karyotyped (Warburton et al. 1987a). A first normal karyotype was followed by a second normal karyotype about twice as often as would be expected for maternal age.

Concordance between repeated miscarriages has also been found for gestational age and stage of development. The later in gestation the first miscarriage had occurred, the later it tended to be in subsequent miscarriages (Warburton and Fraser 1964). According to morphologic studies of repeated losses in 28 couples, miscarriages also tend to be concordant in broad terms (prefetal versus fetal) for developmental stage (Poland et al. 1977).

The available evidence suggests that these concordances for gestational age and stage of development are a manifestation of chromosomally normal miscarriage. Repeated losses of chromosomally normal conceptions late in gestation seem to constitute one typical form of recurrence. In the New York City study, in which the index miscarriage was karyotyped, chromosomally normal losses occurred later in gestation in women who had had three or more repeated miscarriages than in women who had had only one (Strobino et al. 1986a). Such late losses tend to be fetal. (A degree of uncertainty must be allowed. We drew attention in Chapter 7 to the possible lag between the age when development ceases and the gestational age at which the conceptus is expelled; the available data use gestational age alone to describe the stage at which loss occurred.)

RECURRENCE LINKING MISCARRIAGE AND PRETERM DELIVERY

In the light of the concordance of repeated late chromosomally normal miscarriages, one would naturally look to such miscarriages to establish a further link with premature birth. Fetal miscarriage and premature birth differ principally, one might suppose, in their viability at the point gestation ends, a difference governed by the length of their tenure in the uterus. Thus, if some disorder predisposes a woman to provide a short-ened tenure, the pathological processes either on the maternal or the fetal side might well be the same whether she yields up the fetus before or after the gestational age threshold that divides miscarriage from birth.

Miscarriages and prematurity have, indeed, been linked in several studies. Prematurity is operationally defined sometimes in terms of ges-tational age, sometimes in terms of birth weight, and sometimes in terms of both together. Most studies have examined only one of these compo-nents of prematurity (Macnaughton 1961; Warburton and Fraser 1964; Pantelakis et al. 1973; Keirse et al. 1978; Alberman et al. 1980) leaving unanswered whether the primary association is with curtailed gestation or intrauterine growth retardation. Only a few studies have examined repeated miscarriage in particular (Pantelakis et al. 1973; Keirse et al. 1978; Alberman et al. 1980).

Three studies did separate preterm delivery from intrauterine growth retardation. As one might anticipate, repeated miscarriage was found to be connected primarily with preterm delivery (Papaevangelou et al. 1973; Pickering and Forbes 1985; Strobino et al. 1986a). A connection with low birth weight cannot be ruled out, however. In one study, in women who had had repeat miscarriages, birth weight was lowered in both their preterm (<36 completed weeks) and term infants (Strobino et al. 1986a).

The connection of miscarriage with preterm births does, as expected, seem to be limited to miscarriages late in gestation. In one result, the risk is confined to miscarriages at 6 months of gestation or more (Warburton and Fraser 1964). In another result, however, the risk was apparent in the second trimester (Keirse et al. 1978): a raised rate of preterm births was found in women with even one miscarriage in the second trimester; with multiple second trimester losses preterm birth rates rose further. By contrast, in women with miscarriages solely in the first trimester, the preterm birth rate was not raised.

Preterm births themselves tend to repeat, as we discuss in detail in Chapter 15. These findings taken together support the idea that pre-term birth and late miscarriage, most likely of a chromosomally normal fetus, may have a common pathogenesis. From these findings that raised risks of miscarriage or preterm birth attend chromosomally normal losses late in gestation, one cannot freely extrapolate to the risks that attend chromosomally normal losses early in gestation. These and other data suggest a dissociation of the risks after early losses from those after later losses.

Many causes have been suggested for recurrent miscarriage in gener-al. Plausible common causes that could link preterm births and chro-mosomally normal miscarriages in particular fall into two classes: anatomical factors such as incompetent cervix, and physiological factors that might initiate premature labor. It is widely held that an incompetent cervix is a cause of repeated miscarriage. An unbiased test of the hypothesis in which observers are blind to knowledge of the outcome in terms of untimely delivery is yet to be made, however. Hence the magnitude and even the existence of the risk remain in doubt (reviewed in Warburton and Strobino 1987).

Many of the same maternal characteristics under suspicion as risk factors for miscarriage in general are obviously also under suspicion for repeated miscarriage. Any such characteristic that persists or any exposure that tends to be continuous could underlie recurrences. The list of potential influences includes chronic diseases, progesterone deficiency, uterine abnormalities and adhesions, chronic or repeated infections, psychologic characteristics, and environmental exposures such as smoking and drinking alcohol (reviewed in Simpson 1986; Warburton and Strobino 1987).

Few of these factors have been examined in relation to the recurrence of miscarriage. In the New York City study, the question of recurrence was examined in women with three or more miscarriages ("repeaters"). They were compared with two groups: (1) women with only one miscarriage and at least one prior birth ("sporadics") and (2) women who, though of similar gravidity to the repeaters, had had three or more births. A large number of factors were tested, including many of the characteristics and conditions listed. Only two—cervical incompetence and a longer time to conception—were consistently associated with repeated miscarriage (Strobino et al. 1980b, 1986a).

IMMUNOLOGICAL MECHANISMS

Immunological mechanisms in reproductive loss were first established with Rh incompatibility. Hydrops fetalis, erythroblastosis fetalis, and recurrent pregnancy loss late in gestation characterized the condition. Later, ABO blood group incompatibility was also shown to be sometimes pathogenic to pregnancy. Interest was further stimulated by the demonstration that desensitization could deflect the consequences of Rh incompatibility (Freda and Gorman 1962; Clarke et al. 1963).

The underlying assumption was that mother and fetus were naturally compatible. Incompatibility was dangerous and to be prevented, and the success of this work in preventing the abnormal rejection of the conceptus was a triumphant answer to the question. Peter Medawar (1964) turned the question on its head. He suggested that the mammalian embryo or fetus could be considered, by abstraction, as an allograft on the uterus. In this model, what must be explained is the normal retention of the conceptus in the face of the necessary genetic dissimilarity of the fetal graft and the maternal host. The fact that the conceptus is not rejected has intrigued immunologists ever since.

Four mechanisms were proposed early on (Billingham 1964): that the uterus is a "privileged" site and will accept grafts, as does the cornea; that the placenta is free of histocompatibility leukocytic antigens, hence does not provoke a maternal reaction; that barriers interposed between uterus and embryo prevent graft–host reactions taking place; and that hormonal influences, especially progesterone, damp down immunological responses.

Up to now, no firm evidence has been forthcoming for any of the four hypotheses. Workers in the field of recurrent reproductive loss have given most attention to the third idea, namely, that an interposed barrier or blocking factor prevents rejection. We discuss briefly two lines of clinical investigation around this idea (reviewed by Mowbray and Underwood 1985; Simpson 1986; Faulk et al. 1987; Beer et al. 1987; Scott et al. 1987). One line follows the assumption that the conceptus is rejected in error because the maternal tissues, and specifically the uterus, fail to recognize the fetal allograft. The second line follows the assumption that the conceptus is rejected primarily because maternal blocking factor to bar rejection is lacking.

Interpretation of these investigations is hampered by our incomplete understanding of the immunology of continuing or normal pregnancies. Further, the expectation must be that effects will best be detected in chromosomally normal miscarriage, a study requirement that can be met in only one series (Lauritsen et al. 1976). All other observations derive from losses that were not karyotyped. A distinction that has been made more often is between so-called primary and secondary recurrent miscarriage. Primary recurrent miscarriage refers to repeated losses occurring early in gestation, with no pregnancies culminating in births. Secondary recurrent miscarriage refers to repeated losses occurring late in gestation with at least one pregnancy culminating in a birth.

Maternal recognition of the conceptus as foreign is seen by some as the primary or possibly the only step in preventing its rejection. Early in pregnancy, maternal lymphocytes supposedly recognize the trophoblast and protect it; the basis for recognition is thought to be incompatibility between maternal and fetal histocompatibility leukocytic antigens (HLA). According to some reports, couples subject to primary recurrent miscarriages more often share specific HLA antigens (e.g., at the DR and DQ loci) than do couples with a normal reproductive history (McIntyre et al. 1986; Coulam et al. 1987). The speculation is that the antigens of the trophoblast are not sufficiently different from those of the woman to permit recognition. This proposition locates the source of the loss in a particular mating couple; risks of loss for a woman would be expected to differ depending on her partner (Coulam et al. 1986).

The second line of investigation focuses on the so-called blocking factor thought to interpose between the reactions of the uterus to the embryo. To prevent the immunologic rejection of the conceptus, activation of the blocking factor is required. Blocking factor can be demonstrated experimentally by the one-way mixed lymphocyte culture (MLC) reaction. In the normal reproductive immune response, irradiated lymphocytes from the mate who is the genitor tend to stimulate a vigorous response from the lymphocytes of the pregnant woman herself.

The demonstration of this response depends on the culture of maternal lymphocytes under different conditions. Culture in the serum or plasma of an unrelated third person, or of the woman herself when she was not pregnant, apparently stimulates a vigorous response. Culture in the woman's own plasma taken during pregnancy, however, appears to suppress the vigor of the response (McIntyre and Faulk 1979; Faulk et al. 1987). The distribution of this blocking factor among women at different risk is concomitant with what might be expected if the factor could protect a pregnancy from rejection. Reportedly, it is present commonly in multigravidae, inconsistently in women with recurrent losses, and not at all in nulligravidae. These distributions have not been tested to the extent that a causal connection can be claimed.

Ideas differ about the way a blocking factor might work. Some investigators, as mentioned before, emphasize maternal recognition of the foreign graft as a first and necessary stimulus to blocking, and hence blocking is linked to HLA sharing between couples. Blocking activity seems to be a complex matter, however, and some work suggests that it may not be specific to the partner of the pregnant woman. Circulating blocking factors were not found relevant to the success of pregnancy in a prospective observational study of recurrent miscarriage. Although well-controlled, it must be admitted that numbers in this study were small (Sargent et al. 1988).

A third line of investigation for recurrent miscarriage sidesteps the question of blocking: it postulates that the direct immunological response of the woman to the nonmaternal constituents of the trophoblast is in some way inappropriate (Mowbray et al. 1983). Secondary recurrent miscarriages have been attributed to this type of direct and inappropriate immune response on the part of the woman. It seems that couples with secondary recurrent miscarriages do not share components of the HLA complex more often than couples with term births. On the other hand, with such miscarriages, cytotoxins against the paternal lymphocytes are reported to be found more frequently in the maternal circulation than with term births (McConnachie and McIntyre 1984; McIntyre et al. 1986; Coulam et al. 1987; Faulk et al. 1987; Sargent et al. 1988).

The implications for treatment presumably differ according to which theory is at issue, that is, whether the mechanism relates to failure to activate a blocking mechanism because of undue compatibility in the antigens of the cells of the woman and her partner (and hence the conceptus) or, alternatively, whether the direct reaction of maternal antigens to the trophoblast is inappropriate. In order to stimulate antigen activity for the prevention of primary recurrent miscarriages, women in one program have been immunized sometimes by lymphocytes from their partners (Mowbray et al. 1985) and sometimes by leukocytes from other donors (McIntyre et al. 1986).

The rationale for these postulated mechanisms is not always clear. No consistent experimental or epidemiological support is available for any of them. At this juncture, treatments founded on one theory or another must be considered experimental.

FAMILIAL AGGREGATION IN MISCARRIAGE

Recurrent miscarriage might express a genetic factor. Such a factor might manifest in familial aggregation or in higher risk of miscarriage for mating pairs who are kin. When chromosomally normal losses recur, potential genetic mechanisms in the conceptus include homozygosity for lethal recessive genes or autosomal dominant genes (reviewed by Mac-Cluer 1980). In the woman, a possible mechanism is homozygosity for recessive genes that increase the likelihood of reproductive loss. When chromosomally aberrant losses recur, various genetic factors related to the liability to nondisjunction have been postulated but not demonstrated (Alfi et al. 1980; Jackson-Cook et al. 1985; Spinner et al. 1986).

Couples who are kin provide circumstantial evidence on the likely contribution of autosomal recessive defects to miscarriage. When the several studies are considered together, rates of fetal loss among inbred and genetically unrelated couples do not differ. Various interpretations can be made of these observations. The role of recessive gene defects in recurrent losses could be very small or absent; the effects of such gene defects might manifest in the unobserved subclinical phase; or the genetic similarity between inbred conceptuses and the woman might have a protective effect.

Familial aggregation in miscarriages has rarely been examined. In addition to genetic mechanisms involving lethal defects or inherited anomalies of anatomy or function of the maternal reproductive tract, environmental exposures shared by family members could produce aggregation within families. In one study (the National Collaborative Perinatal Project), the rate of miscarriage was positively correlated in pairs of sisters but not sisters-in-law (Naylor and Warburton 1974).

In the New York City study of miscarriages, the chromosomal characteristics of index cases were linked to the frequency of reproductive loss in relatives. Although at this stage the analyses are not complete, they are mentioned here because the data are unique and as fully analyzed as any other relevant data sets in the literature. The studies of repeated chromosomally normal miscarriage in the New York City sample discussed earlier led to the a priori hypothesis that, if familial aggregation was present, it would be a phenomenon of chromosomally normal miscarriages.

The rates of miscarriage in first-degree relatives (as reported by the study subjects) of chromosomally normal cases, compared with controls, were higher for mothers, sisters, and sisters-in-law (which is to say brothers). In these same kin of chromosomally aberrant cases, the rates of miscarriage, in accord with the hypothesis, were more like those for trols (Lee and Kline 1988). Since the raised rates in the chromosomally normal were not confined to female relatives, inherited defects of the reproductive system of the women are an unlikely source of the association.

Factors underlying aggregation within families probably differ from those producing recurrences within a sequence of pregnancies of individual women. Chromosomally normal cases who reported a fetal loss in their relatives had had no more repetitions of miscarriages than chromosomally normal cases who reported no fetal losses in their relatives (Lee 1988).

RECURRENCE OF TRISOMY

Certain forms of Down's syndrome are known to be the result of genetic transmission from a parent. A rare fertile person with Down's syndrome resulting from either trisomy 21 or an unbalanced rearrangement involving chromosome 21 may transmit the syndrome. Also, an unaffected person with a balanced rearrangement involving chromosome 21 may transmit the translocated chromosome in a manner that results in imbalance and Down's syndrome. Inherited unbalanced rearrangements involving extra chromosomal material of other chromosomes, such as 13 and 14, also occur.

Chromosome 21 is involved in all cases of Down's syndrome. Trisomy 21, the defect in the great majority, sometimes recurs in successive births. Only 5 per cent of all cases have the translocation form; of these about three-quarters arise de novo and, not being inherited, do not recur within the sibship in which they are initially observed (Hook 1981a).

Women under the age of 30 years who have a trisomy 21 birth are at increased risk of trisomy 21 in subsequent births undertaken before the age of 30. The increase in risk is at least 15-fold (Warburton 1985a) and perhaps as much as 30-fold. In contrast, when the subsequent pregnancy occurs at 30 years or later, the risk among women with a previous trisomy 21 birth is no greater than expected for the women's age at the subsequent pregnancy (see Table 9-1). Data are not available in the literature to test the possibility that the risk of Down's syndrome birth at later ages differs according to the age of the woman at her first trisomy 21 birth.

Not so many observations in births have been made that sampling fluctuations can be ruled out. Amniocentesis provides another data source and far larger numbers of chromosome aberrations, since the population is selected precisely for the risk of aberration. The risks at amniocentesis are in accord with those at birth (Table 9-1). In women who had a trisomy 21 birth before age 30, the risk of trisomy 21 at amniocentesis was raised four to five times overall. If subsequent amniocentesis was also done before 30 years of age, the risk is raised eightfold. As with births in women who had had a trisomy 21 birth at age 30 years and later, at amniocentesis after a trisomy birth at 30 years or later, no raised risk for trisomy 21 could be detected (reviewed by Warburton 1985a). Here, too, it remains unclear whether the risk of occurrence for a woman under 30 years with a trisomy 21 birth remains high at 30 years and later; effects are modest, and confounding by maternal age cannot be ruled out.

Maternal age does not appear to be the sole factor that underlies repetitions of trisomy. Despite the gaps in confirmatory data across the whole of the relevant age range, these results for the recurrence of trisomy 21 suggest that some individual women or couples carry an increased risk for trisomy 21 pregnancies that persists through reproductive life. That recurrence is dependent on the age of the woman not only at the first trisomy 21 birth but at the second is difficult to reconcile in biological terms. As an explanation, a statistical artifact related to maternal-age risks for nonrecurrent trisomies seems preferable to biological incongruity. At young maternal ages, women with a raised age-independent risk of trisomy 21 comprise a visible proportion of all trisomy 21 pregnancies. At later maternal ages, that proportion could rapidly decrease to the point of statistical invisibility as age-dependent trisomies increase in frequency and overwhelm the small number of age-independent trisomies.

Several speculations have been advanced about mechanisms that could produce a higher risk of trisomy 21 independent of age and persisting throughout reproductive life. Some theories are based on genetic transmission of aberrant germ cells. These include cryptic mosaicism of trisomy 21 cell lines in the parent, or defective genes that predispose to aneuploidy of one chromosome in particular (homoaneuploidy), or of all chromosomes in general (heteroaneuploidy). Other theories relate to in utero survival. The normal rate of attrition of trisomic conceptions in the subclinical or clinically recognized phases of pregnancy might be reduced because of a maternal defect or environmental exposure.

Genetic mechanisms such as mosaicism and genes predisposing to

Table 9–1 Repetition of trisomies (summary of observations)

Study	Age at Prior trisomy pregnancy	Age at Subsequent pregnancy	Number of subsequent pregnancies	Number of subsequent trisomies Observed	Number of subsequent trisomies Expected
Two trisomy 21 births					
Stene (1970)[a]: reanalysis of data					
from Oster (1956)	<30	<30	91	2	0.06
	NA	≥30	244	1	1.33
from Carter and	<30	<30	120	1	0.03
Evans (1961)[b]	NA	≥30	188	1	0.98
Trisomies 21 at birth and subsequent amniocentesis (other trisomies at amniocentesis in parentheses)					
Warburton (1985a)[c]:	<30	<30	1661	13 (5)	1.6 (1.6)
reanalysis of data	<30	≥30	888	6 (3)	2.4 (1.8)
from Stene et al. (1984)	≥30	≥30	922	7 (4)	6.7 (3.7)
Two trisomic miscarriages (Warburton et al. 1987a)[d]					
New York City	<30	<30	8	2	1.4
	NA	≥30	21	11	8.1
Honolulu	<30	<30	9	2	2.2
	NA	≥30	34	15	14.2

[a]Expectations based on 5-year maternal age intervals from Oster (1956) and Carter and McCarthy (1951). Warburton (1985a) provides higher estimates of the expected numbers of trisomy based on Swedish data.

[b]Age at birth of youngest subsequent sib given; all subsequent sibs enumerated.

[c]Expectations for trisomy 21 based on 5-year maternal age intervals below age 35 years and on single year of age beginning at 35 years. Expectations for trisomies 13 and 18 estimated from ratio of these trisomies to trisomy 21.

[d]Expectations taking into account age in single years and location of the study. Expectations based on women with no previous karyotyped miscarriage.

homoaneuploidy would be compatible with recurrent trisomies of the same chromosome. A genetic mechanism leading to heteroaneuploidy predicts, by definition, an increased risk of trisomies of more than one chromosome, or even of other chromosomal aberrations as well. A maternal defect that fails to detect and screen out a particular trisomy in the subclinical or even the clinical phase might well affect other chromosomal aberrations also. Some discrimination between mechanisms might therefore be hoped for from data that yield insight into whether recurrent trisomic pregnancies tend to be of the same or of different chromosomes.

In this regard, amniocentesis data give little guidance. Among women under 30 years of age, at amniocentesis performed because of a previous trisomy 21 birth, the risk of trisomies of other chromosomes, namely, 13 and 18, was raised threefold (95 per cent confidence interval 1.1, 5.5) —distinctly less than the risk of a recurrence of trisomy 21 noted previously, but nonetheless significant (see Table 9-1; Warburton 1985a). This finding suggests a propensity to heteroaneuploidy. Unfortunately, the small numbers and the lack of secure expected rates of trisomies 13 and 18 (Warburton 1985a) make the finding ambiguous.

When we turn to the other available data source, namely, karyotyped miscarriages, some of the ambiguities are resolved and others not. The data source has complexities as well as virtues: karyotyped miscarriages add to the heterogeneity of the trisomies observed and at the same time provide insight into it, including the phenomenon of heteroaneuploidy. Many trisomies that do not survive either to the time of amniocentesis or of birth are brought into the spectrum; sometimes trisomies of chromosomes that do not appear at all in data from other sources are seen.

Until recently, instances in which karyotypes of two miscarriages in the same woman were available for analysis comprised 87 pairs in all. Analysis of such pooled data, few in number and without the needed background information, can be misleading. We first examine these data to elucidate the analytic pitfalls. Correlations seemed to exist, on the one hand, between chromosomally normal pairs and, on the other, between chromosomally aberrant pairs. The aberrant pairs, however, were not restricted to the same type of aberration (Boué and Boué 1973a; Kajii et al. 1973; Alberman et al. 1975; Lauritsen 1976; Kajii and Ferrier 1978). From previous chapters, it is apparent that such correlations do not discriminate between risk attributable to chromosomally normal or to chromosomally aberrant miscarriages; either one could produce the results.

Collateral data gave some support to the inference that correlations among repeat pairs reflected the recurrence of chromosomally normal losses (Alberman et al. 1975; Boué et al. 1975; Lauritsen 1976). Thus, in women with a known chromosomally normal miscarriage, the frequency of miscarriages either before or after the index event was raised. At the same time, data from one of these studies, in London, supported the parallel inference of the recurrence of trisomic conceptions. Thus there appeared to be a raised risk of Down's syndrome births before and after trisomic miscarriages (Alberman et al. 1975; Alberman 1981a). The London observation was not replicated in three other series, however (Boué et al. 1975; Lauritsen 1976; Warburton 1985a).

Studies of correlations between karyotypes in paired losses do not lend themselves to ready inferences about the processes producing the correlation. By definition a sample of repeated miscarriages that have been karyotyped is selective; it is limited to women who have experienced one miscarriage, undertaken at least one more pregnancy, and then experienced another loss. Thus, concordance in karyotypes between two miscarriages might arise simply from highly selective sampling for already known risk factors. For example, the strong association between maternal age and trisomy could itself produce a concordance for trisomy in repeated miscarriages. Women with a first trisomic miscarriage tend to be older. They are older still in subsequent pregnancies, and thus at even greater risk of a second trisomic conception that will result in miscarriage.

A full understanding of correlations between karyotypes from repeated miscarriages thus requires knowledge of how the rates of pregnancy and of miscarriage vary in relation to the outcome of previous pregnancies, the karyotype of these previous pregnancies (whether births or miscarriages), and maternal age. It also requires knowledge of the distribution of karyotypes among miscarriages to women of the same age.

The ideal cannot be attained. We have already seen that data about reproduction subsequent to a karyotyped loss are limited to the observation that the risk of miscarriage is higher after a chromosomally normal than after an aberrant loss. A guide to interpreting data from repeated miscarriages, however, can be found in estimates of the expected distributions of karyotypes among miscarriages by maternal age. In light of the small number of cases in the several early studies, it is perhaps not surprising that in deriving expected frequencies adjustments for maternal age were not carried out. The combination of two later and larger series of repeat karyotyped miscarriages—148 women in Honolulu and 125 women in New York City—have since provided the necessary data and analyses (Warburton et al. 1987a).

Data from nearly 5000 karyotyped miscarriages were used. The expected odds of chromosomally normal, trisomic and other aberrant karyotypes at miscarriage were estimated, taking into account maternal age and reproductive history. The risk of repetition of a trisomic miscarriage was not significantly raised above expectation. After a first trisomic miscarriage, the odds of a second was 1.3 times that expected (95 per cent confidence interval 0.7, 2.1). For women who were still under 30 years old at the second miscarriage, the same risk held (odds ratio = 1.3, 95 per cent confidence interval 0.4, 4.5). The result is not, on the face of it, compatible with those we described for trisomies at amniocentesis or at birth. The number of women with two karyotyped miscarriages before 30 years of age is only 17 (see Table 9-1). Yet the upper 95 per cent confidence bound of 4.5 for the odds ratio excludes the eightfold risk for trisomy 21 at amniocentesis observed in women under 30 with a previous trisomy 21 birth.

A possible explanation for the divergence of these findings in miscarriages from those in births and amniocentesis is that recurrence is specific to trisomy 21 (in other words, there is homoaneuploidy for chromosome 21). The sample of karyotyped miscarriages, despite its size, provides too few cases to test the specificity of trisomy 21 recurrences: among women with repeat karyotyped miscarriages in New York City and Honolulu, trisomy 21 was found at the first miscarriage in only four, and only one woman was under 30 years at the time of the second karyotyped loss.

To conclude, from the live birth and amniocentesis data we can infer that some couples carry a greater risk of homoaneuploidy in the form of repeated trisomy 21 pregnancies. On the other hand, from the miscarriage data we may infer that the same does not hold for heteroaneuploidy; there is no evidence of a raised risk of repetitions for all trisomies in general. The number of instances of repetition is small; hence they do not flatly contradict the possibility, suggested by the amniocentesis data cited previously, that for some couples a higher risk of heteroaneuploidy may exist.

Recurrence in trisomy 21, it has been suggested, might be the result of mosaicism; on this theory a cryptic trisomic cell line might be transmitted by a parent not manifestly affected by Down's syndrome. Trisomy 21 mosaicism in parents of Down's syndrome offspring has been estimated as between 2.7 and 4.3 per cent (Uchida and Freeman 1985). Of 10 mosaic parents described, 2 had more than one child with trisomy 21. Such findings could be accounted for by a high risk of trisomy 21 pregnancies when one member of a couple is mosaic. With a hypothetical probability of the order of 50 per cent, the trisomy 21 recurrences observed in the amniocentesis data could be accounted for by trisomy 21 births to only a small number of couples (perhaps 1.3 to 3.3 per cent) in which one partner is mosaic (Warburton et al. 1987a).

Other mechanisms, such as a rare but persisting environmental exposure, might also produce an increased risk of trisomy 21 in all pregnancies of certain couples. Under such circumstances, it would not be possible to determine whether the exposure led to an increased risk of trisomy 21 at conception or to an increased rate of survival into the phase of clinically recognized pregnancy. One might suppose that an environmental factor that altered the rate of subclinical loss would not discriminate between trisomies of different chromosomes. If this supposition is correct, then the absence of recurrence at miscarriage of trisomies regardless of the chromosome involved argues against an environmental factor that discriminates against subclinical loss of trisomy 21 in particular. The argument does not weigh against an environmental factor acting to produce recurrence at conception, however.

III Later Gestation

10 The Separation of Entities: Preterm Delivery, Low Birth Weight and Maturity

> Conception (in contrast to the fully public fact of birth) suggests not only the unknowable but the forbidden: our birth dates are matters of public record but our dates of conception are permanently shrouded in mystery.
>
> Joyce Carol Oates

Infants born well before their due date of delivery have always been recognizable—excepting a quickly grown few—by their small size alone. Writers have emphasized that the same care is needed for the small infant whether preterm or ill-grown (Tow 1937). Hence much medical literature on premature infants has obscured the distinctions between preterm delivery indicated by gestational age, on the one hand, and smallness indicated by birth weight, on the other.

The conflation of these separate dimensions is apparent from early writings on the subject before 1800 to the present day. Indeed, until the late nineteenth century, infants were seldom weighed at birth. Early obstetric texts (e.g., Mauriceau 1683; Lobb 1747; Smellie 1766; Hamilton 1785), all of which hardly mention birth weight, took the average weight to be an amazing 12 or 13 pounds. A correct range of weights was first reported in Gottingen in 1753, and in London in 1786 (cited by Cone 1961). In Paris in 1815 Friedlaender reported birth weights of 7077 newborns (Friedlaender 1815); these appeared, in the first such data published in the United States, in an 1836 textbook (Dewees 1836). In 1835 Adolphe Quételet, a founder of biological statistics and auxology, reported on the growth of infants weighed at birth and followed into childhood (Quételet 1869). By 1852, routine weighing of infants to monitor breastfeeds and growth was being advocated (Guillot 1852).

The availability of the birth weight datum did not abate the conflation of gestational age with size. For instance, 15 very small infants were described as a group of prematures (Cullingworth 1878), in what was possibly the first use of the term in this sense (Oxford English Dictionary, suppl. 1982); at least 1 of the 15 was full term and growth retarded.

By the end of the nineteenth century, a change is detectable: some obstetricians began asserting independence for the condition of prematurity defined by preterm delivery. In 1902, Pierre Budin defined prematures as infants born during or before the thirty-sixth week of gestation. William Ballantyne, in an address in Edinburgh in the same year, made his main theme the unready state of the preterm infant for extrauterine life. Writers in the following two decades maintained the point (Hess 1922). A further distinction was drawn, by George Newman in 1906 in a study of infant mortality, between prematurity and immaturity, the latter to "include all those conditions of congenital disability other than prematurity. . . ." We shall see that immaturity, too, has not been consistently defined.

The emerging separation of the two criteria for prematurity was not long insisted on. A proposal that prematurity be defined by a birth weight of 2500 grams or less, made by Arvo Ylppö in 1919, quickly gained currency. As a result, in the 1920s and for some decades thereafter, the distinction between age and size at birth was largely suppressed in clinical and statistical practice. Only scattered intimations of discomfort with the single parameter of size appeared in the literature, for instance in the work of Charles Peckham (1938a,b). In 1950, the report of a World Health Organization committee recommended Ylppo's birth weight criterion as a standard for either "prematurity" or "immaturity," without distinguishing between the two terms (WHO Technical Report Series 1950). Because the proposal was eminently practical in the circumstances of the time, especially for vital and hospital statistics, it soon gained wide acceptance.

The growing interest in birth weight coincided with changing patterns of survival. In western Europe, infant mortality had begun a rapid decline at the turn of the nineteenth century (at least a half-century later than adult mortality). At first, the burden of mortality in childhood shifted to the latter part of infancy. Later, after the First World War, pediatricians were surprised to find that seasonal peaks of mortality from summer diarrhea had virtually disappeared (Gale 1945). As other infectious diseases too had declined and epidemic patterns changed, the burden of the residual infant mortality had shifted still further towards the earlier months of life. By the mid-1930s, in the United States more infant deaths occurred in the first month of life than in the next 11 months of the first year. In England and Wales likewise, half of all infant deaths occurred in the first month, and by the mid-1950s, two-thirds (Figure 10-1). Among first-month deaths, an increasing proportion occurred in the first week. In a continuing trend in developed countries, "prematures" (defined by weight) formed a steadily rising proportion of these deaths among the newborn.

This concentration of deaths among the newborn made obvious the public health import of low birth weight for infant mortality. New York City began the trend toward routinely recording birth weight for the

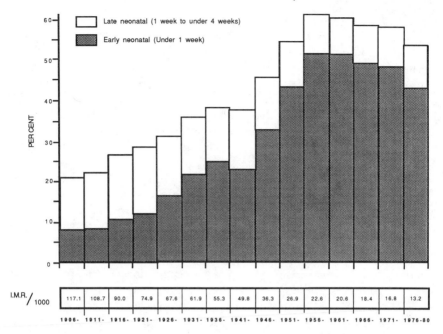

Fig. 10–1 Infant mortality by age at death: changes during this century in proportions of first-year deaths occurring in the first month and the first week of life. (Data, for England and Wales, from Macfarlane and Mugford 1984)

general population. A special confidential section was added to the birth certificate in 1938, in which the birth weight datum was first collected and coded with other medical information. New York State, California and others followed suit. National analyses in the United States, the first of which was in the 1950s (Shapiro and Unger 1954) still required a special undertaking until 1959. In Britain from 1945, local health authorities recorded low birth weight (<5½ pounds) on local notifications of live births to medical officers of health and, from 1955, on notifications of stillbirths. In 1975, birth weight began to be recorded on the birth certificates of the national registry system so that national analyses no longer required a compilation of local data of varying reliability and little depth (Macfarlane and Mugford 1984).

The World Health Organization, from its perspective as an international agency for public health, recognized a need for simple, practical and standard indicators of health in the populations of the world and promoted their use. As noted, in 1950 birth weight was chosen as the indicator of prematurity and slowly became a part of vital records in many countries. Some of the limitations on the generality of birth weight as an indicator were not yet apparent. In less developed countries, few data were available that could clarify the role of birth weight in infant mortality, and the issue is only now being sedulously researched.

From a parochial as well as a broad public health perspective, birth weight made for a ready index of prematurity. In hospitals and clinics, balance scales provided a reliable and accurate measure of weight that nurses or other staff could obtain quickly and simply. For home deliveries—and even in the United States a minority of births took place in hospitals as late as the 1930s—spring scales, if less accurate than balance scales, were easily carried into homes. Indeed, from the middle of the nineteenth century some hospitals had adopted the practice recommended by Guillot and recorded birth weight routinely. For instance, in Montreal University Lying-in Hospital, the records extend from 1851 (Ward and Ward 1984). On the Johns Hopkins obstetric service in Baltimore, it was possible to analyze birth weight (as well as other dimensions of the newborn infant) in consecutive deliveries from 1896 to 1932 (Peckham 1938a,b).

The practical grounds for the gradual adoption of birth weight as a criterion of prematurity do not entirely explain the longstanding disregard for a more accessible, more direct, and no less simple criterion, namely, the interval from date of last menstrual period to the date of delivery. One reason for the failure to apply length of gestation as a criterion is that a proportion of women are uncertain of the date of the last menstrual period or mistaken about it. These uncertainties were expressed in obstetric writings as long ago as 1671. "Women themselves, especially young ones of their first child are so ignorant commonly, that they cannot tell whether they have conceived or not, and not one in twenty almost keeps a just account, else they would be better provided against the time of their lying in, and not so suddenly be surprised, as many of them are" (Sharp 1671). Doubtless, precise dating of the last menstrual period could not have been widely practiced until calendars and literacy were widespread.

In modern times and in literate societies, doctors and midwives continued to mistrust estimates of length of gestation at delivery based on the date of the last menstrual period. As is natural to clinicians, the deviations from normality of individual cases remain vivid in the storehouse of impressions out of which clinical lore is woven. Thus, a sense of many individual errors in estimating the date of the last menstrual period has tended to override the actual norms of the collective experience of the population at large. These norms, in any event, did not become directly accessible to clinical practice until the site of delivery, shifting from home to hospital, was no longer dispersed among midwives and general practitioners.

As a result, in the individual case obstetricians have been accustomed to rely on their own clinical estimates of the duration of gestation. On birth certificates, too, the record of the length of gestation at delivery at first depended on the obstetrician's clinical judgment. Such judgments are liable to be shaped by clinical preconceptions about duration of pregnancy, as well as by the size, appearance and behavior of the infant

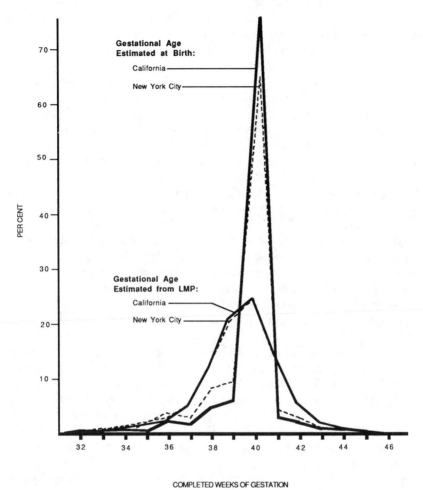

Fig. 10–2 Distribution of gestational age at birth (New York City and California): (a) by mother's history of last menstrual period; (b) by clinician's judgment at birth. (Adapted from Hammes and Treloar 1970)

at birth. The practice resulted in a distribution of durations of pregnancy concentrated at 40 completed weeks, with very little dispersion around the peak. The familiar bell-shaped distribution for length of gestation did not emerge from the data until estimates based on the mother's reported dates for the last menstrual period replaced the obstetrician's judgment (Figure 10-2). Baltimore, New York City, and California took this step in 1957.

The wide and even dispersion of gestational length based on women's reports suggested that menstrual dates had greater biological validity than they had been credited with. Evidence in support of this suggestion came from longitudinal studies (Treloar et al. 1967a). The menstrual cycles of a cohort of 2700 women were followed over many years. Recruited in college, first in 1934, the women kept diaries over an average of 25,803 person-years, and had 2083 pregnancies.

The understanding that in the majority of pregnancies menstrual histories were substantially accurate was slow to dawn and to be applied in epidemiological studies. In England as early as 1951, the consistency of such data had been demonstrated by Thomas McKeown and his associates (McKeown and Gibson 1951); 17,000 births for the year 1947 in Birmingham, England, analyzed to excellent purpose over the years, were compared with 12,000 births in Germany (Hosemann 1948). Indeed, these British writers inveighed against the neglect of gestational age and the thoughtless application of birth weight as a universal, all-purpose parameter. Both parameters were needed, they argued, to study etiology, to predict outcome, and to provide appropriate care. Their analysis of the distributions and divergencies of perinatal mortality in relation to the two parameters still stands as an informative model. Low and normal birth weight do not exactly coincide with any dichotomy that separates preterm and term delivery (Figure 10-3).

Some of the tardiness in the use of the gestational age measure might be explained by the impact of contemporary and subsequent studies that underlined the dramatic contribution of low birth weight as an antecedent of mortality in the newborn (Peckham 1938a,b; Baumgartner et al. 1950; Baird and Thomson 1969; Bergner and Susser 1970; Shah and Abbey 1971; Chase 1972). Birth weight, regardless of length of gestation, was shown to account for somewhat more than 90 per cent of the variance in perinatal mortality. Length of gestation, with birth weight controlled, accounted for 4 to 6 per cent of the variance (Susser et al. 1972).

Birth weight is the final common pathway for the expression of many factors embedded in the social and biological processes leading to birth. Adjustment for birth weight alone proved sufficient to account, in a statistical sense, for the twofold excess of perinatal mortality of blacks over whites in New York City from 1958 to 1961 (Bergner and Susser 1970). Although in such analyses some problematic aspects of standardization for birth weight tended to be ignored (Wilcox and Russell 1983a), these do not detract from the ultimate predominance of birth weight in relation to mortality. Birth weight was also emphasized in many studies as an antecedent of developmental morbidity later in life (Birch and Gussow 1970; Thomson 1983).

As a matter of epidemiological practice, then, the utility of birth weight as a variable for purposes both of predicting outcome and of controlling confounding had served analysts with great efficiency. Length of gestation fell into the shadows as an epidemiological variable. In comparisons of populations, adjusting for birth weight alone pro-

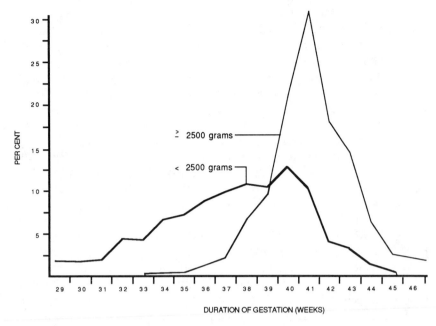

Fig. 10–3 Overlap in definitions of prematurity: per cent births ≥2500 g versus <2500 g, by length of gestation. (Adapted from McKeown and Gibson 1951)

vided good control of confounding by virtually all the factors antecedent to birth weight, whether they were socioeconomic, ethnic or nutritional (Paneth et al. 1982a).

An exemplary application has been in international comparisons. The international ranking of the United States in material wealth and technical resources is not matched by a corresponding ranking for newborn mortality rates. This low ranking has been a longstanding public health concern (e.g., Shapiro and Moriyama 1963). It was therefore a surprise when, with birth weight adjusted, newborn mortality in the United States turned out to be lower than in any other developed country (Lee et al. 1980). In other words, the poor ranking of the United States with birth weight unadjusted was predominantly a matter of disadvantageous birth weight distributions. Logically, this finding directs concern about perinatal mortality in the United States to the causes of low birth weight rather than to deficient medical care for the newborn.

Similar analyses of U.S. national newborn mortality with birth weight standardized had a bearing on medical care. Improvements over time could be seen to be owed mainly to factors over and above birth weight, and not to changes in the birth weight distribution and the socioeconomic and demographic factors that underlie it (Lee et al. 1980; Kleinman 1982). Among these factors, improved newborn medical care was a strong candidate, if not the only one. Again, in a demonstration of the effectiveness of intensive care for small newborn infants in New York City, adjusting for birth weight was the keystone in the control of selective factors governing the use of different types of hospitals (Paneth et al. 1982b).

In striving to understand better the connection between birth weight and mortality, statisticians and epidemiologists have sought to identify what is optimal in terms of outcome and to segregate what is "normal" from what is "abnormal." Some have devised statistical models to describe the distributions of birth weight, sometimes in relation to length of gestation and sometimes not (Karn and Penrose 1951; Yerushalmy 1967; Anctil et al. 1964; Ashford et al. 1969; Goldstein and Peckham 1976; Hoffman et al. 1977; Wilcox and Russell 1983b,c).

One proposed model, derived by the use of probit analysis, divided the birth weight distribution around 2500 grams. As perinatal mortality declined with increasing birth weight, the decline in the mortality curve became steeper above that point (Ashford et al. 1969). A subsequent model divided the distribution into two overlapping components: one "predominant" component is normally distributed around mean birth weight, a second "residual" component is confined to the tail of the distribution and comprises an excess of very low birth weight infants (Wilcox and Russell 1983b). In our judgment, statistical models for the most part have yet to be translated into practical terms that discriminate between the antecedents or the consequences of the birth weight classes identified in the models.

In current perspective, indeed, the emphasis on birth weight could be said to have been exaggerated. As a matter of logical inference, an emphatic role for birth weight in newborn mortality and morbidity does not require the displacement of length of gestation as another important factor. Length of gestation, taken as a measure of fetal age, is the necessary antecedent of the fetal growth that produces birth weight. Only in special circumstances could one consider reversing the logical order of the two variables of fetal age and fetal growth—for instance, parturition could be accelerated or delayed because of large or small fetal size, respectively; or a small and seriously impaired infant might be delivered prematurely. With the causal structure in mind that fetal age is the antecedent of fetal growth, it becomes evident that fetal age deserves equal attention as a subject of study in its own right. That is, one needs to understand how preterm delivery comes about as much as what its consequences might be. In this regard, both epidemiological and clinical needs are served by improved precision in measuring fetal age. As we discuss in the next chapter, ultrasonography is a technique that contributes to precision.

Along with length of gestation and birth weight, "maturity" offers still another dimension of the newborn infant by which to characterize prior prenatal development and, possibly, developmental prognosis. It is commonsensical to expect that a premature infant would be "unfinished" in various ways, or that it would be still primitive in its neurological responses. In the 1960s and 1970s, some students of early human development, still implicitly discounting length of gestation as a measure of age at birth, turned to the notion of a biological clock that more or less strictly governs the unfolding of development. Thus, they sought to substitute clinical or biological measures of maturity for chronological measures of age. When these measures are used as a guide to the age as well as the developmental stage at birth of the newborn infant, it is essential that the observations be described in terms separate from gestational age and birth weight. In practice, the need for this separation has been largely ignored, even by research workers. The result has been to renew the conflation of indices that has so troubled the analyses and the understanding of the developmental phenomena observed at birth.

To assume the identity of maturity and true gestational age is to court circularity and obscure the nature of the interrelations of maturity, gestational age, and birth weight. One example comes from a careful study of the neurobehavioral responses of preterm infants, at birth and at a supposed postconceptional age of 40 weeks (Aylward et al. 1984). Gestational age at birth, not chronological but assigned from the Dubovitz maturity scale, correlated with infant responses at 40 weeks. An interpretation that "gestational age," so defined, influences later neurobehavioral response would be vacuous, in that the observed correlation is not between age at birth and later development, but between development at birth and later. Better understanding of maturity will elude us until the relationships among indices are separately analyzed and compared in many different groups.

Still another elaboration of criteria for prematurity was the introduction of the concept of intrauterine growth retardation (McBurney 1947; Gruenwald 1963; Anctil 1964; Battaglia and Lubchenco 1967). Gestational age as denominator and infant weight as numerator are combined to create the variable. The advent of this concept in epidemiology only in the mid-1960s suggests that the phenomenon was not easy to operationalize. Since Jacob Yerushalmy and his colleagues (1965) quantified the variable, clinicians have given it close attention as a prognostic criterion. At the same time, attention has been diverted from the task of establishing the independent effects of gestational age and size that compound the criterion. Cecil Drillien (1957), in an early case-control study, concluded that ". . . prematurity on a weight basis was a mixture of two categories, early and small," and that each had different causes. To our contemporary way of thinking also, we need to understand the separate roles of age and size no less well than their derivative in growth rates (Susser et al. 1972; Thomson 1983). In the next three chapters, we review our understanding first of preterm delivery resulting from shortened gestation, and then of small size resulting from slow growth.

11 Preterm Delivery:
I. Indices and Enumeration

Epidemiological studies with a calculated focus on the duration of gestation and on preterm delivery have been few in number. Even those few were seldom technically accomplished. Aside from the slow historical evolution outlined in the previous chapter, the problems of measuring the variable of interest (Keirse 1979) have deterred researchers.

From either a biological or a clinical standpoint, it is an open question whether a natural dividing line between preterm and term deliveries exists. It follows that when gestational ages are cast in classes as term, preterm, and postterm, some arbitrariness about dividing lines is unavoidable. Of more concern is inconsistency in the definition of classes. These have differed from one learned body to another, from one country to another, and within the same official international body from one decade to the next. Further problems arise with that minority of cases in which the size of the infant seems markedly discordant with its reported gestational age. In one approach, all large discrepancies are imputed to measurement error (Milner and Richards 1974). The untoward result is to close off investigation of the alternative explanation of abnormal growth rate.

We mentioned, in the previous chapter, that problems exist in measures of maturity, and in the use of physical, physiological, and neurodevelopmental assessments that stand in for gestational age and prematurity. When such problems of determining prematurity or postmaturity are resolved, preterm infants still include cases heterogeneous both in cause and in outcome. Loose terms and definitions add to these impediments to understanding. In this chapter, we deal with the issues of the measurement and categorization of preterm delivery and the consequences for interpreting reproductive loss, and also with the relations of gestational age to developmental age.

ESTABLISHING DATES

The exact day of fertilization is seldom known, except for such unusual circumstances as artificial insemination, in vitro fertilization, and exposure to insemination on no more than one dated occasion in a given cycle. The most precise available indicator of date of ovulation from which to calculate date of delivery is usually obtained by way of Naegele's 1812 calculation from a definite history of the date of the first day of the last menstrual period (LMP). Under favorable circumstances—women "certain" of their dates who delivered infants of 3000 grams or more—the mean length of pregnancy in a recent and sufficient sample was 284 days, with 9 out of 10 terminating within 23 days on either side of the mean, and about 2 out of 3 terminating within 15 days of the mean (Andersen et al. 1981a, 1981b).

In some women, the first day of the last menstrual period gives an imprecise estimate of the day of ovulation. Uncertainties arise in women who are lactating but not menstruating, after a recent miscarriage or delivery, and for more obscure reasons. Variations in the length of the menstrual cycle—especially the first phase between the first day of menstruation and ovulation—may produce erroneous estimates, although such variation should not exceed 5 days (Birkbeck et al. 1975). Constant and marked irregularities of the menstrual cycle, however, may render the date of the last menstrual period unobtainable or, when it can be obtained, invalidate it as a pointer to ovulation.

After conception, cyclical bleeding at the anticipated time is sometimes mistaken for the last menstrual period and so defers the estimated date of delivery beyond the true date by the length of the cycle. This classification error overestimates preterm deliveries. On the other hand, if an anovular cycle or a subclinical loss precedes the cycle of conception, the estimated date of delivery would be advanced by the length of the cycle. This classification error overestimates postterm deliveries.

Despite these problems, a history can usually establish, if not the exact day, at least the week when the last period began. Care and timeliness in history-taking shortly after the first missed period diminishes uncertainty with dates. Thus, in the United States a diary study of menstrual cycles afforded a test of the reliability of the date of last menstrual period as an indicator of conception, albeit in a population selected for college education and assiduous diary keeping. Dates taken from the diaries were compared not only with the dates elicited by a single private obstetrician (Treloar et al. 1967b), but also with those elicited for public clinic deliveries (Hammes and Treloar 1970). In neither case did the clinical records differ appreciably from the diaries.

In Aberdeen, Scotland, among 55,000 unselected maternities on the obstetric services of the city, the date of the last menstrual period was known in 75 per cent, approximated in 15 per cent, and not known for

10 per cent. When dates were imputed for uncertain cases from the mean for known birth weights, inclusion of these approximations caused no irregularity in the curves based on "certain" dates (Thomson et al. 1968). In nearly 1 million births in California and Georgia, when dates were likewise imputed in 14.8 per cent (in California) and 21.8 per cent (in Georgia), their inclusion did not alter the patterns or the direction of the neonatal mortality rates (Binkin et al. 1985). In both states, infant death rates were somewhat higher for cases in which the gestational age was unknown. This follows at least in part because records most often tend to be incomplete for stillbirths and very early neonatal deaths.

When a menstrual history is taken well into pregnancy, or at some time after the birth, the date of the last menstrual period elicited may be "uncertain" for as many as 20 per cent of cases. The epidemiologist must then resort to other estimators of the date of conception. Clinical measures—audibility of the fetal heart, the height of the uterine fundus, and the mother's sensation of quickening—have been assessed for this purpose. None of these signs taken individually gives as good an estimate as do the reports of women certain of their dates. Taken together, however, the approximation has been found to be no worse than a known date for the last menstrual period (Andersen et al. 1981a, 1981b).

Women who do not provide menstrual dates for the record are likely to differ from those who do both in physiological and social characteristics (Hall et al. 1985). The dual nature of these characteristics is likely to be compounded in estimates of last menstrual period and length of gestation. Thus, physiological factors—the recency of a previous pregnancy, lactation and oral contraceptive use, and the woman's health and nutritional state—influence menstrual histories. Several social factors—social class, ethnicity, migration, and the woman's age—influence these physiological factors. At the same time, these social factors and others, such as home language, affect the personal interaction between obstetrician or midwife and the pregnant woman, and thereby the precision of the menstrual history. Such a complex of linked physiological and social factors readily leads to confounding in interpretations of the risks and determinants of preterm delivery.

Unambiguous menstrual dates are at least matched by ultrasonography in predicting delivery dates. For term deliveries there tends to be good agreement between the two methods, if not on either side of term (Kramer et al. 1988). The clear advantage of ultrasonography for the purpose of establishing dates is largely confined to cases in which menstrual dates are uncertain. Crown rump length (CRL) and biparietal diameter (BPD) are the most useful estimators. Both crown rump length before the twelfth week and biparietal diameter before 24 weeks (usually 13 to 20 weeks) predict the date of delivery as exactly as impeccable dates for the last menstrual period (Lancet 1986). For term pregnancies, however, ultrasonography has not been shown to do any better than menstrual histories. Thus, in one study, neither a single measure of biparietal diameter in the twenty-sixth week nor repeated growth-adjusted sonographic age methods (GASA) improved on reliable menstrual histories (Simon et al. 1984).

The earlier ultrasonographic criterion (CRL before the twelfth week) does better than the later one (BPD at 13 to 20 weeks). This result accords with and complements our understanding that third trimester growth rates vary and account for the differences in birth weight that occur regardless of length of gestation (Smith 1947; McKeown and Record 1952; Gruenwald 1966a,b). Presumably, in the first several weeks of development, individual tracks for growth rate have not yet been established, and variation from one individual to the next is small.

Assessment of the overall benefits and costs of routine early ultrasonography must weigh—besides its precision in predicting an expected date of delivery—its contributions to clinical certainty in such other matters as the viability and anatomical integrity of the fetus. Precise knowledge of fetal age can be important in a number of clinical situations. The stage of gestation matters for the timing of procedures for prenatal screening and intervention, for instance, in the sampling of maternal serum for α-feto-protein, of chorionic villi or amniotic fluid for chromosomal aberrations, and of fetal blood for genetic disorders. The age of the fetus is a crucial factor when premature delivery threatens, or when induction of labor before term needs to be considered because of complications such as diabetes, hypertension of pregnancy, growth retardation, and the breech position.

The capacity of ultrasound imaging for dating of fetal age might not recommend it for routine clinical use on these grounds alone. The results of randomized controlled trials of routine ultrasonography, taken separately or together, have been judged indeterminate (Thacker, 1985). Even with uncertain dates ultrasonography has not been shown to exceed the reliability and validity of multiple and carefully elicited clinical signs for predicting delivery dates. Ultrasonography would seem to have a palpable advantage in such cases, however, in providing a single reliable measure. Thus, when ultrasonography is available—as it is increasingly in the United States in the private offices of obstetricians as well as hospitals—a clinician might have reason to use the technique. Caution is in order. Ill effects from exposure have not been so thoroughly explored as to be ruled out entirely (Neilson and Hood 1980; Lancet 1986).

The epidemiological grounds for systematic ultrasonography are different from the clinical grounds and, perhaps, more cogent. The argument in favor relates to a clinically important minority of cases in which reported menstrual dates do not agree closely with ultrasonography. A well-documented study (Kramer et al. 1988) assumed, for the purpose of evaluation, that ultrasonography was the more valid criterion: biparietal diameter at 16–18 weeks was taken to be the "true" estimate of date of conception. For babies delivered at term according to ultrasonography, the date of delivery predicted by menstrual dates was in agreement in 95 per cent of cases. Before term and especially after term, however, agreement was much less good. For births delivered preterm, the menstrual date systematically underestimated gestational length and also overestimated preterm delivery: 12 per cent were actually term births according to the ultrasound prediction. For births delivered postterm, the menstrual date systematically overestimated gestational length and also postterm delivery: 78 per cent were term births according to the ultrasound prediction. The consistency and the causes of these discrepancies have not been established. A strong case can be made for research to elucidate them so that informed clinical decisions can be made.

The need sometimes arises, perhaps more often for research than for clinical purposes, to fix a date of conception from available data relating to menstrual history, ultrasonography, and clinical assessment. Coding rules provide an epidemiological guide to such decisions. In a study of poor black and Hispanic women in New York City selected for high risk of preterm delivery, the patient's report of the last menstrual period was selected as the criterion of choice in 84 per cent of cases, the sonogram was selected in 13 per cent, and clinical assessment in 3 per cent (Thaul 1988). Decision rules for estimating delivery dates have also been formulated by others (Hall et al. 1985).

ESTABLISHING CATEGORIES

For the separation of term from preterm births, a threshold of 38 completed weeks was recommended by the American Academy of Pediatrics (1967). Other organizations and other countries have made other choices. A World Health Organization publication approved by the International Federation of Gynecology and Obstetrics (WHO–FIGO 1977) tried to bring order and consensus with standard definitions using days or *completed* weeks. Three categories were created for gestational length at delivery, namely, *preterm* (<259 days or <37 completed weeks) *term* (259 to 293 days or 37 to <42 completed weeks) and *postterm* (>294 days or ≥42 completed weeks). Before that time, the literature is pervaded by studies of preterm delivery defined according to the arbitrary choice of the investigator.

Even after the 1977 definitions of preterm birth had specified completed weeks, confusion persisted. Thus, the same publication, in recommending a criterion for term delivery of 37 completed weeks or 259 days, at the same time obliterated the 37-week threshold by recommending the use of 2-week gestational-age intervals that spanned the thirty-sixth to thirty-eighth completed week. From the perspective of the epi-

Table 11–1 Number of fetal deaths and live births during each completed week of gestation beginning at 20 weeks, New York City, 1984

	Fetal death	Live birth
Week of gestation		
20	35	35
21	42	49
22	54	71
23	49	89
24	46	143
25	28	152
26	29	178
27	21	222
28	35	274
29	28	372
30	29	446
31	27	545
32	23	758
33	35	1099
34	30	1751
35	41	2714
36	32	4322
37	34	7974
38	46	15327
39	51	24652
40	46	24818
41	38	14506
42	20	7087
43	16	3007
44+	12	2347
Total	847	112938

Source: Data from J. Kiely, personal communication.

demiologist dealing with large populations, observations coded in intervals marked by single completed weeks of gestation or single days are certainly preferable. This at once removes issues of comparability arising from incompatible categories, and permits flexibility in analysis.

Problems of classification and comparability often follow from the elementary fact that numerators in population rates are always smaller than denominators. Consequently, changes or errors in numerators have greater impact on rates than changes or errors of the same size in denominators. When large classification shifts impinge on small numerators, comparability can be severely impaired. The problems arise with categories at both the upper and lower bounds of gestational age for a given outcome (Table 11-1).

At the upper bound for preterm births, categorizations of gestation by week that neglect to specify completed weeks can disagree by as much as

6 days. Often births in the thirty-seventh week of gestation—days 252 to 259—have been classified as term and not preterm. If the 7974 live births *during* the thirty-seventh week in New York City in 1984 had all been classified as full term, 11.7 per cent would have been designated preterm, in contrast with the 18.8 per cent so designated when births after 37 completed weeks (≥259 days) were classified as full term. In addition, such discrepancies in classification are not random with respect to the age and weight of infants assigned to each class: at birth, the largest proportion of preterm births subject to misclassification as term births is always at the upper margin of the preterm class. Late in gestation, the fetus in utero may be gaining as much as 20 grams daily (Birkbeck et al. 1975). Thus, this nonrandom error in classification, by excluding the heavier infants from the preterm class, can lead to a significant downward bias in estimates of the weight of preterm births.

Category problems similar in principle arise with preterm births at the lower bounds of gestational age. At earlier ages, preterm births must be distinguished from miscarriages. For comparisons of rates of live preterm births, the choice of the lower cutoff point for gestational age has no great import. The choice does have import for comparisons of late fetal death rates.

By longstanding convention, 28 completed weeks of gestation was the dividing line separating stillbirths from miscarriages, on the assumption that earlier births were nonviable. It followed that preterm births included all those occurring between 28 and 37 completed weeks, and the numerators for mortality rates were calculated within these limits. In recent years, however, the proportion of infants delivered before 28 completed weeks and pronounced alive at birth has been rising. A downward shift of the threshold for viability to accommodate the increasing though still small number of infants born alive before 28 weeks causes no more than a minor rise in the rate of live preterm births: in New York City in 1984, the proportion born preterm was 17.9 per cent after 28 completed weeks, 18.5 per cent after 24 completed weeks, and 18.7 per cent after 20 completed weeks.

For rates of late fetal and newborn mortality, a downward shift in the dividing line has greater impact. Above 28 completed weeks of gestation, the numerators of these mortality rates are small. Below the 28-week threshold, many deliveries are stillborn or die soon after birth. These losses, added to a small numerator, substantially enlarge it but do not proportionately enlarge the denominator: in New York City in 1984, the proportion of stillbirths as the threshold is moved earlier in gestation was 0.5 per cent after 28 completed weeks, 0.6 per cent after 24 completed weeks, and 0.7 per cent after 20 completed weeks. At the maximum, this change brings about a 40 per cent increment, as can be calculated from the data in Table 11-1.

Conversely, with upward shifts of the boundary dividing miscarriages from stillbirths, the reclassification of stillbirths into the miscarriage class does not substantially affect the residual miscarriage rates. In the gestational intervals beyond 20 weeks, fetal deaths are few compared with earlier stages of gestation. Hence their reclassification as stillbirths removes a trivial proportion from the numerator of miscarriages: in New York City in 1984, given a miscarriage rate among all pregnancies up to 20 completed weeks of 12 per cent, the rate would be 12.1 per cent up to 24 completed weeks, and 12.2 per cent up to 28 completed weeks.

Classification has been affected by other changes over the years. Health records bear mightily on the public health. To provide knowledge that can guide policy, records must change as circumstances change. Thus, practices in recording births for vital statistics have not remained constant. Some of these changes aim to improve the competence of records and statistics for describing the outcome of births that are very early or very small. In developed countries, especially since the 1970s, infants born at early gestational ages have survived increasingly. In 1977, therefore, the World Health Organization published a recommendation (WHO–FIGO 1977) that national statistics should include all infants, alive or dead, of more than 500 grams in weight, or 25 cm in length, or 154 days (22 completed weeks) in gestation.

At the same time, it was recognized implicitly that, in most countries, many births so early in gestation would be missed. For this reason, the recommended standard for international comparisons was less inclusive, namely, all births more than 1000 grams weight, or 35 cm in length, or 196 days gestation (28 completed weeks). In the United States, most states now aim to be more inclusive than either of these standards, and they register pregnancy terminations down to 140 days (20 completed weeks). In New York City all terminations are supposed to be registered, regardless of length of gestation. There, as elsewhere, registration or notification is least complete the earlier the gestational age.

The historical changes in reproduction and in mortality among very early and very small births also draw attention to the need for refining categories of fetal loss during pregnancy and at birth. In the present era, perinatal death rates have reached very low levels compared with the past. At the same time, rates of infant death after the newborn period had begun to decline sooner and did so faster. Consequently, as Figure 10-1 shows, the residue of perinatal deaths at term has come to constitute the greater proportion of infant losses.

Further advances in understanding depend on refinements of the constituent elements of perinatal loss. For instance, among late fetal deaths, a distinction needs to be made between prepartum and intrapartum deaths, because they carry different messages for prevention. In less developed countries, a large component of late fetal deaths comprises intrapartum deaths, which points to the process of delivery. In developed countries, the case is the opposite. Newborn death rates in the

1980s in the United States have declined at a rate faster than ever before. The same may be true, we suspect, of intrapartum fetal deaths, but may not be true of prepartum fetal deaths. Through the 1970s in the United States, by far the largest component—four-fifths of the total—was prepartum fetal deaths (Kiely 1983). From a world perspective on late fetal deaths, the appropriate focus for prevention thus shifts from the delivery process in less developed countries to prepartum fetal deaths and preterm live births in developed countries.

In summary, with *fetal death rates*, refined analyses can be markedly affected by the gray areas at the bounds of the gestational age definitions. The number of fetal losses is clearly increased when births very early in gestation and at very low weights (*intermediate fetal deaths*) are included with later fetal deaths to form an enlarged numerator. If enumerated, the shifts make a distinct difference to stillbirth rates but not to miscarriage rates. All these rates are subject to classification errors, particularly as gestational age boundaries shift or are imprecisely defined. If drawn from routine statistics, the estimated rates are also beset by simple gaps in recording and enumerating of relevant data and events.

With *preterm deliveries*, we saw that a lower boundary between miscarriages and preterm delivery that is late in gestation rather than early ignores few live births but a substantial number of fetal deaths. By contrast, an upper boundary between preterm and term delivery that is early in gestation rather than late—for instance, when infants born in the thirty-seventh week are counted not as preterm but as full term—sizably reduces both the rate of preterm live births and the mean birth weight among them, because of the sharp rise in births and the somewhat lesser rise in birth weight as pregnancy nears term.

GESTATIONAL AGE AND REPRODUCTIVE RISKS

Live-born infants delivered very early in gestation are of great clinical concern. They are at imminent risk of death and, if they escape death, of severe neurological impairment. Much of the sharp increase over time in the survival of small infants is surely owed to modern techniques of intensive care at delivery and in the newborn period. Modern intensive care can have an impact sufficient to alter population mortality rates. In New York City, small infants (<2250 g) born in hospitals where modern newborn intensive care was available had survival rates 30 to 40 per cent better than those born where it was unavailable (Paneth, et al. 1982b).

The results of intensive care are made problematical by conflicts of value. On the one hand, physicians bound by Hippocratic tradition do all they can to ensure survival. On the other hand, some parents and the public interest may weigh the burdens and the costs of lifelong handicap more heavily than the added numbers of healthy children among the survivors.

With regard to impairment rates in survivors, intensive care may act in more than one direction (Kiely et al. 1981). Very small preterm infants are at high risk of brain impairment. Whether the impairment eventuated before, during, or after parturition may be crucial. It is entirely likely that intensive newborn care increases the chances of survival of infants born impaired, and so adds to the prevalence of handicap. At the same time, it is equally likely that intensive care reduces the incidence of impairment in those born unimpaired, and so subtracts from the prevalence of handicap.

Infants are most often assigned to intensive care based on the single criterion of birth weight, and not length of gestation. Very low birth weight (VLBW) is sometimes defined as less than 2000 grams, sometimes as less than 1500 grams. Among these births, all technically at high risk based on one or the other criterion, neither birth weight nor gestational age, taken alone, encompasses all infants at high risk (see Figure 10-3). Moreover, the proportions of infants identified as high risk by each of these classifying criteria differ between blacks and whites and between girls and boys. Figure 11-1 shows the correspondence of mean birth weight with completed weeks of gestation, in New York City in 1984, separately for live-born infants of black and white parentage and of each sex.

When the effect of birth weight was held constant in data from the 1960s, gestational age at delivery accounted for a relatively small proportion of the variance in perinatal mortality—about 5 per cent in an analysis of several data sets (Susser et al. 1972). The same relationships hold in newer data (Figure 11.2). Of course, shorter gestational age is itself a cause of low birth weight, and that part of the contribution of gestational age to mortality is removed by a standardization procedure. Aside from this contribution through birth weight as an intervening factor in the causal chain, the effect of gestational age on mortality was seen only between about 36 and 40 weeks of gestation. During that gestational interval, mortality risk was raised when gestational age was prolonged for a given birth weight (i.e., growth was retarded), and also when it was abbreviated (i.e., growth was accelerated).

Taking each ethnic and sex group separately, at virtually every gestational age interval heavier babies do better. Perinatal mortality is highest at the lowest weights and decreases exponentially. This relationship holds, regardless of length of gestation, up to an optimum weight in the region of 3500 grams, after which the rates again began to rise. The point has been illustrated in different ways (Hoffman et al. 1974; Goldstein and Peckham 1976).

These generalizations hold true *within* an array of ethnic and sex groups. In comparisons *between* ethnic and sex groups, however, a given

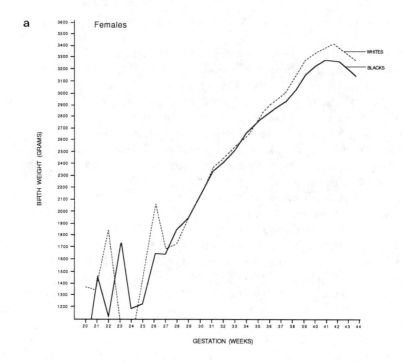

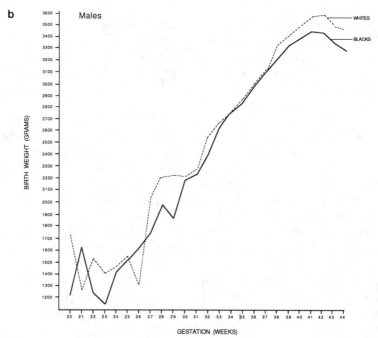

Fig. 11–1 Birthweight by gestational age in liveborn infants: (a) females, blacks and whites; (b) males, blacks and whites; (c) blacks, females and males; (d) whites, females and males. (Data for New York City, 1984, from J. Kiely, personal communication)

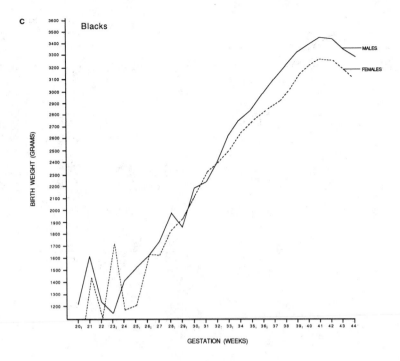

c

Blacks

BIRTH WEIGHT (GRAMS)

MALES
FEMALES

GESTATION (WEEKS)

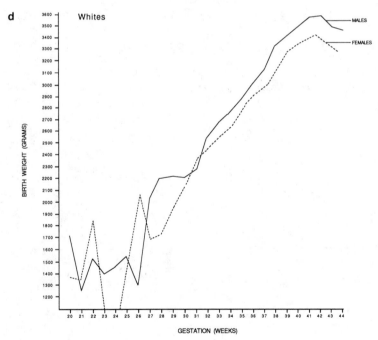

d

Whites

BIRTH WEIGHT (GRAMS)

MALES
FEMALES

GESTATION (WEEKS)

185

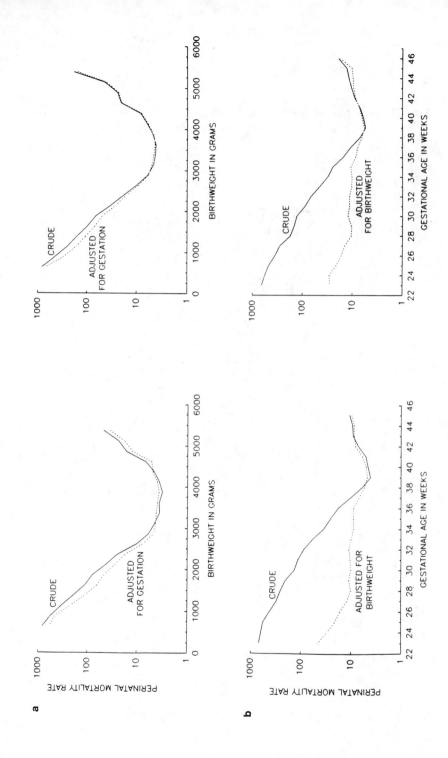

birth weight at a particular gestational interval does not always give rise to the same level of perinatal mortality in each group. In other words, ethnicity and sex are indicators of effects on mortality over and above those of birth weight and gestational age. Conversely mortality, as well as its complement in hardiness and vitality, reflects more than postconceptional age or size at a given age. To explain mortality, therefore, we need to consider developmental parameters that are not entirely measured by the age and size of the infant. This conclusion returns us to the concept of maturity or developmental age.

DEVELOPMENTAL AGE AND GESTATIONAL AGE

Developmental age is an observed state of development, whether somatic, neurologic, physiologic or behavioral. The norm for developmental age at birth is set by the average range of observations around term. Departures from the norm are generally taken to indicate advanced or retarded development. Considerable differences in developmental age are to be expected at different gestational ages, since intrauterine development is comparatively rapid. During gestation, the cartilage of the ear, the fissures on the palms and soles, the readiness of the cardiac respiratory apparatus to function independently, and the maturation of the neuromuscular system each follows a regular developmental sequence. Systematic observations on births in which menstrual dates were "certain" have permitted norms of development to be refined and established for given gestational ages.

A variety of indices and scales have been created to capture infant maturity. Prenatal indicators, before the birth weight could be known, were biochemical; they were used to guide the clinical management of delivery. Postnatal indicators, when the birth weight was known, tapped various dimensions of development. Structural scales of maturity largely depended on anatomy and physical form (Usher et al. 1966), functional scales on neurological responses (Andre-Thomas et al. 1960; St. Anne Dargassie 1966; Brazelton 1973; Prechtl 1977), and others combined structural and functional elements (Dubovitz and Dubovitz 1981). These indices were quickly adopted by neonatologists as indicators of the condition and appropriate treatment of the infant in the newborn period and, to a lesser degree, of the prognosis for development. Some analysts emphasize the norms of these scales as a guide to an infant's age and

---

Fig. 11–2 Unique contributions to perinatal mortality of birth weight over and above duration of gestation and vice versa (log linear analysis of births to New York City whites and nonwhites, 1978–1984). (a) Perinatal death rates by birth weight, crude (—) and adjusted for duration of pregnancy (...). (b) Perinatal death rates, by duration of pregnancy, crude (—) and adjusted for birth weight (...). (Data provided by Kiely, personal communication)

developmental stage; others emphasize the deviance from norms as a guide to possible neurological and behavioral disorder.

In the previous chapter we noted the frequent substitution of developmental stage for age, and the circularity that follows in describing age-specific norms of development. For the analyses of antecedent risk factors, too, the use of maturity scales at birth as surrogates for gestational age can invite errors of interpretation. To substitute a maturity scale for gestational age is to assume that both the true and the substitute measures vary concomitantly within each subgroup analyzed. This is not always the case.

Evidence that measures of development do not correspond with post-conception age in a way that is consistent—across ethnic groups, sex, age at birth, and health status—can be compiled from various sources. Numerous comparisons, for different countries, peoples and circumstances, provide examples of group-specific departures in the developmental phenomena around birth or later at given postconception ages.

Sex is one such criterion that differentiates between chronological and developmental age. At the same gestational ages for singletons, girls are smaller and yet more mature than boys, and they have a survival advantage made even more notable by adjustment for their lower birth weight (Skovron 1982). A biochemical indicator of these sex differences is the lecithin/sphingomyelin ratio, which is taken to be a sign of maturity and is a useful predictor of respiratory distress syndrome (Torday et al. 1981). The appearance of ossification centers is taken to be an indicator of developmental maturity that is, to some extent, independent of chronological age. On this ground, too, girls are ahead of boys of the same gestational age, for instance, as indicated by radiographs of the cuboid bone (Christie et al. 1941).

Ethnicity or race is another criterion that differentiates between chronological and developmental age. In Uganda, for example, African infants compared with infants of expatriate European women were functionally more mature in terms of their neurological responses at birth (Geber and Dean 1957). In later studies in Uganda, African infants at birth were also found to be physically more mature in terms of such physical signs as skull hardness, lanugo hair, nail length, nail texture, and breast size (Parkin 1971).

Ethnicity and race are complex variables. The demonstration of a negroid/caucasoid difference in one culture or society is not necessarily general to other societies and, when measured in functional and not physical terms, may indeed not be independent of culture and social factors (Susser et al. 1985b). Nigerian neonates, for example, were found to have scores on the Dubovitz scale quite compatible with European norms (Brueton et al. 1973).

In the United States, several studies have compared blacks and whites on developmental measures. An early comparison of classification centers in the cuboid bone found that these centers had appeared at younger gestational ages in blacks than in whites (Christie et al. 1941). The general pattern suggested by the assembled results of such comparisons is that, at birth and through the first postnatal year, black infants are functionally in advance of white infants. Throughout this period of development, size as well as gestational age is a powerful determinant of cognitive function and behavior (Rush et al. 1983), and should be taken into account in all such comparisons. When such adjustments are not made, measures of development that reveal functional differences in favor of blacks are likely to understate their advantage, because at birth and for some time thereafter black infants are smaller than white infants of the same gestational age.

The most systematic comparisons so far stem from the follow-up of a large cohort of preterm infants; interrater reliabilities were established and the range of results fully reported (Aylward et al. 1984). We have already noted, however, that in this series age at birth was assigned, not from gestational age, but from a developmental score. The comparisons of blacks and whites might be assumed, from the generalizations in the preceding paragraph, to understate functional differences in favor of blacks and overstate those in favor of whites. The trends support the differences reported from previous smaller and less systematic studies. At an estimated age of 40 weeks after conception, black infants had more mature neurological control: spontaneous motor movements of the legs were stronger and more flexed; resistance was greater against passive movements of the shoulders, elbows, wrists and knees; and arm control was more vigorous.

We conclude that, although in many groups the functional norms for developmental and gestational age coincide, in others they may not. The divergence between these measures sometimes matters for clinical judgments of the current condition and prognosis of a child at risk; it always matters for scientific judgments about the nature of group norms and differences and their causes and consequences. If black infants are indeed more mature than white infants of the same gestational age on scales of neuromuscular maturation, and if girls are more mature than boys of the same gestational age in terms of the sphingomyelin/lecithin ratio, then these items bear differently on the prognosis for these comparison groups. We take the question of appropriate norms somewhat further in Chapter 14.

From the clinical perspective on preterm births, in which prognosis is all-important, it is possible but not proven that developmental age predicts survival and subsequent development with a precision as great as or greater than gestational age. From an epidemiological perspective on preterm births, in which a search for determinants of variation in gestational age at birth assumes central importance, we urge that the determinants of any endpoint need to be sought in their own right. The substitution of developmental age for gestational age can be justified only when their correspondence has been established. Indeed, in the matter of prognosis, too, although each criterion of development seems to have a similar degree of utility, the same correspondences need to be established.

12 Preterm Delivery: II. Risk Factors

Useful observations on determinants of preterm delivery that lie beyond the range of immediate precipitating events during pregnancy are hard to come by. Because of the problems of measurement, definition and categorization described in the preceding chapter, even different incidence rates of preterm delivery (North 1966; Kaminski and Papiernik 1974; Bjerre and Varendh 1975; Fedrick and Anderson 1976; Kaltreider and Johnson 1976) are difficult to compare directly. The few case-control studies of risk factors in preterm delivery that we have discovered differ in the categories used for both preterm delivery and birth weight.

One cohort study provides a starting point (Fedrick and Anderson 1976). The study population comprises 17,000 singletons born in one week in 1958 in Britain. The definition of preterm was "delivered of a liveborn or stillborn infant [after 28 completed weeks and] before 37 weeks after the LMP, which weighed less than 2500 grams and showed no maceration or major congenital defect at birth." Because of the exclusion of both preterm births of more than 2500 grams and births in the thirty-seventh week, this definition gives a frequency lower than the total of preterm births according to the most current definition. In the event—with multiple births, induced deliveries, macerated stillbirths and congenital malformations excluded—the population yielded only 283 preterm births, a low rate of 1.67 per cent.

Preterm delivery had several associations with the social and personal attributes of the mother: out-of-wedlock birth, low social class, young maternal age, maternal smoking and low prepregnant weight. A number of obstetric factors were also associated, for instance, prenatal bleeding before the third trimester, and also a previous history of prenatal bleeding and other adverse outcomes such as preterm delivery, perinatal loss or low birth weight.

These results share with all others the difficulty that many of the factors studied are associated with each other. In the absence of logically structured multivariate analysis—indeed, often in its presence—the independence of their effects cannot be established. Only three among all the factors—low social class, a history of adverse outcomes in previous pregnancies, and bleeding during pregnancy—appear consistently in several studies. For example, the raised risk of preterm delivery at young ages contradicts some other studies, which is not to say it is in error. Sometimes the risk has been higher not for younger but for older women, sometimes it has been bimodal with a tendency toward a j-shaped curve, and sometimes an association with maternal age has been present only for girls under 17 years of age or has not been present at all (see also Chapter 16). Low maternal prepregnant weight is another factor, found in this study but not consistently in others, that probably poses a valid risk (see also Chapter 15). To achieve a better grasp of the existing literature, we proceed to examine the nature of the risks one by one, proceeding from broad group factors to individual factors.

SOCIAL CLASS

This variable invokes the broadest societal environment. Such an encompassing variable poses severe design and analytic problems for the researcher. These problems have been dealt with at length elsewhere (Susser et al. 1985b; Liberatos et al. 1988); they involve problems of concept, of operation and practice, and of interpretation and inference. Nonetheless, the discovery of an association with social class can have overriding social, public health and etiological significance, and in consequence such associations are prime activators for further research to elucidate that significance.

Low social class (whether defined in terms of occupation, income or education) uniformly heightens the risks of preterm birth as well as of retarded fetal growth and perinatal loss. The ways in which social class comes to be connected with any one of these adverse outcomes have so far proved difficult to unravel. In the United States in particular, ethnicity is a major confounding factor. Black women are generally of lower social class than white women. As we discuss later, they also have both a shorter average period of gestation and an excess of preterm delivery. A social class effect that is independent of the effects of ethnic status is therefore not easily estimated.

Nevertheless, social class gradients persist in situations in which no appreciable ethnic differences have existed. In the years after World War II in Aberdeen, Scotland, a strong class gradient was found in the presence of minor if any ethnic differences (Butler and Bonham 1963). The existence of a social class gradient calls for an intensive search for those factors contained in the class complex that might explain the disparities. High on the list are all those other factors associated with preterm delivery that might mediate the relationship. The many possibilities include cigarette smoking, maternal size, physical work, psychosocial stress and nutrition, all factors we consider individually later in this chapter. We turn now to ethnicity and race.

ETHNICITY AND RACE

Duration of gestation varies among ethnic and racial groups. In the United States, black women deliver on average a few days sooner than do white women (Taback 1951; Henderson 1967; Alexander et al. 1985) and have about twice as many preterm offspring (National Center for Health Statistics 1982; Paneth 1986; Shiono et al. 1986b). In the United States, as mentioned earlier, race and ethnicity are in many respects surrogates for social class and for differences in social situation and behavior. With all ethnic differences in outcomes, therefore, separation from these social variables requires close attention.

The confounding of race and class can be illustrated in myriad ways. Throughout the United States, blacks are at a socioeconomic disadvantage. In occupation, education, and income they are less well-off than whites. Complete control of these social differences between ethnic and racial groups almost certainly has not been achieved by any study of reproductive outcome carried out so far. For example, the same number of years of education does not signify the same quality of education for different groups; the educational impact of the years spent in poor schools and in well-endowed private schools are hardly comparable. Some of these questions are now under investigation (Hogue et al. 1987).

The disadvantage of blacks and of the poorest classes in the incidence of preterm delivery may be greater than suspected from data collected without special care. In these groups, histories of menstrual dates are more often uncertain than in better-off groups. These uncertain histories, in turn, are more often followed by preterm deliveries than are histories giving certain dates (Binkin et al. 1985; Geronimus 1986). The exclusion of histories that cannot be classified is bound to produce an apparent incidence of preterm deliveries that is lower than the true incidence.

The fullest analyses so far used a cohort of more than 28,000 predominantly middle-class women in a California prepaid health plan (Shiono et al. 1986b). Odds ratios were adjusted for many potential confounders (maternal age, education, marital status, employment, parity, previous miscarriage and induced abortions, smoking and drinking during pregnancy, time of entering prenatal care, and infant sex).

With whites as the reference group, the respective relative risks of preterm (<37 completed weeks) and very early delivery (<33 completed weeks), respectively, were 1.79 and 2.35 for blacks; 1.40 and 1.31 for Hispanics (mainly Mexican-American); and 1.40 and 1.10 for Asians.

The risk ratios were little altered by the exclusion of cases with such known antecedents or accompaniments of preterm delivery as antepartum bleeding and premature rupture of the membranes. The covariation between the rates of preterm delivery and the position of each ethnic group in the social hierarchy of the United States is striking. This pattern suggests that with adjustments for more refined social measures, preterm delivery differences between blacks and whites are likely to be diminished.

To conclude our discussion of the ethnic and social class gradients for preterm delivery, there is no doubt that in the United States, with its marked ethnic mix, such gradients are prevalent. Britain and France have less ethnic admixture, but the ethnic differences are in the same direction and the class differences are sharp. Refined study and analysis to discover their source has been insufficiently applied to these differences.

CIGARETTE SMOKING

Smoking is a factor that could contribute to the social class gradient for preterm delivery. The smoking habit, so intimately personal in a physiological and psychological sense, also has intimate ties in a social sense, as mentioned in Chapter 8. As it has changed forms, customs, and mores over the centuries, tobacco smoking has come to pervade every segment of society at one time or another. But this history of distribution has always been socially governed. At different times, different social classes, and within classes different genders, have been most habituated. In recent times, women and children have adopted the habit as men dropped it, and most recently, lower-class women have adopted it as upper-class women have begun to drop it. Finally, it is becoming a scourge of the less developed world including, at the last, its children and its women.

In the 1958 British national cohort study, cigarette smoking has a relative risk for preterm delivery of about 2 (Fedrick and Anderson 1976). In several other studies, smoking has no more than a modest effect on mean gestational length, and sometimes no effect. These studies all exemplify the multiple variable problem. As described in the preceding paragraph, the smoking habit has strong social class and cultural connotations and varies greatly between generations and therefore with age. It also relates to low maternal weight, low birth weight and fetal loss, and miscarriage (Chapter 8). Moreover, the smoking mother is at risk of antepartum hemorrhage and abruptio placenta, both of which pose a major risk of preterm labor and infant death (Meyer 1977). Unless all of these confounding or intervening factors are dealt with by research design and analysis, the exact effects of smoking must remain obscure.

The association of preterm delivery with smoking during pregnancy has, in fact, been estimated with several potential confounding variables controlled. The large prospective study of nearly 30,000 women who used a prepaid health facility in northern California (Shiono et al. 1986c) took into account the use of alcohol, contraceptives, and medications as well as prior reproductive events. For preterm delivery overall (<37 completed weeks), the adjusted odds ratio for smoking was 1.2, a small effect but in that large series statistically significant. For very early preterm delivery (<33 completed weeks), however, the adjusted odds ratio for heavy smoking (≥1 pack per day) was 1.6. The attributable risk of 7 per cent for very early preterm delivery is not negligible in a population sense.

This study also points to some of the intermediate mechanisms that may be involved with smoking. Although smoking was associated with idiopathic preterm delivery (without known precipitating factors), the association was considerably stronger in the presence of antepartum hemorrhage (abruptio placenta and placenta previa) or of premature rupture of the membranes. It is a plausible inference that bleeding and membrane rupture served as the intervening variables between smoking and preterm delivery. The analysis presented does not allow one to deduce what proportion of preterm deliveries might be accounted for by precipitating or accompanying factors of this kind.

OCCUPATION

Occupations may entail physical, mental, and emotional strain; they also entail earnings, social position, and an overriding relationship to the means of production in a society. In this sense, occupation is often a determinant of individual social class, although the converse may also hold. Effective analysis of occupation as a factor therefore needs to be highly specific and well controlled for confounding, a point illustrated in a recent review of work in pregnancy in relation to a range of perinatal outcomes (Saurel-Cubizolles and Kaminski 1986). In addition, physical strain can be considered as a factor in its own right in preterm delivery. For instance, very strenuous physical effort (e.g., long distance running), has been described as a risk factor for shortened gestation (Clapp and Dickstein 1984). Most such evidence remains on an anecdotal level. Work-related effort has received more attention (see also Chapter 8).

Women's work outside the home has been compared with full-time housework as a cause of preterm delivery, and of other adverse outcomes of pregnancy. Good evidence for either situation is lacking, in part because valid comparisons are so difficult to make. In contemporary Western societies, working women can be expected to manifest the "healthy worker effect": a selective bias, self-imposed or otherwise, excludes from employment persons at high risk of adverse outcomes. The sick, the disabled and the handicapped, and those who abuse alcohol or illicit drugs, are less likely to be found among the employed.

Social and self-selection for work goes beyond such specific characteristics. In the developed world, in most social classes, pregnant women who are employed are better educated, better off (precisely because they work), and in better health. On the other side, the full-time housewife, especially in the poorer classes, may be far from at leisure. With strained resources, housework itself and child care can be strenuous, while at the same time the woman may be at hazard from the unknown effects of indoor pollutants from gas ranges, cleaning material, and other sources.

In some societies of the less developed world, selection for employment in an opposite direction may result in an "unhealthy worker effect." A likely example occurs in a study in Addis Ababa of the effects of heavy work during pregnancy (Tafari et al. 1980). The "slave" class of servants did the heavy work and had the adverse outcomes. The mistress class did no such work and had the more favorable outcomes. Whether heavy work or other related unfavorable conditions accounted for the adverse outcome remains an open question.

In studies of risks for reproduction from women's work, therefore, the question of the precise and independent nature of the exposure must be finely focused, as it has been only occasionally (Kaminski and Papiernik, 1974). Some comparisons might usefully be restricted to women in employment. Thus, in groups comparable in social background and demographic characteristics, the effects of occupation might be measured by comparing different kinds of work.

This strategy was used in a French study of women employed outside the home (Mamelle et al. 1984). Detailed histories were taken from women at the time of delivery. Women who delivered before 37 completed weeks of gestation had high scores for so-called occupational fatigue, and they more often worked on night shifts. Cleaners and unskilled workers had the highest occupational fatigue scores; teachers, executives and clerical workers had the lowest; and skilled workers, shopkeepers and medicosocial workers were intermediate.

These fatigue scores were a potpourri, compounded from factors for posture, machine work, physical exertion, mental stress, and physical and chemical exposures. Constructs labelled as mental stress and environmental exposure appeared to contribute most to the excess of "occupational fatigue." The relative risk of preterm birth with a high fatigue score was 2.1 (confidence limits 1.3 to 3.5); with adverse medical factors the risk was only 1.4 (confidence limits 0.9 to 2.2). Occupational fatigue was much more common than medical risk, so that the fraction of preterm births attributable to occupational fatigue was a substantial 21 per cent, compared with 8 per cent for medical risks.

The interpretation of this innovative study is not simple. The occupations that generated high scores are also differentiated by social class. Indeed, from what was said in introducing this subject,occupation may be a consequence of class while at the same time it forms part of the objective conditions that create a social class gradient for preterm births.

On the technical side, the occupation scores compound heterogeneous elements, hindering clear-cut inference of the aspects of the job that might be deemed causal. In addition, confounding by such factors as the workers' perception of the nature and effects of the work, and even the use of tobacco and alcohol, cannot be ruled out. In particular, in a case-control study of any event stressful in itself such as preterm birth, the potential for biased exaggeration of relationships on recall cannot be ignored when histories of exposure are taken after the event.

The investigators later applied the same scales for fatigue to a different series of cases and controls (Mamelle and Munoz, 1987). They obtained only partial confirmation of their earlier findings: machine work and mental stress were again more often reported by cases, but on this occasion not posture nor physical exertion. The score for high fatigue, however, did replicate. The replication strengthens the initial findings although it does not erase the difficulties of interpretation.

Consistency is not sustained overall: in a Washington State population (Meyer and Daling 1985) physical activity did not relate to preterm births; in a very large population in Montreal (McDonald et al. 1988), a fatigue index did relate to preterm births, but weakly so. Reviews of the literature (Kramer 1987a; McDonald 1988) are not decisive on the question, and strenuous physical effort remains a subject for further study. Little research has specified effects of activity at particular phases of gestation. As things are, recommendations and regulations for the workplace must resort to commonsense judgments (American College of Obstetrics and Gynecology 1977).

PSYCHOSOCIAL STRESS

In the case-control study of occupation and preterm delivery mentioned earlier, the mental stress factor had a prominent place in the occupational fatigue score. Although the items labeled under mental stress assume a somewhat arbitrary character, the result reinforces the beliefs of many obstetricians. Mental stress could well have an intermediary role in the relationship of social class or occupation to preterm delivery. Poverty and lower social class situations notoriously engender mental stress (Langner and Michael 1963; Susser 1968; Dohrenwend and Dohrenwend 1969).

In what follows we narrow our concern, by definition, to those forms of mental stress commonly referred to as psychosocial. The adjective implies that the stress has an environmental origin in a person's situation, especially the social and psychological situation. Psychosocial stress in pregnancy has been the principal focus of several studies. Unfortunately, many have lacked a rigorous design and some have also lacked well-tested measures of either the stressors to which women were exposed or the emotional states the stressors supposedly induced. It is perhaps not surprising that the wide range of outcomes examined exhibit a notable lack of consistency in their associations with stressors.

Despite such indeterminate results, the hypothesis that psychosocial factors adversely affect pregnancy cannot be rejected. Aside from human studies, a body of experimental work on rodents and on primates suggests plausible biological pathways. Catecholamines are secreted in response to stress. When administered to the pregnant mouse, they produce uterine vasoconstriction and hyperactivity, which in turn produce fetal asphyxia. Primates stressed during shipment are very likely to abort (Morishima et al. 1978). One early study carried out in Aberdeen, Scotland, related clinical outcome to routine antenatal evaluations of personality and anxiety (Scott and Thomson 1956). The incidence of difficult labor (defined by length of labor, uterine dysfunction, and resort to surgical intervention) was low in women judged well adjusted and with few neurotic tendencies.

An often cited study (Nuckolls et al. 1972) tested the hypothesis that the effect of stressful life events on pregnancy outcome was mediated by the social and psychological support available to the stressed woman. The outcome of interest was defined as "all complications of pregnancy." An interview instrument to assess "favorable psychosocial assets" was administered to women who registered for prenatal care at some time before the twenty-sixth week of gestation. A second instrument, to assess "life change," was mailed to participants in the thirty-second week of pregnancy. Finally, pregnancy outcome was abstracted from hospital records.

For several tests the results were generally neutral regarding associations between life changes and complications. Nonetheless, one selected positive interaction between life changes and slender psychosocial assets caught the imagination of workers in the field. Life changes did relate to adverse pregnancy outcome in women who had a weak network of social supports. In this study, the grouping together of all adverse outcomes including pregnancy complications inhibits inferences about possible mechanisms, and gives no indication of whether there might be specific effects on preterm delivery. Until recently little has been done to test this intriguing if tenuous result.

More recent studies have not greatly improved matters, although some of the issues have been better operationalized (Newton et al. 1979;

Newton and Hunt 1984; Chalmers 1984). A summary of Israeli studies illustrates three separate approaches: one used a retrospective case-control design, one was prospective, and one was ecological in type (Omer et al. 1986). In the case-control study, the cases were hospitalized women with surviving infants who had had preterm or threatened preterm deliveries, and the controls had had term deliveries. Scores obtained at delivery for stressful life changes in the weeks before did not differ for cases and controls. The retrospective coloring that an individual who has had an adverse experience is likely to give to antecedent events that might relate to the experience always poses the threat of bias. In this instance, events reported several months later may pose the larger threat in terms of the accuracy and reliability of the stress scores based on those reports; imprecision in recall may have suppressed such differences as existed. In the prospective study, women who delivered prematurely had slightly higher life event scores and higher anxiety levels during pregnancy than did those who delivered at term. The ecological study used the opportunity of a natural experiment: the pregnancies studied coincided in time with the stressful Yom Kippur war of 1973. No excess in preterm deliveries was discovered.

In three other studies, two prospective and one retrospective, more was done than previously to control confounding by multiple variable analysis. In one prospective study, a modest association was found between life stress preceding the pregnancy and gestational complications; these complications included but did not separate preterm delivery (Norbeck and Tilden 1983). A second prospective study, from Oxford, England, used state-of-the-art measures for life events, social difficulties and psychiatric state as independent variables. The shortcoming in design of this study is the size of the sample; statistical power is insufficient to detect hypothesized effects of quite meaningful size on length of gestation and birth weight (Stein et al. 1987). In a case-control study in the United States, white women with preterm deliveries, but not black women, reported stressful life events during pregnancy and negative attitudes to the pregnancy more often than did controls with term deliveries (Berkowitz and Kasl 1983). One conditional result, for women who had positive attitudes to the pregnancy, was consistent among both whites and blacks and has the ring of plausibility: in this subgroup of women, those who delivered preterm reported more stressful life events than those who delivered at full term.

The results of observational studies taken together are so far indeterminate (reviewed by Istvan 1986). Effects of stressful experiences in pregnancy on the risks of preterm delivery (and of low birth weight as well) have been neither strong nor common. Nor have the few experimental studies reported thus far been any more convincing (Oakley et al. 1986). The problems that have beset studies in this area are not all avoidable, but there is still room for stronger studies to address the questions at issue. For example, the suggestion that a woman exposed to life stress who endures pregnancy in poor circumstances is more liable to have an adverse outcome requires further testing. Any such test might do well to give special attention to women at a social disadvantage who have scant material and psychosocial assets.

The results reported from France (Mamelle et al. 1984) suggest that studies of stress in pregnancy should take account of mental stress arising from work and the occupational environment. In line with this, some French investigators are strong advocates for the importance of such factors in the outcome of pregnancy (Blondel et al. 1987). The legislated rights of pregnant women to long leaves from work are postulated as a main factor in the reduction in the rate of preterm delivery in that country during recent decades (Saurel-Cubizolles and Kaminski 1986; Papiernik, personal communication).

Studies of the relationships with psychosocial stress fare better with prospective than with case-control designs, because of the difficulty of overcoming biased recall among cases. Prospective studies might also have to contend with bias in reporting life events. At the stage of pregnancy when a woman is called on for a history of life events, she could unknowingly already have awareness of a process that will eventuate in adverse outcome, an awareness that could contaminate her account of them.

NUTRITION

A good number of studies of nutrition in pregnancy, both observational and experimental, take birth weight as the outcome (Susser 1981; Rush 1982). By contrast, few take preterm delivery as the outcome. This is perhaps to be expected, since the nutritional hypotheses that spring to mind most readily concern the primordial connections of food and growth. Reports of the acute wartime famines of Leningrad in 1943 and Holland in 1944–45 showed that infants exposed prenatally were certainly born underweight (Sindram 1945; Antonov 1947; Smith 1947).

The Leningrad famine persisted for 3 years and reached more profound depths than the 6-month long Dutch famine. In the later stages of the siege, infants were born prematurely as well as being growth retarded. The Dutch famine, although less severe, is much more extensively documented; from these data, it is apparent that the effects of exposures limited to early and to late pregnancy differ. Premature birth and growth retardation were effects that could be differentiated in this way. At the height of the famine, exposure in the third trimester shortened gestation by an average of about 4 days. No excess of preterm deliveries (<37 completed weeks) could be detected. Presumably the 4-day shortening occurred equally over the main birth weight distribution.

Exposure in the first trimester during the same period of intense famine, however, produced no detectable shortening of mean gestational length but an excess of preterm births. The effect of starvation early in gestation in precipitating delivery was apparent in relatively few cases. Presumably this was a severe effect with a threshold confining it to one extreme of the distribution of births (Stein et al. 1975a).

Neither shortened gestation nor the excess of preterm deliveries with severe famine lends itself to extrapolation to more usual circumstances. In developed countries, the forms of undernutrition that might occur among the poor and the lower social classes are much milder. In less developed countries, although famine is a hazard, the chronic malnutrition that pervades many communities differs from famine both in the nature of the dietary deficiencies and in its lifelong character. A variety of studies, however, support indirect inferences that bear on the relation of nutrition to preterm delivery.

In an early case-control study of 1953–55 births in Edinburgh, small preterm infants as well as growth-retarded infants were more often born to women whose parents were of low social class. A nonsystematic exploration suggested that maternal nutrition as indicated by maternal size was a possible intervening factor in preterm births (Drillien 1957).

Maternal weight has obvious nutritional implications. This factor has been examined extensively in relation to birth weight and to some degree also in relation to preterm delivery. Low prepregnant weight has been found to be an antecedent of preterm delivery at several times and places—in Britain in the national birth cohort study discussed earlier (Fedrick and Anderson 1976), in France (Kaminski et al. 1973), in Canada (Meyer et al. 1976), and in the United States (Edwards et al. 1979).

Somewhat more direct evidence comes from an evaluation in the United States of the national Women, Infants and Children (WIC) program. In this program, food coupons for the purchase of food supplements had been given to women and children who attended prenatal and well-child clinics and who fell below a specified threshold of poverty. In one large-scale ecological analysis of pregnancy outcome, fewer preterm deliveries were found in those areas across the country in which greater use of the program had been made (Rush 1988). In less developed countries, support for a direct effect of nutrition on preterm delivery comes from two studies (Pebley et al. 1985; Villar et al. 1986) discussed more fully in Chapter 16.

INFECTION

Maternal infection has been indicted as a cause of preterm delivery. Some indictments are indirect and based on the implications of variation with such factors as sexual behavior and season; others are more direct. We begin with a consideration of the more general factors.

Sexual Activity

As in recent times discoveries have added to the list of organisms found to be sexually transmitted, coitus during pregnancy has come under suspicion as a factor in premature delivery. Sexual behavior is strongly shaped by culture and values; historically it has differed sharply among social classes, ethnic groups, age groups, generations and, indeed, between the sexes. Plausible hypotheses refer to infections transmitted or provoked into pathogenic activity by coitus, and investigators have sought to connect coitus with higher frequencies of chorionitis in preterm delivery that might result from such infections (Naeye 1979b).

Many of the results reported are clouded by potential confounding. For instance, declining sexual activity as normal pregnancies near full term confuses comparisons with sexual activity in pregnancies that end prematurely; the norm for sexual activity close to delivery in the preterm deliveries relates to an earlier stage of gestation. Thus, case-control and cross-sectional analyses court erroneous comparisons when the "case" is a woman with a preterm delivery and the control is a woman whose pregnancy has proceeded to term. Analysis in the prospective life-table form avoids the problem. Prospective data adequately controlled for changes in coital frequency as pregnancy progresses do not indicate a raised risk (Klebanoff et al. 1984b).

Seasonality

Seasonality in outcome has been taken as a general pointer to the role of infections that flourish more in one season than another. In practice, seasonality is a variable with broad implications for the discovery of a range of etiological factors in health disorders in the population. Sometimes it has been a pointer to the effects of heat or cold on disease, sometimes to social and cultural habits and behavior connected with season. In reproduction the most prominent seasonal effects have related to fertility and, especially in the straitened circumstances of very poor societies, to nutrition and the energy expended by women in the hard work of cultivating the fields. The ultimate objective is to narrow by elimination the range of potential factors that lead to the seasonal distribution of a disorder.

Seasonal effects for preterm delivery have been examined on several occasions. In one study (Cooperstock and Wolfe 1986) singleton low-birth-weight (<2500 grams) deliveries born at 27 through 35 weeks were compared with term deliveries of normal weight (≥2500 grams). Gestational age could be estimated from the date of the last menstrual period recorded during the prenatal period, and hence the births could be assigned to a cohort of conceptions. In addition, the effects of season on fertility and of several demographic factors were taken into consideration. The findings indicated a dearth of preterm deliveries in the spring and an excess in the autumn. This result, reasonably consistent with previous reports, is compatible with the behavior of acute respiratory infections, influenza viruses, and the like (Katz 1953; Hewitt 1961; Brezowsky and Dietel 1967; Keller and Nugent 1983).

Specific Infections

Infections that might cause preterm delivery can be grouped into two broad classes: systemic infections, usually acute, and local infections in the genitourinary tract and the chorion (reviewed in Peckham and Marshall 1983).

With regard to systemic infections, in the less developed world the best available evidence relates mainly to protozoan infections, particularly malaria. We leave discussion of this infection to Chapter 16; here we note only that several observations suggest a link between epidemic malaria and miscarriage or "prematurity," defined in the main by low birth weight (Covell 1950). Extrapolation of such findings to preterm delivery is defensible from studies of fever in miscarriage. Fevers are characteristic of malaria, and reasonably good evidence argues for fever as a cause of miscarriages, early and late (Kline et al. 1985).

In the developed world, the evidence on systemic infection and preterm delivery relates mainly to viral infections. The influenza epidemic of 1918 contributed necessarily to maternal mortality as well as general mortality (Harris 1919); apparently, it also brought on preterm deliveries (Bland 1919). Hepatitis and measles are two other epidemic infections related to preterm birth. In New York City, large-scale studies of notifiable diseases found raised frequencies of "prematurity" (≤ 2500g) with these infections. With rubella infections, no connection with preterm births was found. Low birth weight was connected with exposure in the first trimester, a fact coherent with the known effects of the disease and supportive of the overall validity of these studies (Siegel and Greenberg 1960; Sever et al. 1965).

Maternal infections of the urinary and genital tracts have been reported to shorten gestation by several investigators, but not without contention. Urinary tract infections can be classified by severity as asymptomatic (or covert) bacteruria, acute cystitis, and acute pyelonephritis. Asymptomatic infection has been shown to be widely distributed among fecundable and fertile women. In the United States it has been especially common among young black, sexually active women (Kunin et al. 1964); these women are also those at a greater risk of preterm deliveries and low birth weight. Urinary infection is treatable; if causal, it thus presents as an attractive target for the prevention of low birth weight, for instance, by screening all pregnant women for bacteruria.

In the 1960s, bacteruria was found in a number of studies in association with low birth weight and perinatal morbidity and mortality. In a randomized trial, treatment with tetracycline apparently reversed these ill effects (Kass 1960; Elder et al. 1971). Subsequent studies have produced conflicting results both about the relation of urinary infection to birth weight, and about the preventive treatment of urinary infection to avert low birth weight. Points of definition for both outcome and exposure remain at issue. With regard to outcome, among studies that report associations with birth weight the differentiation between shortened gestation and retarded growth is not clear. With regard to exposure, distinctions between the effects of acute episodes of pyelonephritis and cystitis and of mild or asymptomatic episodes of bacteruria are not clear. We concur with the report of a conference of the National Institutes of Health in 1983, from which we quote: "Despite numerous studies, it is currently not possible to state unequivocally whether these infections affect fetal growth or the time of initiation of labor or both" (MacDonald et al. 1983). Equivocal results raise questions about routine screening in pregnancy for bacteruria as a preventive measure. We should also note that, even if bacteruria were shown to cause adverse outcomes, the specificity and sensitivity of a single test and the predictive value of the procedure do not argue for its efficiency.

Vaginitis and cervicitis are, like bacteruria, putative causes of preterm delivery and low birth weight about which there is uncertainty and controversy. The suspect microbial pathogens include chlamydia, trichomonas, mycoplasma and group B streptococcus. Firmly to establish causal effects of these organisms on the outcome of pregnancy has proved no less difficult than with urinary infections; a substantial, indeterminate literature has accumulated for each organism (cited in MacDonald et al. 1983). Thus, the National Institutes of Health Conference on infections of the urinary and genital tracts mentioned previously could be no more conclusive about genital than about urinary infections. Some answers can be anticipated from an ongoing prospective multicenter study of the outcome of genital infection and its treatment in pregnancy sponsored by the National Institute of Child Health and Development.

ADVERSE REPRODUCTIVE HISTORY

In epidemiological studies it has seldom been possible to specify histories of low birth weight in terms of their origin in preterm delivery or growth retardation. For this reason, the association necessarily reported most often is with previous low birth weight. The association of preterm labor with previous adverse reproductive experience, cited previously from the national British study (Fedrick and Anderson 1976), nonetheless finds support in several subsequent studies. In particular, a sufficiency of Norwegian national data indicate that prior preterm delivery is a significant factor in pregnancies that end prematurely (Bakketeig 1977). The more prior preterm infants that are born to a woman, the greater her risk in a current pregnancy (Bakketeig et al. 1979). The reported association of preterm delivery with histories of perinatal loss can be taken to be part of the same complex.

The individual risk carried by women who experience repeated preterm deliveries may have a familial element, as we consider further in Chapter 15. Thus, sisters but not sisters-in-law have been found to have similar risks of preterm labor (Johnstone and Inglis 1974). For the present, the genetic or environmental factors that might underlie this familiality are unknown. Whatever they may be, familiality does not rule out the possibility of some persisting environmental factor as the cause of recurrences of preterm delivery. Indeed, even the possibility that a first preterm delivery itself sets the conditions and raises the risk for a subsequent one cannot be ruled out.

COMPLICATIONS OF PREGNANCY AND MATERNAL MORBIDITY

The factors in preterm delivery most easily studied are those that emerge as health disorders of the pregnancy or of the pregnant woman. In any respectable obstetric service, such data are systematically recorded and readily accessible, and they provide the bulk of the available observations on preterm delivery.

Many complications of pregnancy can precipitate preterm delivery. The uterus itself is a factor in complications. Thus, a known antecedent factor in maldevelopment of the uterus is prenatal exposure to diethylstilbestrol (see Part I), and these malformations are accompanied by high rates of preterm delivery and low birth weight (Barnes et al. 1980; Herbst et al. 1980).

Placental problems—abruptio placenta, placenta previa, and premature rupture of the membranes—often set off a chain of events in which the risk of prematurity and perinatal death or subsequent developmental impairment tends to be high.

Preeclamptic toxemia or, in its early manifestation, *pregnancy hypertension,* appears most often as a rise in blood pressure late in the second or in the third trimester. In parallel with rising blood pressure, the growth of the fetus tends to be slowed and the pregnancy to terminate prematurely. The relationship seems to be curvilinear, in the form of a j-shape: with hypotension and growth retardation, preterm delivery is also somewhat more frequent (Friedman and Neff 1977). Since the risk of perinatal death generally rises with both growth retardation and preterm delivery, affected offspring seem to be in double jeopardy.

Induction of labor before term has been orthodox obstetric practice for such maternal conditions as severe toxemia of pregnancy, congestive heart failure, and diabetes. In some past series of preterm deliveries, as many as 20 per cent were deliberately induced. Inadvertent induction before term was also common until, with the advent of ultrasonography and biochemical tests of the amniotic fluid, more precise estimates of fetal maturity could be made. In the search for causes of preterm delivery, induction is of little interest. For studies of the consequences of preterm delivery for the infant, however, premature induction offers a fertile field for epidemiological study.

In vitro fertilization, it seems from one report, may raise the risk of preterm deliveries (Australian In Vitro Fertilization Collaborative Group 1985). Among 108 singletons surviving to at least 20 weeks of gestation, 7 per cent were born before the thirty-second completed week, and 15 per cent after the thirty-second and before the thirty-sixth completed week. These high frequencies cannot be evaluated without taking into account both the strong selective factors that lead to the in vitro procedure such as advanced maternal age and nulliparity, and the operative interventions that may follow during pregnancy.

Chronic maternal disorders coincidental to pregnancy are probable factors in preterm delivery. A high incidence of low birth weight has been reported in women with a variety of chronic diseases. The relative contributions of preterm labor and of growth retardation to lowered birth weight in such conditions have been little studied and are uncertain in most of such conditions. The interrelations of the two contributing factors can be complex, especially with metabolic disease. Diabetes mellitus accelerates asymmetrical fetal growth by deposition of fat without any increment in length or organ size. At the same time, the fetus is at high risk of antepartum death and of consequent premature delivery.

CONCLUSION

In concluding this chapter, we must point out that we have not attempted a thoroughly comprehensive review, since several have appeared recently (Kramer 1987b). Evidence from the experimental animal literature is neglected. Some salient epidemiological literature, too, is not dealt with, such as that on multiple births (McKeown and Record 1952; Barron and Thomson 1983; Berman et al. 1987a). Our review has nonetheless made plain the many causal factors in which resolution cannot be reached. Sometimes the uncertainties reside simply in lack of adequate definition of outcomes of pregnancy in reports of studies, or of adequate refinement of outcomes in the design of studies. In truer measure, the uncertainties are inherent in the development of the field of reproductive epidemiology. As the scope of the problems at issue becomes more focused and questions narrower, the broad strokes that served to connect crude measures of attributes and exposures with undifferentiated outcomes no longer suffice to advance the field. In the realm of the public health, we need to identify the causes of preterm delivery in their own right. We need also to identify its consequences, not only in low birth weight, but in terms of impairment or retardation specific to this form of low birth weight. In the course of such studies, we shall learn whether the role of mother or fetus is primary, and the circumstances under which the outcome can or should be prevented.

13 Fetal Growth and Birth Weight: I. Indices, Patterns and Risk Factors

Intrauterine growth rates are measured by relating the size of the infant at birth to its putative gestational age. Weight, being the most accessible and reliable dimension of the infant at birth, remains the measure of size commonly used for epidemiological purposes. Calculations of norms for intrauterine growth rates pose or conceal a number of problems.

First, a *state* of the infant at birth, characterized by size, is taken to imply a *rate* of growth over the preceding time period beginning at conception. This rate, if not within the norm, may be retarded or accelerated. The two components of the imputed rate, attained growth and time, both deserve consideration. On the one side, the several dimensions of the size component—weight, length, head size—are not always symmetrical among themselves in their relations to population norms. On the other side, the time component is affected by the problem, familiar from the preceding chapters, of measuring length of gestation: when the date of conception is uncertain, the period of time over which growth has taken place cannot be precise. We expand on these questions under the heading of "Indices of Growth."

Second, the diagnosis at birth of a state of retarded or accelerated growth, in practice, depends on a single set of observations made at an endpoint. The measure of growth rate must therefore average the amount of growth achieved over the whole of the antecedent prenatal growth period. Any irregular or nonlinear progression in intrauterine growth that may have preceded the time of observation is ignored and, in fact, the velocity of fetal weight gain varies during gestation (Figure 13-1). Such irregularities are accorded practical effect in some hypotheses; they are thought to depend on the types of factors at work, and on their timing, duration and severity. We discuss these questions under the heading of "Specific Factors in the Progress of Growth."

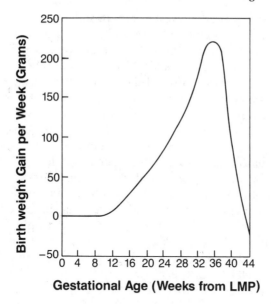

Fig. 13–1 Changing rates of growth from conception to birth. (After Brenner 1976)

INDICES OF GROWTH

A number of problems of inference beset the construction of indices of growth, especially in relation to gestational age. The first involves the assumptions made about past development. In usual practice, as noted, we do not compute a rate of growth over time in order to determine the presence of retarded growth; instead, we impute retardation to age-specific size at birth or at the time of an ultrasonograph. When we interpret a state observed at a given point of time, the imputation carries the hazards of all those inferences about past happenings and their time relations that are made from cross-sectional observations.

To the problem of retrospective assumptions about rates of growth, one must add the problem of the extent to which these cross-sectional observations could be selective and biased. Much of our knowledge depends on the compilation of consecutive cross-sectional observations of infant size beginning at the earliest gestational ages at which infants are born viable, and continuing to the latest gestational ages at which delivery occurs. At any gestational age, these observations rest on a sample selected—by the operation of many possible but usually unknown adverse factors—from a cohort in utero. It could be a misleading assumption, although it has been a necessary one, that infants delivered prematurely are representative of the total cohort of births of the same gestational age, that is, both those expelled from the uterus and those that still remain to be delivered. The advent and proper application of new imaging techniques, however, can produce longitudinal observations that clarify interpretation. Recent ultrasonographic studies of fetal growth in utero suggest that the assumption of representativeness is not unreasonable (Brenner et al. 1976). Naturally, it can be valid only if the births studied are representative of the population to which the observations are extrapolated.

Postterm deliveries, like preterm deliveries, are also affected by selection. Small size may be one of the selective factors; the smaller the fetus, perhaps, the later it will reach a size sufficient to initiate labor (Thomson et al. 1968; Stein et al. 1975a). Around term (at least in experimental animals), the size of the products of conception seems to contribute to the onset of labor (McLaren and Michie 1963). The earlier delivery of twins compared with singletons, and of triplets compared with twins, conforms with the idea that their large combined weight triggers delivery (McKeown and Record 1952) (Figure 13-2). Postmature survivors also conform. Both body weight and placentae in several data sets are, on average, smaller in postterm deliveries than in those delivered at term: at best, postterm infants are no larger than term infants.[1]

Gestational or fetal age is the index from which the duration of the growth period is inferred. We noted in previous chapters that the reputation of menstrual histories for imprecision is not really deserved: the great majority of estimates of gestational age based on carefully taken dates are adequate, and careful clinical assessment, early pregnancy tests, and ultrasonography help with the uncertain residuum.

Many reports in the literature refer only to low birth weight without specifying gestational age. In terms of consequences, birth weight enwraps a large part of the effects of growth retardation, and some authorities still prefer to focus on it almost entirely (Thomson 1983). The fudging of the distinction between growth retardation and low birth weight within a single population might have little practical import for newborn and child care. Low birth weight owed to retarded growth on the one hand, and to premature delivery on the other, pose risks for perinatal mortality that may not differ enough to matter.

In terms of definition, process and understanding, this analytic imprecision about birth weight does matter. For studies of etiology and their application to prevention, the factors that retard growth need to be distinguished from those that precipitate delivery and cut short the prenatal growth process. In populations exposed to markedly different circumstances, different kinds of intervention may be called for.

In developing countries, for example, growth retardation accounts for a distinctly larger proportion of low birth weight infants than in developed countries (a point discussed in a later chapter). The same is true for

---

[1]Misclassification of term infants as postterm, which one analysis finds to be extreme (Kramer et al. 1988; see Chapter 11), affords another possible explanation for the size distribution of postterm births.

the desperately poor or disadvantaged compared with those better off. For clinical purposes, too, the distinction has uses. Differences in morbidity typify the two forms of low birth weight. Preterm infants are especially liable to such special ills as respiratory distress syndrome and cerebral palsy. Growth-retarded infants seem more liable than preterm infants of the same weight to be retarded in subsequent development and to remain small, especially if the growth retardation represents a congenital or acquired intrauterine pathology.

Departures from symmetry in growth along several size dimensions are also held, in hypotheses proposed by different investigators, to be particular to certain antenatal precursors and also to have particular consequences (Miller and Hassanein 1971; Walther and Ramaekers 1982). It is self-evident that the recognition of asymmetry requires the use of more than one dimension, and indices suitable for this purpose must be brought to bear. Asymmetry among several dimensions of size—especially weight, length and head circumference—is taken to indicate disproportionate growth. Different tissues are affected in a sequence governed by the severity of the growth retardation. Large-scale pathological studies first suggested that less severe degrees of retarded growth involved soft tissue depletion, more severe degrees involved skeletal growth, and only the most severe degrees involved the head and brain (Gruenwald 1966a,b). This sequence was also found in studies of the 1958 British birth cohort (Gruenwald 1963) and the Dutch Famine data (Stein et al. 1975a).

SPECIFIC FACTORS IN THE PROGRESS OF GROWTH

Growth and symmetry are affected not only by the severity of the factors involved, but also by their timing and duration and their intrinsic nature. Through the successive phases of gestation, growth can be regular or irregular in rate as well as in form. Rate and form may be intimately related. With malformations, asymmetry may indicate some intrinsic or acquired impairment in the embryo; conversely, asymmetrical growth may underlie the shape and dimensions of the maldevelopment.

With regard to timing, we referred earlier to the limitations of observations made at a single point in time: a diagnosis of a growth pattern made at birth precludes direct knowledge of irregularities in growth in successive phases of gestation. This is not to rule out indirect knowledge obtained from deductions about development. In the first section of the book, we emphasized that in teratogenesis the timing of changes in the pace of growth may be crucial in determining outcome. For this reason the form a maldevelopment takes can be a marker of the timing of the growth disturbance and hence of the exposure.

Epidemiologists have for long explored discontinuities in growth rate and their contribution to birth weight. For example, the intrauterine growth of twins or triplets apparently starts off similarly to that of singletons. Growth rate decelerates in multiple pregnancies, as we noted before; in the case of triplets their weight curves begin to diverge from those for singletons from the thirty-second week, and in the case of twins from the thirty-sixth week. Postnatally, the individual offspring tend to catch up with singletons. Hence the discontinuity in growth is generally attributed to the physical constraint the uterus places on more rapid growth.

The intrauterine environment influences the birth weight and growth patterns of singletons, too, as do genetic and environmental factors in general. Sex is one expression of the genetic contribution to fetal growth pattern. Boys and girls grow at similar rates until the twenty-eighth week, after which the rate of growth in boys is relatively faster (see Figure 11-1). Boys preserve their faster growth rate for some time postnatally.

We have emphasized the elementary logic that a factor, in order to induce malformation, must act either before or concurrently with the stage in embryogenesis at which the affected organ develops. If a factor is to induce symmetrical growth retardation, one might deduce that it would act throughout pregnancy and possibly before. If a factor is to induce asymmetrical growth retardation (in the absence of malformations), one might deduce that it would act in the latter half of pregnancy, when the greater part of prenatal growth takes place. Since growth is involved, it is to be expected that most salient evidence comes from studies of nutrition and nutrient supply. The controlled conditions of animal experiments help to bring order into human observations relating to these factors.

Nutrient Deficiencies

The exact nature of the factors that lead to growth retardation—for instance, whether nutrients are depleted by local vascular supply (Gruenwald 1966a) or by deficient maternal intake—has been thought to influence symmetry (Rosso and Winick 1974). The difference in antecedent factors has not in itself been shown to be material. Regarding uterine blood flow, experiments in rats suggest that maternal blood volume may be a crucial variable in fetal growth: this is a topic at present under active investigation (Rosso, personal communication). Most experimental evidence is in line with the idea that restricted blood supply reduces body weight and length but spares head and brain in an asymmetrical growth pattern (Cheek 1968). The additional hypothesis that, in the presence of unrestricted blood flow, a depleted supply of nutrients from the mother symmetrically retards the growth of the whole organism, including the brain (Wigglesworth 1964), on the other hand, lacks experimental support. In experiments with ewes, exquisite control was achieved over the nutrient supply to fetuses removed from the uterus by supplementing input (by intragastric intubation, for example) while sustaining vascular connections between fetuses and ewe (Charlton 1984). As with the restriction of blood supply, the bodies of the lambs deprived of nutrients were small, but the heads were spared in comparison.

In human studies, the timing, duration and severity of a factor can be difficult to separate; situations seldom allow each element to vary separately. With nutritional deficiencies, the circumstances of the Dutch famine did permit opportune studies of the effects on births of timing and severity. With nutritional deprivation confined to the first half of pregnancy, even starvation was insufficient to produce growth retardation (Smith 1947; Bergner and Susser 1970; Stein et al. 1975a). Starvation confined to the third trimester did depress fetal growth, and produced the typical asymmetrical pattern; that is, birth weight was predominantly affected, length less so, and head size the least. Nutritional deprivation during the famine, when quantified, produced graded effects. The lesser degrees of growth retardation were also asymmetrical, and were again confined to third-trimester insults. In other circumstances in late pregnancy, a deficient vascular supply of nutrients might be involved. Thus, in a study of poor black women in New York City, the placental infarcts that occur in the latter part of pregnancy have been found to be associated with asymmetrical growth retardation (Nuchpakdee 1978).

These results do not rule out the possibility that symmetrical stunting could be produced by appropriate timing and duration of a deficiency of limiting nutrients. Timing and duration were crucial in the experiments with pigs conducted by Thomas McCance and Elsie Widdowson (1974). They demonstrated symmetry in the marked and irreversible stunting caused by nutritional deprivation beginning early and sustained throughout gestation. They demonstrated asymmetry in the less severe and reversible stunting caused by deprivation begun at a later stage and then reversed.

In the less developed world, chronic nutritional deprivation is likely to be sustained throughout pregnancy. The predominant form of growth retardation seems to be symmetrical (in Chapter 16 we take up the question again). In the developed world, severe nutritional deprivation sustained throughout pregnancy seldom occurs. The moderate forms of nutritional deprivation that do occur in association with growth retardation have not been shown to cause more than a small reduction in growth, most notably in birth weight (Susser 1981). Thus, the predominant forms of growth retardation are asymmetrical (Gruenwald 1966a,b; Naeye 1981a) and become apparent in the third trimester, as represented schematically in Figure 13-2.

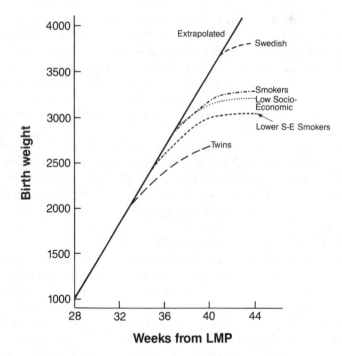

Fig. 13–2 Fetal growth (determined from birth weight) in births from several populations and subgroups: schematic representation of divergence at different stages of gestation from extrapolated linear growth curve. (After Gruenwald 1966)

Smoking

In the developed world, maternal cigarette smoking is the most consistent and widespread, and one of the most potent, of known environmental determinants of fetal growth retardation (Simpson 1957; Butler et al. 1972; Abel 1980). The typical effect on birth weight ranges from 150g to 250g. The vulnerable period is in the latter part of pregnancy; the offspring of women who quit smoking before mid-trimester seem to be unaffected (Butler et al. 1972; Hebel et al. 1988). In the light of the notion that symmetrical growth retardation is the result of factors acting early in pregnancy (Campbell 1976; Villar and Belizan 1982b), the supposedly symmetrical effect on growth retardation (Hardy and Mellitz 1972; Davies et al. 1976) of a factor that seems to act in the latter half of pregnancy is unanticipated and calls for more study.

The placenta, which is large relative to the fetus, is an exception to the symmetry. The relatively large placenta has been attributed to physiological compensation by the mother for hypoxia induced by smoking. Anoxia in the latter part of pregnancy may not be a sufficient explanation for the effects of smoking on fetal growth, however. In a number of studies (Rush 1974; Davies et al. 1976), but not in others (Anderson et al. 1984), diet has seemed to interact with smoking to affect birth weight. In the New York experiment with prenatal diet supplementation, the off-spring of heavy smokers seemed to be protected by diet supplementation from the weight decrement seen in unsupplemented smokers. In that study, at least part of the effect of smoking seemed to be mediated through maternal weight gain (Rush 1974). Since smoking and under-nutrition during pregnancy, taken separately, do not produce identical results, there is room for complementary biological action. Cigarette smoking releases many chemicals, produces high carbon monoxide levels, constricts vascular flow, and damages the placenta, any or all of which could reduce nutrient supplies to the fetus and exaggerate a primary depletion of food supplies. This hypothesis, and several other aspects of the effects of smoking, are in need of further exploration.

Alcohol Abuse

A consensus now allows that heavy prenatal exposure to alcohol can produce the effects described as the fetal alcohol syndrome. The pathognomonic triad of the syndrome encompasses two somatic effects—growth retardation and dysmorphic facies—together with mental dullness. Quantitative and qualitative aspects of the relationship need further clarification. Frequencies and risks are not well established. Such cooperating factors as cigarette smoking have generally not been ruled out, and the probable role of individual susceptibility remains to be demonstrated. The timing and duration of the exposure necessary to produce the fetal alcohol syndrome is also not yet clear.

A case can be made that the somatic effects of growth and form reflect two independent manifestations of alcohol abuse: disturbed organogenesis early, and slowed fetal growth later. Alternatively, by analogy with the severe prenatal nutritional deficiency in pigs reported by McCance and Widdowson (1974), both effects could be expressions of the same growth disturbance, with the form governed by the stage of gestation. Against a disorder of organogenesis is the weak and inconsistent evidence that maternal alcohol abuse is associated with any malformations or anatomical disorders besides the fetal alcohol syndrome facies (Mills et al. 1988). Against a unitary underlying disorder of growth must be set the inconsistency across studies with which delayed fetal growth attends heavy alcohol use (reviewed in Stein and Kline 1983; Ernhart et al. 1985). This inconsistency, however, might be the result of variations in the timing, the dose, the type of beverage, and the characteristics of the women. Separately or together such factors might mediate the effects of maternal alcohol use on fetal growth rate.

Altitude as a Risk Factor

Very high altitude has a relative risk for low birth weight not exceeded so far by any other well-measured specific factor. Since it is a general

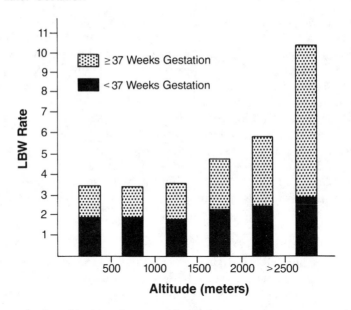

Fig. 13–3 Altitude and birth weight: rates of low birth weight (LBW < 2500 g) and preterm deliveries (<37 weeks gestation) at different altitudes among births selected for low risk of growth retardation. (After Yip 1987)

ecological attribute of the physical environment, there is no escaping its effect for women who dwell at high altitude.

Early studies that pointed to altitude effects—in the mountains of Colorado, the Andes, and elsewhere—were vulnerable in varying degree to confounding (Macfarlane 1987). Several potential confounding factors were removed from account in a study of birth certificates for 13 million infants born in the United States from 1978 to 1981 (Yip 1987). The study population was large enough to confine analysis to homogeneous strata. The analysis dealt only with births to white women of ages and socioeconomic groups that were optimal for reproduction in terms of ethnicity, education, and marital status. At the high altitudes of 2500 to 3100 meters, mean birth weight was reduced by 10 per cent compared to altitudes under 500 meters; the risk of low birth weight (with 2500 grams as the lower common threshold for normal birth weight) rose to threefold. As altitude increased, the effect on birth weight grew stronger, exceeding a simple linear relationship to produce a marked reduction in the highest mountain regions (Figure 13-3).

The effects on birth weight can be safely attributed to fetal growth retardation. The length of gestation was affected but little, and the rise in the frequency of low birth weight with altitude was notable among term infants born at 37 completed weeks of gestation or later. Other data from Colorado (Unger et al. 1988) show that the slowing of fetal growth apparently begins after the thirtieth week. In this respect, the effect is similar to that with maternal smoking. The reduction in the fetal/placental ratio also resembles the effects found with maternal smoking; placental weight is not reduced to the same degree as birth weight (Kruger and Arias-Stella 1970). In theory, the timing of these effects on growth should produce asymmetry in fetal growth, but we are aware of no data with which to test the theory.

CONCLUSION

In this chapter, we have considered variation in growth associated with maternal nutrition, parental cigarette smoking, the use of alcohol, and residence at high altitude. [In later chapters we discuss the sex of the offspring, parity, ethnicity (Chapter 14), familial factors (Chapter 15), possible effects of the age of the mother (Chapter 17), and maternities in less developed countries (Chapter 16)].

To summarize the effects of specific factors on the progress of growth, our review shows that the patterns of intrauterine growth have several determinants. Uterine capacity is the main limiting factor for multiple births; growth is constrained as their total fetal size exceeds that of singletons in the later phases of pregnancy. Inherent growth potential different for the fetuses of each sex is a main factor in differentiating the patterns of boys and girls, which also diverge in the later phases of pregnancy. With acute food deprivation, maternal smoking, and residence at high altitudes, simple nutrient deficiencies and anoxia alone may be enough to damp down the trajectory of growth from about the thirtieth week of gestation.

These patterns correspond to the model of intrauterine growth retardation shown in Figure 13-2; for all, we would expect birth weight to be the dimension most affected, and length and head circumference less so. With smoking and altitude, however, the patterns of placental growth are distinct, the probable expression of anoxia: growth is not depressed to the same degree in the placenta as in the fetus, and the fetal/placental ratio is reduced compared with the norm. With chronic malnutrition the growth pattern seems to differ from that in acute malnutrition; slowing of growth appears to occur more often in mid-trimester and to affect all the dimensions of growth symmetrically. With maternal alcohol abuse, a small infant is typical of the fetal alcohol syndrome; besides this feature, evidence about particular growth patterns is not strong, and for the present we may judge it indeterminate.

Although many research papers have dealt with other possible influences on intrauterine growth, few factors are sufficiently studied to be useful in terms of interventions and prevention. A comprehensive survey of the literature (Kramer 1987a,b) concludes that the only influences on fetal growth retardation deemed "causal, important and modifiable" are, before conception, young maternal age and low prepregnant weight and, after conception, caloric intake, weight gain during pregnancy, and cigarette smoking. We would add altitude and, for the less developed world especially, malaria. There are grounds also to consider aspects of diet that may not act through maternal weight (Rush et al. 1980).

Nevertheless, even in developed countries, little-understood connections with social inequalities persist and some may prove modifiable in the long term. For fetal growth retardation as for preterm delivery, these include all the aspects of social class reviewed in the previous chapter—strenuous physical work and occupational fatigue, psychosocial stress, and availability and use of medical care.

14 Fetal Growth and Birth Weight: II. Norms and Thresholds

Fetal growth rates are stated not in absolute but in relative terms, as deviations from some accepted norm. What that norm should be for groups with weight distributions that differ from the optimum or the mean in given populations, however, is not self-evident. A section on establishing norms is devoted to these issues. Even when a norm is agreed on, we may ask how much deviation constitutes abnormality of a degree that calls for efforts to prevent or treat. In the section on the threshold for growth retardation we consider this problem. Each of these seemingly simple issues has aspects that prove to be complex and substantive. We deal with each in turn, although not equally.

ESTABLISHING NORMS

We turn now to consider reference norms for fetal growth. A central question asks what an appropriate standard might be against which to measure departures from normality in population subgroups or risk groups that differ from the mean or optimum for the population at large.

"Norm" and its derivative "normal" have several meanings. In a *statistical* sense, the norm delimits the modal area of variation on a measure; the limits of this mode are derived from the distribution of the measure in a population—particularly the average values and the standard deviation, which is the dispersal of individual values around the average. In a *clinical* sense, the norm distinguishes all that is unimpaired, functioning and well from all that is impaired, malfunctioning, and ill. The *social* sense, in which different norms denote behavior that is actual, expected, or ideal, does not concern us here.

In the first part of the discussion, we keep to the statistical sense. The question is focused on the selection of an appropriate population or subpopulation on which to base the average intrauterine growth rates and the measures of their dispersion. This is a theoretical question that has considerable practical implications.

A clinical diagnosis of fetal growth retardation is given heuristic meaning by relating it to prognosis. Outcomes relevant to the diagnosis include fetal and newborn mortality, newborn morbidity, and neurodevelopmental impairment, disability and handicap. To illustrate, perinatal mortality provides a criterion of outcome that is convenient, significant and widely reported on. In general, poorer prognosis for survival in the perinatal period follows slower growth; the lower the weight attained for any gestational age, the greater is the probability of death.

Since fetal growth has significance for outcome, to establish a norm for fetal growth is, in addition, to influence what the reference standard for that outcome should be. Further, to establish a norm for subpopulations that differ from the general is to accept a higher or lower reference standard for fetal growth in that population. In allowing a different standard we discourage comparisons based on the standard for the general population, we promote expectations of outcome in relation to that standard for the subpopulation, and hence we run the risk of condoning inappropriate expectations for the subpopulation.

The appropriate choice of norms for fetal growth, it is evident, is not a straightforward matter. For the purpose of choosing a norm special to a population or population subgroup for prenatal growth rate—that is, for birth weight specific to gestational age— we propose a single criterion: the distribution of birth weight for gestational age should differ immutably from that of the comparison population.

The argument that a distribution is immutable is an inductive one and difficult to sustain; strong grounds are called for to support the idea of immutability. The argument for an unmodifiable distribution would be supported, for example, if it were robust to the challenge of multiple and widely divergent environmental conditions. It would also be supported by a relationship of outcome to prenatal growth rate unique to a subpopulation: one might seek for unanticipated ways special to the subpopulation in which outcomes like perinatal vitality and mortality or developmental maturity relate to gestational-age-specific birth weight.

It should be at once apparent that the question of modifiability differs according to the stage in the life cycle and the stage in a given reproductive episode. Before any conception as well as after, there is no modifying the genetic and environmental conditions that shaped a parental generation. Once pregnancy has supervened, there is no modifying the conditions antecedent to the pregnancy that shape the development of the fetus. In this regard, the obstetrician and the midwife in clinical practice and the epidemiologist concerned with intervention in populations stand in different relationships and face different problems.

In obstetric practice, a logical approach to selecting growth norms is to accept the condition of the woman at the point she enters care as a given. The purpose of all diagnosis, and of the screening functions of prenatal care, is primarily predictive: the train of consequences invoked by the diagnosis on the screen points the way to appropriate activity. It may be appropriate not to act at all, or merely to ensure that no harm is done, or to reassure. Nonetheless, the preferred mode of activity is to prevent, and the next is to cure. It is worth noting that the presence of unmodifiable antecedents that retard growth does not preclude action that is effective in alleviating the consequences of such unavoidable growth retardation. Unmodifiable antecedent maternal attributes set limits, indicate risks, and prescribe targets against which to evaluate the effectiveness of intervention for the obstetrician. For the woman already pregnant, unlike such modifiable factors in growth retardation as diet and smoking, these antecedent attributes entail only watchfulness.

In the short term, then, in the immediacy of prenatal care, action to prevent growth retardation can be directed only to *postconceptional* risk factors. The optimum achievable norms for intrauterine growth on a service, therefore, may with reason refer to births within the service. Among relevant postconceptional factors in growth retardation some, such as smoking, hypertension, preeclampsia, are known and modifiable; in some populations and with some forms of dietary supplementation, it has also proved possible to some degree to modify low prepregnant weight and low maternal weight gain. By this logic, women who experience such known and preventable adverse factors are best excluded from the population that constitutes the statistical base for the norm.

In the long term and for research and public health purposes, we want to generate norms from a wider perspective than a service for women already pregnant can provide. Such norms should take account of *preconceptional* risk factors, not all of which need be regarded as forever fixed, either for individual women or for groups. Contrasts between the growth rates of males and females, on the one hand, and between the offspring of primigravidae and multigravidae, on the other, illustrate some of the issues.

Sex

From about the 28th week of gestation onwards, we noted earlier, the male fetus is heavier than the female for given gestational age at birth (see Figure 11-1). Yet the sexes are often combined in a single gestational-age-specific birth weight distribution. In such a distribution, any birth weight threshold for growth must assign more girls than boys to the category of growth retardation.

Across the sexes, however, girls in comparison with boys flout the rule that perinatal mortality is greater where gestational-age-specific birth weight is lower. At term, girls are lighter than boys by an average (in New York City) of 150 grams. Yet girls have a considerable advantage over boys in perinatal survival. This advantage holds at all gestational ages. Some but not all of the female advantage can be attributed to the fact that, given the same birth weight, the average girl must be older and more mature than the average boy. When the age advantage is allowed for by adjusting for the sex difference in birth weight, the chances of survival remain better for girls than boys. There are no grounds for suspecting differences in the environmental conditions of gestation for the two sexes. It follows that girls possess an advantage over boys in intrinsic viability. This advantage might inhere, in part at least, in one or other of the developmental characteristics that differ between the sexes, for instance, those indicated by fetal lung maturity.

An intrinsic difference in the birth-weight-specific prognosis of the sexes can be taken as added support for the view that the divergence in the birth weight distributions of the two sexes is immutable. The sense of an intrinsic sex difference is reinforced by the fact that the growth of female infants does not catch up to that of males in several postnatal months (Cawley et al. 1954). Thus, there are good grounds for believing that the differences between the sexes—in gestational-age-specific birth weight, in gestational-age- and birth-weight-specific perinatal mortality, and in postnatal growth—are intrinsic to the genome of the fetus. Logically, this justifies separate norms for each sex.

Parity

Mean birth weight for primiparous births is consistently lower than for multiparous births. If primigravidae and multigravidae were combined in a single distribution, a bigger proportion of the offspring of primiparae than of multiparae would be defined as growth retarded. In the instance of parity, however, we argue that grounds for the immutability of birth weight distributions with parity are not sufficient to support the use of different norms. Certainly, the conditions of primiparity and multiparity are, like sex, unmodifiable in themselves. Yet a sense of mutability pertains to two collateral facts. The first is that systematic differences in the mean birth weight of women of different parity are largely mediated by the mutable variable of maternal weight (Love and Kinch 1965; Weiss and Jackson 1969; Rush et al. 1972). It is reasonable to believe, therefore, until proved otherwise, that to modify the distribution of maternal weight by parity will modify the distribution of birth weight by parity. The second and consonant fact is that in firstborn infants, unlike female infants, postnatal growth accelerates to overcome within a few months their size disadvantage compared with those born later (Cawley et al. 1954).

For possible support of the fundamental criterion of a unique distribution, we again look to perinatal mortality. In this regard parity, in contrast with sex, falls in line with the general rule: the difference in prognosis between the offspring of primiparae and multiparae is accounted for by birth weight. That is, no factor inherent in multiparity acts in its favor over and above birth weight. Whatever the parity, therefore, birth weight predicts mortality across parities with equal exactitude. That a given birth weight carries the same prognosis for mortality irrespective of parity in this instance offers no indication of uniqueness in the distributions of birth weight by parity. Further, we know of no other features unique to birth weight distributions by parity, although we are not aware of any concentrated effort to test the question.

These observations lead, by our criterion, to grouping birth weight distributions regardless of parity. This decision does not exclude interest in birth-weight-specific mortality rates for comparison with other parity groups, but it guards against the suppression of modifiable differences between groups by the use of different norms. In other words, it is fair to suppose that the mortality risk with parity is a function of the variation of birth weight and is modifiable. A modifiable risk offers a prospect of prevention, and not a yardstick against which to view departures from normality.

Race and Ethnicity

From these two straightforward examples for deriving norms, we proceed to the more complex. Into the 1960s in New York City, infants designated as white and black differed in their patterns of birth weight relative to gestational age. Mean birth weights among blacks were greater than those among whites up to about 30 weeks of gestation; in the remainder of pregnancy they were lower. For that great majority of births that occurs around term, therefore, black infants were on average smaller than white infants. It follows that at any given birth weight toward term, black infants tended to be of greater gestational age than white infants. This advantage in age may be reflected in an apparent advantage in the maturity of their behavior at given birth weights (see Chapter 11). With regard to perinatal survival, however, any advantage derived from the greater gestational age and the apparent maturity of black infants was confined to lower birth weights.

Despite this mortality advantage at the lower birth weight ranges, blacks have had overall perinatal mortality rates nearly double those of whites during the 1960s and since in New York City. Their disadvantage could be entirely explained (in a statistical sense) by the fact that the proportion of infants of lower birth weight was larger for blacks than for whites, so that larger numbers of black than white infants were at higher risk of perinatal death (Bergner and Susser 1970). In the light of the adverse perinatal mortality rates that ensue from the low birth weights of black infants at gestational ages above 30 weeks, their third-trimester fetal growth rates can properly be regarded as suboptimal.

It has been argued, to the contrary, that birth weight distributions—by sex, race, ethnicity and so on—are intrinsic and hence unmodifiable. This argument rests on the fact that the birth weight optimal in terms of mortality maintains a fairly constant position in relation to the mean; in all groups studied, the optimum weight is always greater than the mean weight. In population groups of different mean birth weight, the curves of their birth weight distributions can be made to coincide simply by shifting the position of the mean so that they fall at the same point (Wilcox and Russell 1983b,c). This coincidence leads readily to the notion of birth weight distributions intrinsic to each group.

We do not find these arguments from statistical modeling in themselves persuasive of the existence of intrinsic differences (which may of course exist). Thus, recent data from New York City challenge the assumption because they suggest that the patterns of ethnic differences for birth weight may be changing. In 1984, birth weights of black infants born before 34 weeks were no longer higher than those for white infants (see Figure 11-1), as they had been in earlier decades. This point is not yet conclusive; for example, the ethnic mix included under the rubrics for black and white may no longer be the same. Also, related changes in perinatal mortality are still to be analyzed.

The notion of intrinsic differences between blacks and whites has been taken to support the additional idea of a fixed threshold value that divides normal from low birth weight. If such a threshold exists, it argues against the use of standardization in comparing the effects of birth weight between groups. Standardization then obscures intrinsic population differences that govern mortality and development.

Nonetheless, we cannot allow that standardization for birth weight is any less justified in the comparison of perinatal mortality between groups than it is, say, for age in the comparison of postnatal mortality between groups. In New York City in the period 1958–61, perinatal mortality for blacks, standardized for gestational age, was lowest in the birth weight range 3000 to 4000 grams; for whites it was lowest in the range 3501 to 4000 grams (Susser et al. 1972). The upward shift in the birth weight for black infants seen in data of the 1980s may well have reduced the earlier differences. These results suggest that, although the optimal mode could be somewhat lower for blacks, the optimal range of birth weights for black and white infants might be quite similar (see Figure 11.2).

Regardless of the appropriate statistical model for birth weight, the disadvantageous black perinatal mortality rates found throughout the United States are not wholly intrinsic. By ordinary procedures of analysis, the main black disadvantage is in infants of normal birth weight and above. The effect of applying the model of a fixed threshold for low birth weight is to shift the disadvantage and the focus of attention from normal to low birth weight infants.

In either case, the existence of a real disadvantage is made plain by various observations. For one thing, comparative rates changed over time (Kessel et al. 1984). For example, in 1939–40 in New York City, in contrast to the data of 20 years later cited previously, neonatal mortality for low-birth-weight infants was equal in blacks and whites (Baumgartner et al. 1950). Some factor other than an intrinsic race difference must have been operating. For another thing, at any one time and within the black population, differences between social classes are in the direction expected from social position.

Ethnic disparities in birth-weight-specific mortality are quite likely to be a consequence of social disparities in the quality of medical care. Several kinds of evidence point in this direction: in 1939–40 in New York City, birth-weight-specific perinatal mortality was higher for blacks than for whites in the city taken as a whole, but not in teaching hospitals taken separately. Indeed, in a special service for low-birth-weight infants, survival for black infants was consistently superior (Baumgartner et al. 1950). At the Johns Hopkins Hospital from 1896 to 1936, likewise, under equal conditions of medical care mortality in low-birth-weight infants was lower for blacks than for whites (Peckham 1938a,b).

We take the position, for all of these reasons, that stronger evidence is needed to justify different norms for blacks and whites. What must be demonstrated are differences in the prenatal growth rates of blacks and whites that are intrinsic and independent of mutable personal and social attributes. If stronger grounds for such differences exist, and they are found to signify unique prognostic differences in themselves, the case for separate norms would be that much more cogent. In the absence of such evidence, a common norm is more constructive and, we think, more informative.

Altitude and Norms

Altitude is not, of course, an intrinsic factor but an immutable ambience. For that subgroup of women tied to a place of residence, it is unavoidable. On the grounds of inescapable effects on prenatal growth, population subgroups defined by the high altitudes at which they dwell qualify in terms of our logic for separate norms. It follows that the outcomes of pregnancies with respect of size, mortality, development, and the effectiveness of care deserve to be judged against standards that pertain to the special experience of women who live at high altitudes (see Chapter 13).

In Colorado in past decades, the risks of perinatal mortality were raised concomitantly with the growth retardation they experienced, as might be anticipated from the strong relationship of mortality to birth weight overall. These findings, it seems, focused attention on this adverse outcome to good effect. Concurrently with the advent of modern methods of newborn intensive care and their regionalization in the state in the mid-1970s, a dramatic decline occurred in infant mortality. The change was most marked at higher altitudes and among low-birthweight infants. Among full-term infants of normal weight (≥ 2500 grams) and preterm infants, the decline was much less marked; hence, we may infer that full-term growth-retarded infants obtained the main benefit. Remarkably, these recent data show that Colorado has improved on the infant mortality rates of the United States as a whole (Unger et al.1988). The full drama of these changes over time, it will be apparent, emerges only from analyses within the state of Colorado.

Our justification for a separate norm for high altitude rests on the unavoidable effects of an ambient environment. In the Andes, an additional justification could be advanced if, as some suggest, evolutionary adaptation has taken place among the Indian peoples who have long dwelt at very high altitudes (Haas et al. 1980; Beall 1981). Studies suggest that their infants, unlike those of peoples who more recently came to live there, are not of low birth weight; surprisingly, they further suggest that birth-weight-specific mortality is generally better at high than at low altitudes.

If these findings hold, they would provide a rationale for a different norm because of the intrinsic character of the population. Under the difficult circumstances of these investigations, however, we can be even less certain of the absence of confounding by social factors than in the analyses discussed earlier of supposed intrinsic racial differences in the United States.

Appropriate Norms

Here we summarize our arguments on the setting of separate norms for fetal growth. The question of appropriate norms arises with every group variation in mean birth weight; for the offspring of women of different social classes; for those of women who are underweight at conception; for those whose mothers are of different ages, or who were themselves born of low birth weight; for multiple births, and so on. Whether we should discriminate between groups in choosing norms is, we suggest, in most instances best governed by modifiability and the prospects for prevention. In the light of the foregoing, to set up a separate statistical growth norm for a subgroup is to accept that the factors involved are intrinsic or otherwise immutable. A different norm should be eschewed when it is believed that intervention might achieve modification, even when success in doing so is not yet apparent.

The application of this principle differs with the population at risk, especially in terms of the advent of pregnancy. Before conception, the prevention of growth retardation can be an overall objective: a common norm indicates which groups are most in need of attention. After conception, it is reasonable to accept separate norms for preconception factors that produce different birth weight distributions. Prevention of growth retardation can be the objective for the range of factors operating within the prenatal stage, for example, by the cessation of smoking; here, no separate norm is called for. A second objective can be to prevent adverse outcomes in groups already at risk of growth retardation, for example, through use of intensive care; here, separate norms could aid in the evaluation of intervention programs.

On these principles, we would seek separate norms for singleton and plural births as well as for each sex. We accept a separate norm as appropriate because it is practical; the overall disadvantage of plural births in birth weight seems to be beyond the reach of modification. Plural births carry a very high mortality risk overall because of the low average birth weight of the individual offspring. A higher mortality risk for individual twins does not obtain within given birth weight and gestational age groups: with birth weight controlled, members of twin pairs have an advantage in perinatal survival over singletons, just as girls do over boys. Unlike births of different sex, with plural births relative maturity might entirely explain their better birth-weight-specific survival rates. In any event, there is no prospect of overcoming the overall disadvantage of retarded growth in plural births. We argued earlier that we can accept a separate norm for altitude also, because there is every reason to think that the concomitant growth retardation is not modifiable. On the other hand, we would not seek separate norms by maternal age, including very young ages, or for social disadvantage.

With ethnic and racial diversity of all kinds, an intrinsic origin for variations in birth weight distributions and in birth-weight-specific mortalities, though by no means ruled out, is not proven. Until proved otherwise, an appropriate norm for a subgroup of the population should reflect the optimal growth rates in the general population expressed in gestational-age-specific birth weight distributions. In some instances, as with the unique and tenacious differences between the sexes, one may insist on a sex-specific fetal growth factor of genetic origin. For many other subgroups, the argument that observed distributions are optimal for them is a step into teleology.

Generally, within populations and across populations, bigger babies do better up to the optimum weight at term. To reach a firm conclusion about the optimum for each population or subgroup, the distribution for each needs to be studied individually. In some cases, attributes of the mother may constrain the intrauterine growth of the child. Among plural births, such constraint seems apparent from their preterm delivery, from the small size of the individual infants compared with singletons, and from their rapid postnatal catch-up growth (McKeown and Record

1954; Cawley et al. 1954). Maternal size, in terms of height, weight, or both, and including weight gain during pregnancy, is another such attribute. As we discussed before, parity can be seen in the same light.

Clearly some of these maternal conditions can be seen as preventable. Childhood diet combined with exposure to infection limits the growth of millions of future mothers across the world. Increased maternal size, we suspect, might account for one of the first documented instances of substantial increase in birth weight in a population over time, which was reported from Japan (Gruenwald et al. 1967).[1]

Finally, using the criterion of the immutability of growth rates, we conclude that we have good reason to designate three circumstances—sex, plurality and altitude—in which special norms for fetal growth might usefully be based on a subpopulation. Where mutability is not foreclosed, to set up separate norms for a subgroup could do the group a disservice; attention might be turned away from the optimum growth rates of the population at large and from the possibility of attaining them. Even some of the preexisting conditions that set limits to the possibilities of promoting fetal growth might yet prove to be modifiable.

THE THRESHOLD FOR GROWTH RETARDATION

To avert fetal growth retardation is an objective, not in its own right, but because of demonstrable effects on survival and development. This requirement leads us directly into the problem of how to establish criteria for designating the state described as growth retardation. Having chosen an appropriate norm, we must ask what degree or form of deviation from that norm should be described as growth retardation, and what action should follow. The lesser issues revolve around the form for a quantitative statement: should the cutoff point be stated in absolute terms of birth weight for gestational age, or in percentiles or standard deviation units determined from population or subpopulation distributions (Villar et al. 1986). These issues need not detain us except insofar as they bear on the greater issues that revolve around the purposes of making the diagnosis.

In trying to decide about purposes, we come at once upon two distinct perspectives, one for the hospital and one for the population at large. In dealing with growth retardation, hospitals typically select infants for intensive and highly specialized care because low birth weight puts them at high risk of fatality and subsequent handicap. Intensive care, though

[1]This example, we should note, was based on a hospital study that could be confounded by changes in hospital usage over time, in terms of social class or other factors that influence birth weight. In the United States, changes in birth weight over time have been demonstrated at national and state level (Chase 1972, 1977; Kessel et al. 1984), but they are of nothing like the same order of magnitude.

costly, does not involve large numbers. An absolute value of birth weight is usually chosen as a cutoff point. In developed countries, a value below 2000 grams encompasses 1 per cent or fewer of all births. The intensive medical care devoted to these high-risk infants has a palpable effect on their chances of survival, although we do not yet know what the effect of such care is on subsequent neurological impairment.

For the population at large, by contrast, we have a more diffuse but more ambitious goal, which is to reduce the overall rates of perinatal loss and impaired development. Despite the very high relative risk for perinatal death in the lowest birth weight categories, in the community as a whole by far the greatest number of deaths—and the greatest attributable risk—occurs among the much larger population of infants of normal birth weight. Moreover, the birth weight that is optimal for perinatal mortality is well above the mean; any level below the optimum entails a raised risk of perinatal mortality. The importance of considering the total birth weight distribution was well illustrated in the mortality experience of black infants and of plural births in New York City. We noted the advantage of both black and plural births in birth-weight-specific mortality at low birth weights. This advantage hardly begins to offset, in either group, the disadvantage of a high frequency of low birth weight among them.

From the community perspective, then, what matters most in fetal growth retardation is not where the cutoff point is drawn, but the distribution of suboptimal growth rates throughout all gestational ages and up to the optimal birth weight. Optimal birth weight for mortality is likely to be in the region of 3500 to 3900 grams, and optimal gestation around 39 to 41 weeks. The exponential decrease of perinatal mortality with birth weight up to the optimum (Susser et al. 1972) indicates that any gain in birth weight in the range up to the optimum is worthwhile. Analysis of New York City birth data in the late 1970s suggests that for every 100-gram decrease in birth weight the risk of a newborn death in the first 28 days of life increases by 40 per cent; likewise, the risk of a stillbirth increases by 25 per cent (Kiely, personal communication).

Prospect for Intervention

It follows that one can hope to make an impact on perinatal mortality rates at a population level through any measure that raises mean birth weight. Widespread health education, attention to the diet of growing children and pregnant women, and serious antismoking measures might all reduce perinatal mortality. If 40 per cent of pregnant women smoke cigarettes, a 25 per cent increase in the overall frequency of low birth weight (<2500 grams) can be expected. This birth weight loss, one may assume until shown otherwise, will have the same significance for mortality as birth weight has in general. Cigarette smokers carry an excess perinatal mortality risk of about 30 per cent. By eliminating cigarette smoking in the estimated one-third of pregnant women in New York City who currently smoke during pregnancy, we could hope to reduce overall perinatal mortality by about 10 per cent. In the developed world, because of the present-day distribution of the smoking habit, the chief beneficiaries would be the socially disadvantaged. Should it be confirmed that smoking and social disadvantage interact to produce adverse effects greater than their sum, the effect of eliminating smoking might be still greater. In the less developed world, the cigarette smoking plague is being energetically promoted by the tobacco industry and is beginning to impinge on women on a larger scale.

Despite the problems of measurement and definition to which we have drawn attention, intrauterine growth retardation should not be dismissed as an imprecise, ambiguous, or unimportant descriptor. At the same time, the use of birth weight simplifies matters from a pragmatic if not from a theoretical and research standpoint. Birth weight serves community health purposes well. In individual infants, low birth weight and especially very low birth weight is the best available predictor of perinatal problems. In populations, birth weight is the strongest possible indicator of perinatal mortality risks; it accounts for 90 per cent or more of the variance in perinatal mortality.

15 The Family Factor in Birth Weight

Among the progeny of a single family, the resemblance in size at birth (as indicated by birth weight) is greater than in unrelated individuals. This familial resemblance is not the expression of any simple mode of genetic inheritance. Here we probe the extent to which the causal factors might be genetic or environmental, and whether the resemblance resides in fetal growth or in length of gestation. For this purpose, we consider familial resemblances for different kinds and degrees of kin to the extent that data are available. Comparisons can be intragenerational or intergenerational, and the point of departure can be the relatedness of parents or offspring. Within a single generation, resemblances can be compared among progeny who might be full sibs, or monozygous or dizygous twins; resemblances can also be compared among the progeny of a single mother and more than one father, or the converse, who are either maternal or paternal half-sibs. Between generations, resemblances can be compared among parents and their offspring, likewise on the maternal and paternal sides. Some pedigrees are capable of enormous expansion, but epidemiological or population data seldom go beyond the first-degree relatives of the nuclear family, although a few encompass cousins.

PARTITIONING THE SOURCES OF VARIATION

Birth weight has been analyzed by partitioning variance among a number of factors (see Table 15-1). Following the Mendelian model, the "fetal genotype" is presumed to encompass the whole of the paternal contribution together with an equal maternal contribution. Additional maternal contributions are assumed to arise during gestation, when the conceptus is largely insulated from the father. These contributions have been divided into permanent and temporary elements.

Table 15–1 Estimates of the components of variance in birth weight

Source of Variance	Morton (1955)	Penrose (1954a,b)	Rao et al. (1974)	Robson (1978)
Genotype of fetus	−0.09	0.16	0.08	0.10
"Permanent" maternal factors	0.28	0.20 ⎫	0.49	0.24
"Transient" maternal factors	0.37	0.32 ⎭		0.20
Random environment	0.44	0.32	0.43	0.46

Source: Modified from Morton, 1977.

Permanent maternal factors include both the genetic make-up of the mother as childbearer and her own nurture, nutrition, and general developmental experience. Among these, the stature attained by the mother in adulthood has a prominent place. One indication of the consistency of a major maternal role and a minor paternal role in birth weight turns on the relationship of paternal height to birth weight. Birth weight correlates with the height of both parents. The height of parents is correlated, however, because of assortative mating. The underlying similarity in the correlations of birth weight with the height of each parent depends on the association of birth weight with maternal height. When maternal height is held constant, the corelation of birth weight with paternal height is much diminished while, when paternal height is held constant, the correlation of birth weight with maternal height persists unaffected (Cawley et al. 1954).

Temporary maternal factors are not fixed by genes or prior experience and can be changeable from one pregnancy to the next. Examples are maternal age and parity, length of gestation, and smoking and drinking behavior. In this light, it need not be surprising that correlations for birth weight are higher among adjacent sibs than among sib pairs in general (Table 15-2). Some of these temporary maternal factors, if not permanent, are persistent. One might assign social environment and occupational status to this class, as well as the enduring physical environment of a place of residence and persisting habits of diet and smoking. Another group of temporary maternal factors changes in orderly progression, as do birth order and maternal age. Other temporary maternal factors are, like many obstetric complications, transient and sporadic.

An index of permanent maternal factors has been derived from the variance common to sibs when at least three births have intervened between them (Morton 1977). All estimates of variance in birth weight from this model agree in assigning the proportions in descending rank order to random environment, temporary maternal factors, permanent maternal factors, and the fetal genotype, which combines the paternal and maternal inheritance.

INTRAGENERATIONAL SIMILARITIES

Sibs

Human studies of birth weight that yield data on sib pairs are summarized in Table 15-2. A first set of studies deals with the resemblance in birth weight between pairs of full sibs. Intraclass correlations for full sibs

Table 15–2 Correlations of birth weight between full sib and half sib pairs

Description of sample (N pairs)	Correlations (r)	Source
Full sibs		
Edinburgh, live births		
parity 0 and 1 (454)	0.53	Donald 1939
parity 0 and 2 (135)	0.44	
parity 1 and 2 (191)	0.62	
London, *survivors*		
parity 0 and 1 (891)	0.41	Karn and Penrose 1951
parity 0 and 2 (228)	0.44	
parity 1 and 2 (314)	0.47	
London, *survivors* (adjusted for sex and parity) (386)	0.50	Robson 1955
Japan, *survivors*		
adjacent sibs (367)	0.52	Morton 1955
1 sib apart (654)	0.42	
2 sibs apart (153)	0.36	
adjacent sibs with 1st cousin parents (442)	0.48	
Birmingham, live births (5042) all sibs	0.50	Record and McKeown 1969
Aberdeen, *survivors* (4229)		
unadjusted	0.47	
adjusted (for parity, sex, gestation)	0.53	Billewicz, 1972
adjusted (nullipara excluded)	0.56	
adjusted (for parity, sex)	0.49	
adjusted (nullipara excluded)	0.52	
unadjusted (nullipara excluded)	0.51	
Australia, *survivors* (adjusted for sex, parity, gestation, maternal height)		
198 siblings in 41 families	0.56	Tanner, Lejarraga, and Turner 1972
London, *survivors* (adjusted for sex, parity, gestation, maternal height) 49 siblings in 15 families	0.53	Tanner, Lejarraga, and Turner 1972
Half sibs		
Japan, *survivors*, adjacent sibs		Morton (1955)
maternal (30)	0.58	
paternal (168)	0.10	

Source: Adapted and expanded from Robson 1978.

range from $r = 0.36$ to 0.62, with the median around $r = 0.50$. Correlations are higher if other known sources of variation in birth weight are taken into account. For instance, sibs necessarily differ in birth order, and may also differ in such antecedents of birth weight as sex, prepregnant weight of mother, and mean length of gestation. For like-sex dizygous twins, when all these extraneous factors are automatically controlled, the correlation rose to $r = 0.59$ compared with $r = 0.41$ to 0.47 in sib pairs in the same series of births (Penrose 1954a,b).

The contribution of the mother predominates in these sib resemblances. Mendelian or multiple gene models of the inheritance of a trait, except for those linked to the X chromosome, assume an equal contribution from both parents. In this central aspect, the correlations for birth weight do not fit conventional models. At first sight, fathers make a minor contribution, if any, to the resemblances in birth weight among their offspring. The predominance of the mother is seen in the contrast between correlations, on the one hand, for half-sibs with the same mother ($r = 0.58$), and on the other hand, for half-sibs with the same father, $r = (0.10)$ (Morton 1955). Studies of the offspring of identical twins (maternal cousins de jure, who are de facto genetic half-sibs) also provide good grounds for attributing to the mother a large part of the effect of birth weight common to maternal sibs. These studies show strong correlations for birth weight on the maternal side only (Nance et al. 1983).

Cousins

Another approach to familiality in birth weight is to seek similarities between cousins. Here too the paternal contribution appears to be minor. For example, in one study birth weight among the offspring of sisters correlated $r = 0.135$, and among the offspring of brothers $r = 0.015$ (Robson 1955). The inference that the transmission is genetic should not be hasty. *Permanent maternal factors* have been taken to represent the maternal genotype (Robson 1978). Yet sisters may resemble each other in reproductive performance not only because they share genes, but because they share prenatal and postnatal experiences.

The permanent maternal environment imposes similar intrauterine advantages and constraints on sisters, regardless of what the origin and source of the maternal physique or metabolism might be, and these could be transmitted again through the intrauterine environments of their offspring, who are compared as cousins. Postnatal environment, too, might similarly affect the growth and ultimate size of sisters and, through that pathway, also affect the weight of their offspring in similar ways.

Resemblances among maternal cousins in birth weight are not accounted for solely by maternal size. Among maternal cousins in general, the resemblance in birth weight holds up even when the height of the sisters who gave birth to them is controlled. This persisting resemblance does not rule out other possible effects of the "permanent" grandmaternal environment on the phenotypes of their daughters as childbearers.

Equally the resemblance could stem from grandparental genes expressed in those phenotypes. Such genes on the maternal side can be transmitted from grandfathers as much as from grandmothers. In postnatal life, the dominant maternal influence on growth seen during the intrauterine period diminishes as offspring grow older. Hence the contributions of the mother and the father to the size of their offspring are expressed differently at different ages. In individuals followed from birth, birth weight has been found to correlate with adult height, with r = 0.1 to 0.2 (Langhoff-Roos et al. 1987). Although at birth a paternal influence on infant size is hardly detectable, the height of offspring after adolescence reflects a maternal and paternal genetic contribution in equal part.

INTERGENERATIONAL STUDIES

The question of the role of fetal genes in birth weight is a complicated one that needs to be reconsidered. An obstacle to assessing that role has been a lack of necessary data; the birth weights of parents have only rarely been available for analysis in relation to their progeny. A number of data sets have lately been assembled that permit the study of similarities in birth weight between mothers and their children. In four series—two in the United States (Hackman et al. 1983; Klebanoff et al. 1984a), one in Hungary (Toth et al. 1983), and one in the Netherlands (Lumey 1988)—mothers themselves small at birth tended to have small babies. In the American studies, in the births to daughters, birth weight was adjusted for maternal stature and gestational length. The correlations between weights of births to mothers and their daughters, although modest, held firm.

Some recent studies in Norway, the United States, and Sweden have made use of paternal as well as maternal birth weight (Magnus 1984a,b; Magnus et al. 1984; Magnus et al. 1985; Sing 1987; Langhoff-Roos et al. 1987). The results of these studies, unlike those that preceded them, point to some role for the fetal genome: the birth weight of fathers as well as mothers related to the birth weight of their infants.

In the Swedish study, parental birth weights were obtained by recall. Although the validity of such reports may seem questionable, checks against the birth records of a subsample showed good agreement between reported and recorded weights (r = 0.91). Maternal weight and height, smoking and infant sex were taken into account in multiple regression analysis. After adjustment, for every 100 grams increase in maternal and paternal birth weight, infant birth weight increased 19 grams and 16 grams, respectively. From these results, the genetic contribution transmitted by the parents through fetal genes was inferred to be small (5.6 per cent) but significant and roughly equal.

At the same time, the role in birth weight of maternal phenotype, over and above the genotype, was also confirmed. As anticipated from previous studies, the birth weight of offspring was significantly correlated with maternal prepregnant weight. Although before adjustment birth weight of offspring had a correlation with maternal birth weight double that with paternal birth weight, the correlation with maternal prepregnant weight accounted statistically for virtually the whole of this difference. Two propositions synthesize these results: first, the adult size of the mother (determined in part by environment, in part by her genotype) influences the birth weight of her infant; second, the mother's own birth weight and that of the father each have separate and similar but smaller influence on an infant's birth weight.

Other evidence also indicates that maternal size can be assigned more importance in birth weight than fetal genotype. In the human species, more than in most, the reserve capacity of the uterus seems to be limited, and maternal size can be taken as an index of potential constraint on fetal growth. Multiple births are the most obvious example of such an effect. The fall-off in the third trimester of individual weights attained as more fetuses crowd the uterus will be recalled from a previous chapter (see Figure 13-2); only after birth can the growth potential of the infant be adequately expressed (McKeown et al. 1976). (In passing, we note that the effect of plurality on birth weight makes twin studies a vulnerable means for resolving sources of variance in the birth weight of singletons).

In summary, maternal phenotype has a predominant role in familial resemblances in birth weight. Maternal genotype contributes indirectly to infant birth weight through this pathway. Parental genotype contributes directly to birth weight through a second pathway, and here maternal and paternal genotypes have a minor but similar role.

RESEMBLANCES IN RATE AND DURATION OF PRENATAL GROWTH

We turn next to consider whether familial resemblances in birth weight are a function of the rate of fetal growth (retarded, normal or accelerated) or its duration (abbreviated or normal length of gestation). From studies of birth weight in offspring of the same generation, it seems that similarities between sibs depend on the rate more than on the duration of fetal growth (Ounsted and Ounsted 1968; Johnston and Inglis 1974). This is not to deny any effect at all of family resemblances on length of gestation. Correlations between sibs range from $r = 0.16$ to $r = 0.22$, less than half the size of those for birth weight with length of gestation held constant (Karn et al. 1951; Billewicz 1972).

The intergenerational studies that link birth weight in mothers and daughters do not similarly report links for length of gestation. This could be for lack of data in some, for lack of the necessary analysis, or by default in reporting when no link was found. We may infer from the reported results, however, that they do exclude an association between the preterm birth of a woman as proband and the preterm birth of her offspring. Mothers themselves born small produced no excess of very low birth weight infants in intergenerational studies in three countries (in the United States: Hackman et al. 1983; Klebanoff et al. 1984; in Britain: Tanner et al. 1972; Ounstead 1968; in Hungary: Toth et al. 1983). Since nearly all very-low-birth-weight infants are born preterm, the maternal genotype can be ruled out as a factor in preterm births—if not in gestation of normal duration.

Other species also provide relevant results. One should keep in mind, however, that the constraint of uterine size is shared with humans by only a few other species. From studies of cattle, it has been suggested that influences on length of gestation include the fetal genotype, along with the sex of the fetus, the maternal phenotype, and the permanent maternal environment (Morton 1977). With cross-bred Angus and Aberdeen cattle, for instance, length of gestation was midway between the mean length for the species of the bull and heifer. In this formulation, the role of the genitor or bull in birth weight depends on the influence of the fetal genotype on length of gestation and duration of fetal growth.

In the famous hybrid equine crosses between Shires and Shetlands (Walton and Hammond 1938), maternal size had dramatic effects on birth weight but trivial effects on length of gestation. Length of gestation is similar in Shetlands and Shires, however, and cross-bred species that differ are more informative. With rabbits and hares, length of gestation depends on the dam, whichever her species (Cawley et al. 1954). Animal models, it appears, have little contribution to make, by direct analogy, to human beings. We noted in Chapter 13, however, the elegant demonstration in mice that the fetal genotype can indirectly influence length of gestation (McLaren 1965). Strains that had typically slow and typically rapid fetal growth rates were cross-bred: in dams with typically slow fetal growth rates, rapid fetal growth triggered parturition early. We also noted that in human beings, a similar phenomenon may occur; as in mice, large fetal size may trigger labor (McKeown and Record 1953; Stein et al. 1975a). From such results one might infer that in humans, too, fetal genotype could have an indirect role in determining length of gestation, provided it is also one of the factors governing fetal growth rate.

The community-based maternity data assembled over many years for Aberdeen, Scotland, by the late Dugald Baird with his colleagues Angus

Thomson, William Billewicz, Raymond Illsley and others have made signal contributions to reproductive epidemiology. They are informative, too, about the intergenerational maternal transmission of both length of gestation and fetal growth rate (Johnstone and Inglis 1974). Cousins who were the offspring of sisters and of sisters-in-law were compared. In a sample in which the index cases were consecutive low-birth-weight infants (<2500 g), familial resemblances in both preterm delivery (<37 completed weeks) and retarded intrauterine growth were greater among maternal than among paternal cousins. Paternal cousins did not differ from the population at large. The results are reminiscent of those for the birth weights of the progeny of identical twins referred to previously. Familial environment must be included as a factor in the resemblance of maternal cousins. Thus, sisters resembled each other and sisters in-law resembled the general population in social matters such as smoking habits and the proportions who could not date the last menstrual period.

THE MATERNAL ENVIRONMENT

The demonstrable influence of the permanent maternal environment on fetal growth must depend on the uterine physiology and structure provided by the mother. We do not know the extent to which this environment inheres in the genotype of the mother. To the extent that it is genetic in origin, the phenotypic manifestation would have to be sex-specific and limited to females. (For example, adult height on the mother's side, and not on the father's side, would be relevant to birth weight. The height of maternal grandparents would also be relevant to the adult height of the mother, and hence to the birth weight of her infant.)

It is equally likely that the mother's own prenatal and postnatal experiences are determinants of the permanent maternal environment she creates for the growth of the fetus. Nutrition in the early life of the mother has been proposed as one such factor in the fetal growth of offspring (Baird 1977). Studies of dogs and rodents have given the hypothesis some backing. Nutritional deprivation in bitches seemed to produce developmental effects in their pups that persisted in subsequent generations (Platt and Stewart 1971). In rodents, nutritional rehabilitation in an affected generation apparently banished the adverse effects on birth weight (but not on brain or behavior) in a subsequent generation (Galler 1979).

In human beings, two quite different studies previously described—one of diethylstilbestrol and the other of the Dutch Famine 1944–45—exemplify maternal transmission of environmental effects. In both studies, environmental insults suffered in utero by female probands appeared to affect their subsequent reproductive performance. Through such two-sided intergenerational connections, effects in the offspring could be linked to events in the pregnancy of their grandmothers. With diethylstilbestrol, for example, in proband mothers exposed in utero, effects included structural anomalies of the uterus but also a raised risk of preterm delivery during their own pregnancies (Herbst et al. 1980; Barnes et al. 1980).

In the Dutch Famine, proband mothers exposed in utero showed effects on the birth weight of their own offspring (Lumey 1988). These effects have thus far been studied only for first births. The effective in utero famine exposure was confined to the first trimester. Thus, exposure of probands in utero solely in the third trimester—which had produced marked effects on their birth weight—did not affect their offspring. Exposure of probands in the first trimester—which had produced detectable effects on preterm delivery but not on birth weight— did affect their offspring: the risk of low birth weight was almost doubled.

In these two examples, the chain of transmission began with sporadic factors that transiently perturbed the proband-to-be during gestation. These perturbations, in turn, seemed to perturb the maternal environment the exposed probands provided for their own progeny during gestation. But from a different perspective, separate effects of sporadic and persistent maternal environmental factors can also be discerned. The presence of intragenerational similarities in both birth weight and, to a lesser extent, length of gestation (Weiss and Jackson 1969: Ounsted 1974; Fedrick and Adelstein 1978; Bakketeig 1977) suggests that fetal growth retardation will recur in a woman's reproductive history.

Such recurrences were clearly present in national Norwegian data in which repeated births to individual women could be linked (Bakketeig and Hoffman 1981; Bakketeig et al. 1986). In sibships of three or more, births small for gestational age and preterm births both tended to recur among women at a social disadvantage in terms of their own education, marital status, and social status or of their husbands' occupations. By contrast, such births tended to occur only sporadically among women at no evident social disadvantage. In one respect, the distribution of growth retardation differed from that of preterm births. Sporadic episodes of growth retardation (but not recurrent ones) tended to follow sporadic obstetric mishaps, for instance, placenta previa or pre-eclampsia.[1] Preterm births were generally less likely to recur in the same woman, but the repetitive episodes of preterm births that did occur were

[1] These patterns, we suspect, go some way toward explaining previous findings from this research (Bakketeig and Hoffman 1983). The risk of perinatal loss was higher for isolated than for repetitive episodes of fetal growth retardation. These results were taken to indicate that individual women had preordained reproductive tracks, deviation from which predicted adverse outcome. It seems more likely that the sporadic obstetric complications associated with isolated episodes of growth retardation carry a substantially higher risk than the persistent adverse maternal environment associated with recurrence.

associated with sporadic obstetric complications such as placental pathology and antepartum bleeding.

We can conclude that intragenerational recurrence, in the sequence of births to individual women, is a feature of length of gestation and especially of intrauterine growth rates. Between generations, a familial factor can be recognized only for intrauterine growth rates. In large part, the repetitive patterns originate in the maternal environment. Some aspects of the intrauterine environment provided by a woman may be the result of genetic factors—for example, those influencing height— but these factors can find expression in birth weight only through the mother. Other aspects of the intrauterine environment provided by a woman are the result of both persistent and transient environmental factors. The existence of such environmental factors opens the possibility of prevention by means of social and medical improvements.

16 Maternity and Birth in Less Developed Countries

In the preceding chapters, preterm delivery, low birth weight, and fetal growth could be treated in the light of extensive available data. Because data and economic development go hand in hand (Susser et al. 1985b), our attention was on developed countries. Sparse data deter consideration of less developed countries. In spite of this deterrent, the issues are too important to neglect.

Statistics for the less developed world are slowly accumulating. The profile of childbearing that emerges will seem familiar to the student of the health statistics of nineteenth-century Europe and the United States. To one unfamiliar with that history and unprepared by it, the data on maternal and infant losses must read like a biblical ordeal: "in sorrow thou shalt bring forth children" (Genesis 3:16). The contrasts between the past and the present of the developed world make more comprehensible, if not more palatable, present-day contrasts between the developed and the less developed world.

MATERNAL MORTALITY

Maternal mortality, in its own right, is not at the center of our brief in this book. In the treatment of reproduction in the less developed world, maternal mortality takes on such proportions and is so closely tied to the outcome of pregnancies that it cannot comfortably be passed over.

In the eye of someone in the developed world, by contrast, pregnancy and childbirth evoke the glow of health. Hazards and danger do not loom large, except perhaps to wary obstetricians, perinatologists and epidemiologists whose function is to avoid them or deal with them when they occur. More and more, the view of childbearing and birth as a natural process is justified by hard statistics. This privileged view is essentially modern. Evangelists for "natural childbirth" began to appear in force in the 1940s (c.f. Dick-Read 1942). The movement had a rational foundation in the sharp decline over time of maternal and perinatal mortality. Obstetric practitioners, with "masterly inactivity" their slogan, had pulled back from the recognized dangers of unnecessary intervention. Antisepsis had controlled puerperal fever; sulfonamides and penicillin had now conquered it.

In the past, lethal episodes—obstructed labor, torrential antepartum bleeding, and eclamptic fits—had accounted for the literal decimation of women in childbirth. Data authenticate the horrors. A volume of formidable cases was recorded by William Smellie (1697–1763), a "man midwife" generally regarded as a founder of modern obstetrics (Smellie 1766). For sixteenth- and seventeenth-century England, a maternal mortality rate of about 250 per 10,000 births has been arrived at by linking the deaths of women and newborn children in parish registers (Eccles 1977). To this estimate must be added the unrecorded deaths of women undelivered, and of those women delivered of unregistered stillbirths. To obtain the risk of maternal death during the full course of a woman's reproductive life, the result must then be multiplied by an average number of births to each woman, which could amount to as many as six or seven (Kendall 1979). Perhaps 10 or even 15 per cent of women died in childbirth.

During the eighteenth century, the obstetric forceps invented and wielded by male midwives is thought to have reduced maternal mortality significantly. In labors obstructed by malpresentations, or by moderate cephalopelvic disproportion in women ill grown or rachitic or the like, it became possible to deliver the child alive or dead and so save the mother. By the nineteenth century, official vital statistics showed rates of maternal mortality in a birth episode reduced to around 50 per 10,000. If by then 3 to 5 per cent of women died in childbirth, that was still a frightening mortality rate.

At the same time, increasingly frequent medical intervention to assist delivery had brought with it a new plague of puerperal sepsis. At special risk were the poorest women confined in maternity hospitals for want of a home. The risk was not limited to them; the lethality of pregnancy and childbirth pervaded the lives of women in the nineteenth century. In real life, famous writers like Mary Wollstonecraft and Charlotte Bronte died of their pregnancies. In fiction as in real life, many children were tragically orphaned at birth and fathers widowed early in marriage.

The lesson of antisepsis read so convincingly by Ignaz Semelweiss in his classic epidemiological studies in the mid-nineteenth century (Semmelweiss 1861; Lilienfeld and Lilienfeld 1977) was slow to be understood. Widespread application followed three and four decades later. Joseph Lister had first to demonstrate the value of surgical antisepsis in the early 1860s; an unremitting advocate, he was quick to see how the fundamental and contemporaneous work on microorganisms of Louis Pasteur abetted his campaign.

The era of safe childbirth that has followed the marked and steady decline in maternal mortality into the mid-twentieth century was probably a function of several factors. Demographic factors reduced family size and the numbers of births at the dangerous extremes of reproductive age. Socioeconomic factors improved the health and nutrition of mothers. Medicine and public health brought advances in prevention, technique and therapy. Although the maternal mortality rates in developed societies were usually well below 1 per 1000 births (e.g., 5 per 10,000 in both Massachusetts and Sweden in 1950), the decline has continued to lower levels (1 per 10,000 in both Massachusetts and Sweden in 1980). With infection under control, early recognition of potential dangers has allowed sophisticated interventions to be brought safely to bear in the hospital setting.

Underreporting of maternal mortality, however, persisted in many countries. In the United States, even now, misclassification has obscured a proportion of maternal deaths (Smith et al. 1984). Whether a death is to be attributed to childbirth or to some accompanying chronic condition is not always clear, especially if death is delayed for an interval after delivery. In developing countries, this is even more true. There, another and greater deficiency in counts is underregistration of deaths, particularly outside hospitals. Even the rates estimated from studies in obstetric hospitals or from special urban surveys tend to the low side. In inaccessible areas undercounting is bound to be marked.

The "sisterhood method" for estimating pregnancy-related deaths (Graham et al. 1988) is evidently sound, simple and cheap, but it is still not widely applied. The method draws on basic demographic estimates obtained from a census or a household sample survey by techniques developed in worldwide population studies over the past 20 years. Questions are asked about the survival of the close relatives of each respondent; from the data on the proportions surviving, life-tables are constructed. Maternal mortality is obtained from the reports of adults about the survival of their adult sisters.

In less developed countries, maternal mortality remains high (Bernard et al. 1984; Rosenfield and Maine 1985; WHO Chronicle 1986; Kwast and Liff 1988). The ranges are similar to those that obtained in nineteenth-century Europe. Reported rates tend to be local. Subject to much unascertainable error, they are most likely to err on the side of moderation. In rural areas of India, Bangladesh and Bali, rates have ranged from 57 to 87 per 10,000 births. In cities, states, and regions where control over ascertainment is likely to be better, rates have ranged from 2.2 in Shanghai to 30 in upper Egypt. In Gambia, preliminary results of a survey using the sisterhood method indicate a probability of a woman dying of pregnancy-related causes of more than 1 in 20 (about 0.055), or a risk 500-fold greater than in western Europe (Graham et al. 1988).

These many tragedies of women, children, and families are not ineluctable. Cuba reports a national rate of 3.1 per 10,000, remarkably low for a less developed country. Cuban vital statistics, on close study, appear to be highly reliable. They provide a case study of sorts of the effects of a concentrated focus on health problems within a sociopolitical system that can be so directed (Stein and Susser 1972; Santana, personal communication).

That the provision of up-to-date antenatal and obstetric care reduces maternal and reproductive loss for those who can gain access to it has long been known. Booked maternities identify women who are likely to have received antenatal care and to have had supervised deliveries. Thus, in the early 1950s, in a domiciliary obstetric service with a heavy emphasis on prenatal care in a poor black urban township in Johannesburg, South Africa, sharp differences were apparent between booked and unbooked cases, and between women in labor who summoned the midwives in good time and those who did not (Stein and Susser 1959). In the late 1970s, likewise, in a hospital in Zaria in northern Nigeria, mortality for unbooked maternities was more than 20-fold that of booked maternities (286 vs. 13 per 10,000). Among the unbooked, deaths were concentrated in the first few hours after admission. The finding suggested that the greater the delay in admitting the parturient, the greater the risk of death (Rossiter et al. 1985).

Access to medical facilities and their timely and appropriate use is not less important than actual provision. The problems of physical distance and dispersal can be overcome by technical means, as by aircraft and radio in Australia and, to a lesser degree, in Kenya. These problems call for substantial economic and administrative resources, which are not to be had for large segments of the people of the less developed world.

In many societies, moreover, tradition and culture can be as much a bar to the free use of services as lack of access and poverty of resources. Among the Beriba people of Benin, West Africa, women are considered courageous if they disguise the fact that they are in labor, deliver their infants in private on their own, and do not seek help before the cord must be cut. Sometimes women fear admission to hospitals, which they see as places of last resort for hopeless cases. Sometimes women freely enter antenatal care, but refrain from using special domiciliary or hospital delivery services, preferring the traditional ministrations of experienced neighbors or relatives (Sargent 1982; Sargent 1985; McCurdy 1988).

In the study of the Johannesburg township referred to above, the result of a preference for the traditional mode was an extremely high perinatal mortality rate for twins. Women were especially forewarned to call early in labor because their twins would need hospital delivery. Many women used the warning to precisely the opposite effect. By forbearing to call at all, they were able to avoid an unwelcome hospital admission as long as an obstructed labor did not prevent delivery at home. Such problems can be directly overcome only by patiently providing well-conceived education and care at the community level. In most countries societal changes in the economy, culture and general education also make steady if indirect inroads on maternal mortality.

Changes in the demographic pattern of childbearing can improve the outlook. Thus, maternal age and parity at birth have been important risk factors for maternal mortality, as they have been for perinatal mortality. Typically, both age and parity curves for maternal mortality have displayed a J shape: the risk is somewhat raised at the youngest ages and among first births, lowest at intermediate ages and parities, and highest at the highest ages and parities. This typical configuration is seen in the data from a computerized network for university hospitals in Indonesia in the period 1978–80. The overall maternal mortality rate was 38 per 10,000 single births. With the reference standard as the age group of 20 to 24 years, the relative risk at ages over 35 years was 4.2 and that at less than 20 years was 2.3. With parity 1 as the reference group, for grandimultipara (parity 5 or more) the relative risk was 2.5, and for nullipara 1.2 (Bernard and Sastrawinata 1985).

Swedish data of the 1930s provide an instructive analogy typical for developed countries of that time (Bernard et al. 1984). With a maternal mortality rate of 32 per 10,000 births (and the reference age group 20 to 24 years), the relative risk was 19.7 for ages 40 years or more, 16.1 for ages 35 to 39 years, and 1.4 for ages less than 20 years. What can be attained under favorable conditions in the present day is exemplified by the maternal mortality rate for 1976 to 1980 in Sweden, which was down to 0.7 per 10,000 (live) births. Notably, the elevated risk for younger women, and hence the J-shaped curve, had disappeared. The relative risk for ages 35 to 39 years (with the reference age group 20–24 years, as before) was 4.2; for ages 40 years or more there were few births and no deaths; and under 20 years of age the relative risk was better than for the reference group (0.7 : 1 deaths among 5144 births; Hogberg 1985).

BIRTH WEIGHT

In many less developed countries, low birth weight is common, as one might expect from the widespread poverty (Puffer and Serrano 1973; Boldman and Reed 1977). A few exceptions to the association with poverty have been reported among certain ethnic groups, for instance, some Native Americans and Alaskan Eskimos, some Moroccans, and some Chinese (Meredith 1970). We shall see that the differences in low birth weight between developed and less developed countries go beyond frequencies. The relative contributions of growth rate and gestational age to birth weight are not the same. The consequences of birth weight for infant mortality overall, and perhaps for postnatal growth, are also not the same.

Distribution of Birth Weight, Preterm Delivery and Growth Retardation

The frequency of live births of 2500 grams or less ranges widely across the world, from 3 to 43 per cent (Villar and Belizan 1982a). In developed countries rates range from 3.6 to 7.4 per cent (since these rates do not vary much from year to year, they can be interpreted as contemporary). By contrast, no less developed country has a frequency of less than 10 per cent. In Cuba, in Argentina and in a number of African countries, reported percentages are in the teens; in Southeast Asian countries percentage rates are in the 20s and 30s; in Guatemala, the rate in one carefully studied rural area is 41 per cent; in Bombay the rate is an astounding 43 per cent. Within societies, variation follows the gradient to be expected from comparisons between countries. A social class gradient is characteristic of low birth weight in the less developed as in the developed world. The poorest people have the smallest babies. The limited data available show a gradient that grows steeper as the gap between the social strata grows larger (Udani 1963; Gebre-Mehdin et al. 1978; Bernard and Sastrawinata 1985).

Both preterm births and fetal growth retardation contribute to the disparity in the frequencies of low birth weight between developed and less developed countries. With regard to preterm births, many data from the less developed world underrepresent frequencies. The counts nearly everywhere are depleted by stillbirths and early neonatal deaths that go unregistered, excepting some special studies that have maintained registries with household monitoring (compare Meredith 1970; Puffer and Serrano 1973). What can be said in most cases in less developed countries, therefore, holds best for surviving newborn infants.

Among survivors in less developed countries, slow fetal growth makes much the greatest contribution to low birth weight (Villar and Belizan 1982b). Thus growth retardation correlates strongly, and preterm delivery hardly at all, with the frequency of low birth weight in the different countries (Figure 16-1). Across developed countries the opposite holds. Growth retardation correlates much less strongly, and preterm delivery very strongly, with the frequency of low birth weight in different countries. It follows that the proportion of low birth weight infants who are born at term varies as the degree of economic development varies. In most developed countries, this proportion is less than half of all low birth weight infants. In less developed countries, the proportion ranges from two-thirds to three-quarters; in two regions with very high frequencies of low birth weight (Western Guatemala and Bombay), the proportion of term babies is more than four-fifths.

Nutrition

Nutrition cannot be ignored as a factor in intrauterine growth rates. In the less developed world undernutrition and malnutrition of every kind and degree are prevalent. Growth retardation is common where nutritional deprivation is also common. Perhaps for these reasons, little attention has been given to malnutrition as an antecedent of preterm delivery (as we noted in Chapter 11). Some authors argue for two nutritional processes. They contend that gestational length attained at birth is most affected by diet during pregnancy, especially in the first trimester, and that fetal growth rate is most affected by diet before pregnancy, especially chronic malnutrition (Drillien 1957). Similar views have been argued from a long-term nutritional experiment begun in the late 1960s in Guatemala. Prenatal supplements were administered and monitored under tightly controlled conditions in six poor rural villages (Delgado et al. 1982). In a fresh case-control analysis comparing normal, growth-retarded and preterm births, preterm births had much the lowest level of prenatal supplementation, especially in the first trimester (Villar et al. 1986). A similar interpretation can be placed on the results of a Bangladesh study (Pebley et al. 1985). In this report, the risk of mid-trimester pregnancy loss was highest when early pregnancy coincided with the season in which food was least available.

The significance of first-trimester exposure is emphasized by a parallel finding on birth weight of the Dutch Famine study noted in Chapter 11. Slowed fetal growth was the predominant effect of starvation in the third trimester; preterm birth was the predominant effect of starvation in the first trimester (Stein et al. 1975a). A number of subsequent studies of prenatal nutritional supplementation seem to be consonant with this result. During pregnancy, nutritional change (mostly after the first trimester) has produced moderate effects on fetal growth. The revised Guatemalan analysis suggests that, in the presence of nutritional deprivation, moderately improved diet in the first trimester of pregnancy might produce greater effects on length of gestation in pregnancy than similar improvements in midpregnancy can produce on the rate of growth. If so, the effects of severe deprivation in later pregnancy, as the Dutch Famine data show, must be counted an exception to the rule.

The social class gradient in preterm births in developed countries, with the highest rates among the poorest classes, also affords a hint of what may exist in less developed countries. In the United States, length of gestation also emerged as a factor responsive to nutrition in the ecological analysis of poor women in a national food program discussed in

A. LESS DEVELOPED COUNTRIES

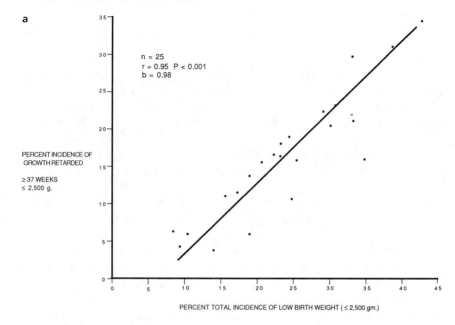

FETAL GROWTH RETARDATION

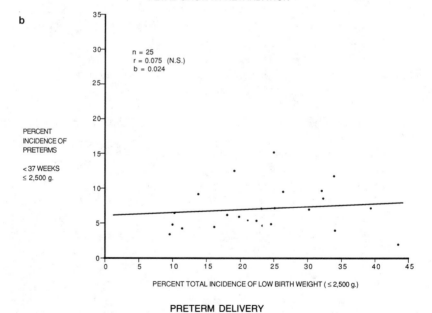

PRETERM DELIVERY

Fig. 16-1 Economic development and antecedents of low birth weight: frequencies of low birth weight (≤2500 gs), correlated with preterm delivery (<37 weeks, ≤2500 gs) and growth retardation (≥37 weeks, ≤2500 g) in (A) less developed countries and (B) developed countries. (After Villar and Belizan 1982)

248

B. DEVELOPED COUNTRIES

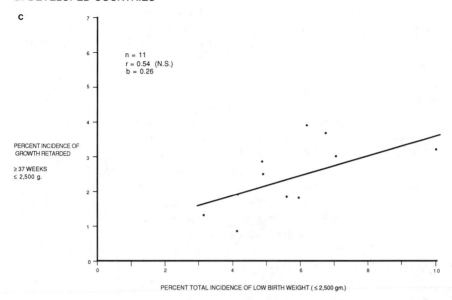

c

n = 11
r = 0.54 (N.S.)
b = 0.26

PERCENT INCIDENCE OF
GROWTH RETARDED

≥ 37 WEEKS
≤ 2,500 g.

PERCENT TOTAL INCIDENCE OF LOW BIRTH WEIGHT (≤ 2,500 gm.)

FETAL GROWTH RETARDATION

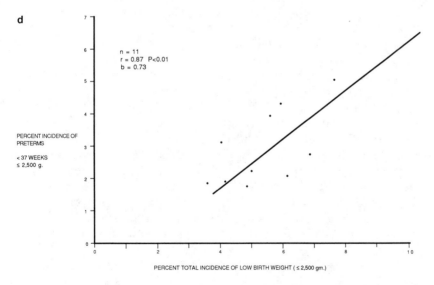

d

n = 11
r = 0.87   P<0.01
b = 0.73

PERCENT INCIDENCE OF
PRETERMS

< 37 WEEKS
≤ 2,500 g.

PERCENT TOTAL INCIDENCE OF LOW BIRTH WEIGHT (≤ 2,500 gm.)

PRETERM DELIVERY

Chapter 11 (Rush 1988). Where physical and economic deprivation exist, psychosocial stress, physical effort, fatigue, and other adverse factors besides nutrition are without doubt magnified. While it is not possible to say what the role of such factors might be in less developed countries, the Guatemalan result underpins that of nutrition.

Infections

Infections in the less developed world also tend to follow patterns distinct from those in the developed world, and some affect reproduction. The most widespread known effects in pregnancy are caused by malaria. Other parasitic infections, especially protozoa and helminths of the intestinal tract, are also widespread in the less developed world and are under suspicion, but only one systematic study exists (Villar et al. 1988). Epidemic malaria in presumably nonimmune populations seems to have striking reproductive effects that contrast with the lesser effects of endemic malaria in primigravidae and the scarcely detectable effects in presumably immune multigravidae.

Early understanding of the role of malaria in pregnancy came from great epidemics in the Punjab in 1908 and in Ceylon in 1934. Marked effects were seen, especially among British colonial women; presumably, they were unprotected by the immunity created by repeated infections from childhood on. Fetal loss rose sharply; in Amritsar in the Punjab, 30 per cent of pregnancies were interrupted, a large proportion attributed to malaria (Covell 1950).

In both endemic and epidemic infections, placental involvement is common and sometimes extensive. Yet even early observers noted discordant effects of malaria in communities in which the infection was endemic. Miscarriage, preterm delivery, and stillbirths were far less remarkable with endemic infections in chronically exposed populations than with epidemic infections in nonimmune populations. Still, in Uganda (Jelliffe 1968) and the Gambia (McGregor et al. 1983), where malaria was endemic, mean birth weight was reduced and the frequency of low birth weight was raised in women with malaria-infected placentas. These outcomes were largely limited, however, to births in primigravidae. In these situations, outcomes such as miscarriage and preterm delivery could not be precisely measured; an indirect estimate in the Gambia suggests that mean length of gestation was reduced in infected primigravidae.

Measles also appears to affect pregnancies differently under different epidemic conditions. In so-called virgin soil epidemics, measles has been associated with raised rates of miscarriage, preterm birth, and perinatal mortality (Christenson et al. 1953; Peart and Nagler 1954; Jespersen et al. 1977). Such effects have not been detected where epidemics are recurrent (Siegel et al. 1966), as they were in the developed world until the advent of the measles vaccine. The post-vaccine situation could possibly pose a fresh risk of virgin soil epidemics. With the herpes virus, primary infections have been associated with fetal complications but secondary infections have not. These observations on malaria, measles and herpes seem to implicate the immune state of the woman as a mediating factor in the outcome of infection in pregnancy.

Human immune deficiency virus (HIV) infection is a modern scourge of the Western World and Africa alike. The effects of the virus on the course of the pregnancy itself, however, are still unclear. Current reports have not suggested anything remarkable in terms of miscarriage, preterm delivery, low birth weight, and neonatal death (Selwyn et al. 1989). Infection in the mother is a known cause of HIV infection in the infant. According to some estimates, rates of transmission of the virus from infected mothers to infants are higher in Africa than in Europe or America. Small series, noncomparable criteria of active infection status, and incomplete follow-up vitiate inference. Whether true differences exist or not, and if they do, whether virus strain, immune state or other factors account for them are matters for speculation as yet unfounded on data.

TYPES OF FETAL GROWTH RETARDATION

In less developed countries, slowed fetal growth appears to differ from that in developed countries not only in frequency but in anthropometric pattern. In a number of studies of poor communities in less developed countries, the large majority of small infants have been found to be symmetrically undergrown. In developed countries (as discussed in Chapter 14) most growth retardation is asymmetrical in that weight is affected more than skeletal structure. The asymmetrical pattern that characterizes growth problems is centered in late pregnancy. The symmetrical pattern, by contrast, is thought to characterize chronic malnutrition that persists throughout gestation.

These patterned differences in growth may be projected into postnatal life. Infants with asymmetrical growth retardation begin to "catch up" in growth and development immediately after birth. Infants with symmetrical growth retardation have been found, in one study, to be delayed in "catch-up growth," even when nutritional supplementation was freely available (Villar et al. 1984). Growth potential was not permanently suppressed. By the third year, differences in height were no longer evident between the growth of children retarded at birth and their peers. Nevertheless, on measures of development the symmetrical group still lagged.

It has been suggested further that asymmetrical growth retardation carries the higher risk of perinatal mortality (Walther and Ramaekers

1982), and that symmetrical growth retardation carries the higher risk of neurodevelopmental impairment in survivors (Villar et al. 1984). A risk of mortality with asymmetrical growth is consistent with several of its causes, which are themselves probably lethal. A risk of neurodevelopmental impairment with symmetrical growth retardation finds some support, though insufficient for a firm conclusion.

In an English study (Parkinson et al. 1981), the onset of growth retardation was diagnosed during gestation by ultrasonography. Developmental delay, especially in boys, persisted up to school age. The earlier in gestation the retardation was observed, the more symmetrical it was, and the longer the delay persisted. In the context of the less developed world, where symmetrical growth retardation seems to be so frequent, the possibility that developmental retardation follows symmetrical growth retardation is especially disturbing. The question needs careful study with refined control for social variables, for its resolution must influence health targets in a major way.

PERINATAL MORTALITY: RISK FACTORS

Perinatal mortality is highly concentrated among the deviant few at the lower extreme of the birth weight distribution. Everywhere most of these are preterm births, but birth weight is the crucial final common pathway in the fatal causal chain (Susser et al. 1972). As birth weight declines from the optimum level for survival, the mortality risk increases exponentially (Karn and Penrose 1951; Shah and Abbey 1971; Susser et al. 1972; Wilcox and Russell 1983b,c). Only around the modal birth weight for the population does length of gestation seem much to influence mortality over and above birth weight, regardless of setting. The distributions of perinatal mortality by birth weight and by length of gestation are not dissimilar in developed and less developed countries (Bernard and Sastrawinata 1985).

The mean or modal birth weight for a given population seems always to be lower than the optimum birth weight for mortality and to bear a constant relationship to it (see Chapter 14). The linear model of Wilcox and Russell (1983b,c), which relates gestational age and birth weight to mortality, is based on this formulation. The model emphasizes the similarity in the shape of the curves for many populations. Because mean birth weight differs across populations, a single model for the distribution of birth weight by duration of gestation should not be expected to fit precisely at all points without shifting the curve to left or right, depending on the mean birth weight. More needs to be understood about the true origin of these birth weight distributions (as we pointed out in Chapter 14) if they are to illuminate the causes of perinatal mortality. In practice, in less developed countries and elsewhere, perinatal mortality probably comprises a combination of constituents before, during and after birth, and a set of causes that differs for each constituent.

Risk Factors

Among less developed countries, Indonesia provides a well-documented and large series of teaching hospital births for the study of prenatal care and other factors. Among term births of adequate birth weight, prenatal care was found to have more impact on perinatal mortality than formal education of the mother (Bernard and Sastrawinata, 1985). Hospital care had substantial benefits on newborn mortality, although little benefit was detectable at birth weights below 1500 grams. In New York City, for both these sets of relationships, the opposite holds; prenatal care has less impact on perinatal mortality than maternal education, and intensive hospital care lowers perinatal mortality among infants weighing less than 2000 grams, but not among larger infants (Paneth et al. 1982).

Again, in the less developed world, with its paucity of proficient midwifery services, intrapartum deaths are likely to account for a much higher proportion of fetal deaths than in the developed world. Among neonatal deaths, birth trauma, neonatal tetanus, malaria and other infections swell the rates. In all these instances, low birth weight infants are likely to be more vulnerable than others. In general, therefore, the combination of high frequencies of low birth weight with the special hazards of less developed countries is bound to exaggerate reproductive loss and produce high mortality rates. The relative weights of all these factors in infant mortality, however, is a more complex matter than it appears on the surface.

Mortality Attributable to Birth Weight

The importance of low birth weight, on its own, when weighed against other factors that affect reproductive loss and development, is not the same in less developed and in developed countries. This kind of question is addressed by the use of *attributable risks;* the difference in consequences is not evident from a consideration solely of relative risks for perinatal mortality.

Low birth weight certainly contributes in an important way to stillbirth rates and to neonatal death rates all over the world. In less developed countries, as we just noted, birth weight predicts perinatal mortality as it does in developed countries. Therefore, we have reason to think that low birth weight, as a final common pathway to perinatal mortality, would account for better than 90 percent of the variance in less developed countries, as it does in New York. One might well add that in less developed countries perinatal losses are substantially higher than in developed countries (Puffer and Serrano 1973).

Yet in less developed countries the *relative* importance of perinatal losses in infant mortality is smaller, nonetheless, simply because they form so much smaller a component of total infant loss. Under harsh environmental conditions, perinatal losses have been seen to comprise less than 1 in 10 of total infant deaths (Stein and Susser, 1958a,b, 1959a,b; Puffer and Serrano 1973; Rush 1987). This balance between perinatal and total infant losses in less developed countries today resembles that at the turn of the century in Britain (see Figure 10-1; Macfarlane and Mugford 1984). Attributable risks convey the significance of these patterns in populations at large: the less the level of economic development, the less perinatal deaths contribute to total infant deaths. It does not follow automatically, when perinatal mortality constitutes the lesser part of infant mortality, that the role of birth weight to total infant mortality can be discounted to the same extent as can the role of perinatal deaths. Low birth weight or the factors that cause it may have effects that persist beyond the newborn period for some time and act on later infant mortality. Thus, in the Dutch Famine, an effect of third trimester starvation and low birth weight on infant mortality could be detected at least through the first 3 months of life (Stein et al. 1975b).

In less developed countries, a question that naturally follows from this finding is what the relative risk of low birth weight might be for the postneonatal mortality of those infants who survive the perinatal period. Given even a modest relative risk, a high attributable risk will follow because of the high frequency of low birth weight. Thus, the answers differ for special groups according to the product of the relative risk and the numbers in the risk group. For instance, very low birth weight infants and twins are two classes at high risk of postneonatal infant mortality, but their small numbers reduce the impact on overall postneonatal mortality attributable to them.

The available data, we remind the reader, are sparse. One study in India gives a good idea of the trends to be expected. An area of high infant mortality (North Arcot) was compared with an area of relatively low infant mortality (New Delhi) (Figure 16-2). In the harsher environment of North Arcot, the overall mortality risk attributable to low birth weight was lower overall than in the milder environment of New Delhi. Among infants of birth weight up to about 2000 grams, the attributable risks as well as the relative risks of low birth weight for infant mortality were equally high in the two areas (Rush 1987). For the much larger number of infants in the 2000- to 2500-gram low-birth-weight range, the risk of dying in the first year of life that could be *attributed* to birth weight was lower in the harsher than in the milder environment. Thus below 2000 grams, the relationship of birth weight to infant mortality produced an identical exponential curve in the two areas: mortality declined equally steeply with rising birth weight. Above 2000 grams, the mortality curves by birth weight for the two areas diverged. In New Delhi, above

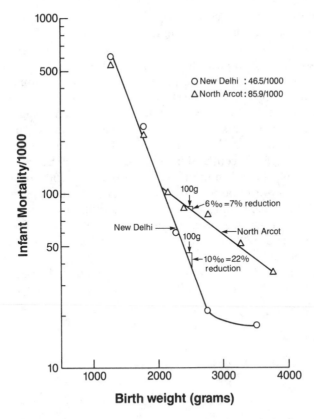

Fig. 16–2 Attributable risks of birth weight for infant mortality with death rates very high (85.9/1000) and moderately high (46.5/1000): birth weight regressed on infant mortality in North Arcot and New Delhi to show (1) equal mortality and equal risks attributable to birth weight ≤2000 g in both areas; (2) higher mortality and lower risk attributable to birth weight >2000 g in North Arcot than in New Delhi. For every 100 g birth weight, respective death rates are reduced 6 per 1000 (7%) versus 10 per 1000 (22%). (After Rush 1987)

2000 grams birth weight mortality continued to decline at the same rapid rate as at lower birth weights; among these infants a regression analysis indicated that a 22 per cent decrement in infant mortality could be attributed to every 100-gram increment in birth weight. In North Arcot, the slope of the mortality curve with rising birth weight above 2000 grams was much less steep; with birth weights above 2000 grams, only a 7 per cent decrement in infant mortality could be attributed to every 100-gram increment in birth weight.

These attributable risks do not settle the question of causes. To reach a secure causal judgment about the exact role of birth weight in post-neonatal mortality is not easy, since the poor circumstances that generate low birth weight in themselves generate infant deaths. Whatever results eventually obtain, we can agree that prematurity in the less developed world entails consequences different from those in the developed world (Villar and Belizan 1982a; Rasmussen et al. 1985).

The broad sweep of the differences with economic development can be briefly stated. In the less developed world, most infant deaths occur not in the perinatal but in the postneonatal period. Compared to the mortality in infants from diarrheal and respiratory diseases, for instance, the mortality directly attributed to low birth weight, preterm delivery, or growth retardation is quite overshadowed. In developed countries, low birth weight has an attributable risk for total infant mortality of at least 45 per cent and possibly more than 50 per cent (Susser et al. 1985b; McCormick 1985); in less developed countries the attributable risk might turn out to be one-half or even one-quarter as great. Finally, we should emphasize that perinatal and postnatal mortality are indices of differences between settings of the most severe order. Equally sharp differences attributable to birth weight in different economic settings are to be expected for outcomes such as morbidity, growth, and physical, psychological, and social development (Rasmussen et al. 1985). The data to test such expectations are still to be collected.

IV Age and Parity

17 Aging and Reproduction: I. Fecundity, Fertility and Gestation

Age as a variable encompasses at least three distinct components (Susser 1968). These three components—intrinsic aging, weathering, and history—all need to be weighed in interpreting any association between reproductive outcome and parental age.

First, age is a marker of the biologic changes that have taken place as a result of intrinsic processes, the unwinding of a developmental clock. Heterogeneity exists in the nature and the timing of these changes.

Second, age is a matter of weathering. The state of the organism at any given age is a product of its experiences from conception to the point of observation. The more time passes, the greater the opportunity is for determining experiences to occur and to work their effects. The greater, too, is the cumulation and variety of other concurrent experiences that might act in concert as cooperating causes.

Third, a given age at any point in calendar time designates membership in a generation or cohort and marks the individual as having lived through a particular historical environment. Members of cohorts born at a particular place and time differ from other cohorts and hold in common a set of life experiences.

Aging should be distinguished from senescence. Aging begins at conception; senescence is a deteriorative process that begins long after conception, although at no single definable point. The ultimate and ineluctable deterioration of the diverse physiological, mental and social functions of individuals begins, for each function, at diverse ages. Further, the norms for senescence in these functions can also be diverse by sex, social group, life-style, and environment generally. Although this chapter (one of two on parental age and reproduction) focuses on the decline in fertility at older ages, it does not entirely ignore youthful reproduction. In older women, biological disadvantage tends to be combined with social advantage. Younger women, in a mirror image, tend to have biological advantage combined with social disadvantage.

Fertility refers to the frequency with which a birth successfully completes the process of reproduction (see Chapter 4). The process has different implications for individual women or couples, and for groups. Couples must accomplish a conception, the woman must sustain the conceptus through the period of gestation necessary to attain viability, and a live child must be delivered. In groups, we may note in passing, successful reproduction requires more than a conception ending in a birth; the offspring must survive until they, in turn, reach reproductive maturity.

To analyze reproductive failure in individuals we need to distinguish, even though we oversimplify, the elements involved. The ovaries have two major interdependent functions. First, they are the locus of production and the repository of female germ cells in the form of ova. Second, they are the source of hormones that regulate the entire reproductive process in interaction with the governing role of the pituitary hormones. The uterus, a target organ that responds to the governance of ovarian hormones, has a main function in nidation; it provides the bed for implantation of the zygote and facilitates passage of the nutrients that sustain the developing organism throughout gestation. In what follows, we speak separately of the function and integrity of ova or germ cells, of the reproductive hormones or endocrine system, and of the uterus.

EXPERIMENTAL BIOLOGY

In several mammalian species, including our own, fertility tends to be low when the capacity for reproduction is first attained; soon thereafter, fertility reaches its highest level, and a plateau is maintained for some time; then fertility declines gradually until it ceases entirely. Various animal experiments with different mammalian species allow us to infer that both uterus and ova play a part in reproductive senescence.

In a paper read to the Royal Society in 1787, the English surgeon John Hunter, a father of experimental medicine, began as follows:

> You will observe that when a woman begins to breed at an early period, as at fifteen, and has her children fast, that she seldom breeds longer than the age of thirty to thirty-five. Therefore, we may suppose either that the parts are then worn out, or the breeding constitution is over. If a woman begins later, as at 20 or 25, she may continue to breed to the age of forty or more. And there are now and then instances of women, who not having conceived before, have had children as late in life as fifty years and upwards. After that few women breed, even if they should not have bred before. Therefore there must be a natural period to the power of conception . . . (Hunter 1787).

In other words, Hunter supposed that the natural limit to fertility was less than the theoretical maximum possible between the childbearing ages of 15 to 50 years. To explore the issue further, he selected two young sows of the same color and size and one boar, all from the same farrow. One ovary was removed from one sow. The spayed sow was identified by a slit cut in one ear; the other he left "perfect." "I had them well fed and kept warm so there should be no impediment to their breeding. And whenever they farrowed, their pigs were taken away at exactly the same age."

Hunter argued that "if conception depended on the ovaria, it was to be expected that the perfect sow would bring forth double the number at each birth, or if she did not, that she would continue breeding for double the time." After eight consecutive occasions, on which each sow produced almost exactly the same size of farrow, the spayed sow simply stopped reproducing. The "perfect" sow continued, and in the end had produced double the number of piglets.

Hunter inferred that the available ova were exhausted. "It seems most probable," he wrote, "that the ovaries are from the beginning destined to produce a fixed number beyond which they cannot go; that the constitution at large has no power of giving to one ovarium the power of populating equal to two. But the constitution has so far a power in influencing one ovarium as to make it produce its number in a less time than would probably have been the case if both ovaria had been preserved."

Since Hunter's time, and particularly since the 1970s, experimental biologists have added to our understanding of the decline of breeding potential with maternal aging (Biggers et al. 1962a, 1962b; Biggers 1969; Maurer and Foote 1971; Finch 1978; Maudlin and Fraser 1978; Gosden 1979). The experiment has not been exactly repeated, but several have tried, like Hunter, to separate the roles of ovaries and uterus. The problem is presently posed rather differently since, as noted earlier, we know that the ovary not only stores the ova, but also acts as an endocrine gland mediating, in concert with the anterior pituitary, the production of estrogen and progesterone. The ovarian hormones are involved not only in the cyclical growth and release of ova, but also in the parallel changes that occur in the myometrium, including the preparation of the uterine lining (the endometrium) for implantation by the blastocyst.

One can restate Hunter's proposition to say that the limiting factor in fertility with aging is the actual number of functional ova that survive to later ages. We now know that, in human beings as in animals, this is not the case. The disappearance of ova is not the primary phenomenon in normal reproductive senescence. One factor, at least in animal experiments, is an impaired capacity of the uterus to support the implantation and retention of the embryo. A second factor is the function of the hypothalamic-pituitary-ovarian axis of the endocrine system that sustains these processes. A third factor is the capacity of the ovum to form a normal zygote that can develop into a healthy embryo and fetus (a subject to which we return in the next chapter). We shall explore what part each of these factors might play.

Hunter's choice of the pig may have been unwise for the purpose of extrapolating to women. Fertility in pigs generally declines not gradually but suddenly. Smaller laboratory animals—mice, rats, hamsters, and rabbits—provide better models for the gradual decline with age in human fertility. Typically, in these animals, the steady decline from peak litter size (the number of births per pregnancy) reached in their prime serves as an indicator of reproductive senescence (Biggers et al. 1962b).

In rodents, the decline in litter size with the aging of the doe seems to result from uterine dysfunction. This can be argued in the first place by exclusion; the decline in litter size appears in the presence of functioning ova. Other lines of evidence support the argument. One consistent finding, for instance, is the presence of excess embryonic loss in aging mice (Finn 1962).

A kind of "cross-fostering" experiment carried out in a number of species demonstrated the uterine role in a positive way. The design ensured that the performance of the doe depended on the uterine function of sustaining the litter during gestation, to the exclusion of the ovum. For example, in rabbits, embryos were taken from donor does that were young, middle-aged, and old, respectively, and transplanted into recipient does similarly stratified by age (Maurer and Foote 1971). Successes with transplants (with the age of the donor held constant) declined with increasing age of the recipients. Thus, it could be inferred, the decline of uterine function of the recipient with age jeopardized the survival of donated embryos.

An aging effect of the ovum existed alongside the decline in uterine function. Thus, in the cross-fostering experiments, the effect of the age of the donor doe was not neutral. Although no difference was found between embryos from the younger and middle-aged donors, embryos from donors reaching the end of the reproductive phase did poorly. Whatever the exact source of this nonlinear age effect, the design of the study precludes a role for the uterus per se.

A localization of uterine dysfunction in these various experiments provides further insight into the problem and also bears on a possible interaction between age and disuse. A characteristic of mice useful in experiments is that the uterus has two horns and, typically, the passage of ova from ovary to uterine horn is ipsilateral. It has been established experimentally that mice kept virgin until late in reproductive life remained fecundable—which attests to the integrity of both ova and endocrine system—and their embryos did not resorb. In mice ovariectomized on one side before maturity, moreover, the uterine horn that remained barren and the fertile horn were similar histologically when examined at older ages (Finn et al. 1963b). Despite this absence of visible cellular change, local dysfunction with aging occurs in ovariectomized mice. In the old but not in the young doe, the ipsilateral horn secluded from implantation by ovariectomy has a reduced capacity to sustain transplanted embryos (Gosden 1979). This reduced capacity can occur independently of ovarian hormones. Thus, localized uterine change with age has been shown also in does maintained on reproductive hormones after oophorectomy. In young oophorectomized does the normal decidual response of the lining of the uterus that anticipates pregnancy could be artificially induced (by injecting oil into the fallopian tubes) (Finn 1966). In old oophorectomized does, no such response could be induced. A decrease with age in estrogen receptors in the uterine tissue might underlie this lack of response (Hsueh et al. 1979).

Hunter's conclusion that reproductive senescence follows the exhaustion of available ova is refuted by other experiments as well. A present-day interpretation of Hunter's results might be that with aging the endocrine function of the single ovary remaining to the "imperfect" sow was insufficient to sustain normal uterine function. In comparable modern experiments, in mice with one ovary extirpated, premature reproductive senescence was manifest in a reduced total number of litters over the life span; at later ages, reproduction failed because the embryos were resorbed. An accompanying decline in number of ova with age does not serve to explain failing reproduction, since many remain in the aging ovary.

That something more than the numbers or even the quality of the ova is involved becomes plain from still other experiments. In these, the ovaries were left intact, but fertilization and implantation were impeded by tying off one fallopian tube. Litter size in these animals was thereby halved, but reproduction continued through the usual reproductive span with no sign of premature senescence (Finn 1963a).

We conclude from this experimental literature that age has strong and consistent effects on reproduction. Deferred implantation also contributes to reproductive failure, but only in interaction with aging. Deferred implantation provides an analogy of a sort with late first pregnancy in women. In mice, the effect of deferred implantation can best be demonstrated when it is local, as with a secluded uterine horn. Reproductive failure with aging in mice first becomes manifest in the resorption of embryos, possibly a local uterine phenomenon. This failure may imply an antecedent role for ovarian or more general endocrine function, but this has not yet been demonstrated.

FECUNDITY AND FERTILITY IN HUMAN BEINGS

Experimental results have not been consistent across all species tested, nor even across strains of the same species. This diversity in patterns of reproductive senescence well justifies the efforts of epidemiologists to unravel age effects in human beings.

Parental age has been studied in relation to several components of fertility. Before we proceed, we return to the definitions of fertility measures given in Chapter 4 and add some new ones.

> *Fertility,* we remind the reader, refers to actual live births to an individual, couple, or population; by contrast, *fecundity* refers to the physiological capacity to conceive and thereby to produce a live birth, and *fecundability* refers to the physiological capacity to conceive, whether or not conception results in a live birth.
>
> *Fertility rates* for any given population take live births over a specified period as the numerator and an approximate population (women of reproductive age, usually 15 to 44 years) as the denominator.
>
> *Crude birth rates* take live births as the numerator and the total population as the denominator.
>
> *Fecundability* is operationally defined as the probability of conceiving during one menstrual cycle in women who menstruate regularly, who engage in sexual intercourse, and who do not practice contraception (see Leridon 1977).
>
> *Recognizable fecundability* takes clinically recognized pregnancies as the numerator, excluding all pregnancies ending within 2 weeks of conception (Bongaarts 1975).
>
> *Conception delay,* ordinarily obtained in special studies, is an index of recognizable fecundability measured by the time that a couple practicing regular coitus without contraception takes to conceive (Stein 1985; Baird and Wilcox 1985; Baird et al. 1986).
>
> *Effective fecundability* takes live births as the numerator; one measure used is the interval from marriage to first birth in noncontracepting populations to estimate the denominator, which is intended as an approximation to the number of menstrual cycles involved (Henry 1957; Leridon 1977). In demographic studies, effective fecundability serves as an operational index of the potential for fertility.

Total fecundability is underestimated by measures of fecundability: they cannot encompass subclinical losses, and early loss in the clinical phase of pregnancy, too, is often either ignored or poorly measured. Total fecundability is even further underestimated because ordinarily no data on the timing of either ovulation or sexual congress are at hand. In practice, then, many demographic studies accept as given the modal conditions governing sexual behavior, the ovulatory patterns, and even the contraceptive norms of the populations under study, and they may not take into account the individual or group variations in these matters.

In considering the relations of parental age to fecundability and fertility, it is useful, first, to consider the maximum number of live births that might be attained in "natural" populations reproducing without voluntary restriction. Age-specific fertility rates have been compiled for a

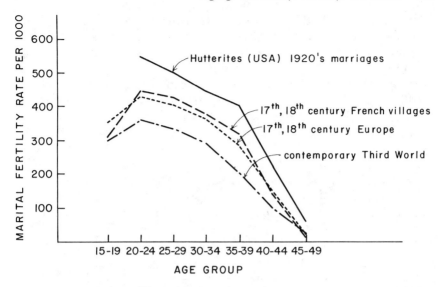

Fig. 17–1 Age-specific fertility in selected populations not using contraception (rates per 1000 married women). (After Stein 1985)

number of such natural populations (Figure 17-1). These populations—seventeenth-century women in Germany and France, contemporary women in Senegal, and a cohort of American Hutterite women who married in the 1920s—supposedly made no effort to limit reproduction. The variation in age-specific fertility rates by time and by place—and surely also by diet and standard of living—is notable. Even more notable is the consistency of the decline in fertility at older ages, regardless of circumstance. Childbearing had virtually ceased by the fifth decade in all except the Hutterites, who were without question the most comfortably off and the best-fed. Even among the Hutterites, fertility in the fifth decade was sharply reduced, by tenfold from the peak at 20 to 24 years.

In the United States and Europe in general, such unrestricted childbearing has not obtained for a century or longer. The decline in average fertility rates has been steady since the last quarter of the nineteenth century, when frequent childbearing throughout reproductive life and improving child survival produced uniquely large families. Very recently, in the 1980s a new pattern of late childbearing has emerged in the United States that turns attention to maternal age. In the vanguard of this change was the "baby boom" generation, the post-World War II birth cohorts which were then moving into their late thirties and beyond.

Several elements affect the childbearing behavior of the baby boom cohorts. Their numbers are large (the result of a rebound in births after the deferred fertility during the disruption of the years of World War II). In youth they were exposed, in the United States as in Europe, to the social and political movements of the late 1960s and early 1970s. Young people grew to adulthood in a climate of profound questioning, and often rejection, of established society and its values. Not least was the economic impulsion that put many women to work, and the determination of many others to enter the world of work and careers equally with men. Finally, the advent and wide dispersion of oral contraceptives, of sterilization that can be performed without hospitalization, and then of legal induced abortion, conferred on this generation a newfound ability to exert effective technical control over their fertility.

Many women of these cohorts deferred marriage until their late twenties and early thirties: thus, rates of childlessness remained high at ages as late as 30 and 35 years and, at the same time, rates of first births rose at ages as late as 30 to 34 years. The trend of the present day toward having first births in the thirties is most marked among well-educated women. Thus far, the generations born after the baby boom seem to be following the example of their immediate predecessors in deferring marriage and childbearing.

The nature of the decline in family size that ensued contrasts with the decline of family size during the latter part of the nineteenth century and the early twentieth century. In that period of relatively early marriage, a feature of childbearing was its compression into an ever-shortening time span. By the middle decades of the twentieth century, childbearing through the whole reproductive period had been compressed into the first 10 years after marriage and, most recently, into the first 5 years after marriage (Aral and Cates 1983; Hendershot 1984; Susser et al. 1985b). With the deferral of childbearing to later ages, biological factors have come to rank along with birth control and social factors as important determinants of family size.

Natural populations shed light on infertility as well as fertility. The risk of childlessness by age of the woman at marriage has been estimated in several historic populations among whom late marriage was relatively common and deliberate fertility control rare (Menken et al. 1986). When women marry in their late thirties or early forties, the data (shown in Table 17-1) suggest that as many as one-third to one-half of those who may desire children will remain childless (Vincent 1950; Henry 1961; Leridon 1977). Historical cases may not fit the case of the modern women of the developed world. Indeed, contemporary as well as historic trends in fertility have stirred controversy about the causes of the shifting patterns in childbearing. Reproduction in recent cohorts has not yet run its course, and there is room for surprises. Women in their thirties

Table 17–1 Childlessness by bride's age at marriage

Age at marriage (years)	20–24	25–29	30–34	35–39	40–44
Per cent childless	5.7	9.3	15.5	29.6	63.6

Source: Menken et al. 1986.

and later who have remained childless or had one child may still desire to bear children, and their childbearing patterns could evolve further in the coming years.

Diverse experiences might advance or delay the onset of infertility. Many modern women are well-nourished and much healthier overall than their forebears, and public health and medical interventions can prevent or treat some of the causes of infertility. On the debit side, in recent decades many women have begun to smoke cigarettes and had multiple sexual encounters. Good nutrition promotes early menarche and may possibly defer the menopause; if so, it could extend the period of fertility. On the other hand, cigarette smoking may reduce fecundity, and hence fertility, in some degree. In smokers, both conception delay and the menopause are affected; the time taken to conceive is lengthened slightly (Baird and Wilcox 1985) and the menopause occurs sooner (Jick et al. 1977; Kaufman et al. 1980; McKinlay et al. 1985). Multiplicity of sexual partners raises the risk of sexually transmitted disease, which can affect fecundity through pelvic infection and hence also reduce fertility (Westrom 1980; Menken et al. 1986).

Infecundity

The median age for the menopause, in the United States today, is about 52 years (McKinlay et al. 1985). An end to menstruation with the menopause almost conclusively indicates infecundability and consequent infertility, but the onset of the menopause and that of infertility are not coincident. Before the menopause, many women experience a phase, lasting 5 to 10 years or more, which we term *functional infertility.*

Functional infertility is a subclass of infecundability in which the clinical conditions for normal fertility appear to be present but are not realized in clinically recognized pregnancies. That is, while sexual activity and menstruation appear to continue normally, both clinically recognized pregnancies and births are reduced in frequency even in women who are not using contraception. Although menstrual cycles are not always accompanied by ovulation (Metcalf 1979), the functional nature of this phase in premenopausal women is indicated by the ova still contained by the ovaries, as seen at menopause in biopsies and autopsies. This physiological condition of functional infertility becomes manifest, demographically, in a decline in effective fecundability. Epidemiology informed by biology is an aid in posing questions about the phenomenon that can be tested in human populations.

First, by analogy with the animal experiments discussed earlier, we may ask whether declining fertility with age is limited by a woman's ability to sustain a pregnancy, or by a couple's ability to produce a viable conception, or perhaps by both. In the sphere of the woman's ability to sustain pregnancy, one looks to the function of the uterus and the hormonal system on which it depends. With depleted functional capability, the risk of miscarriage might be expected to rise with advancing age, and to be manifest especially in the frequency of chromosomally normal loss. On another cue from animal experiments, one might expect a particular risk from the failure of uterine function in a first pregnancy near the end of a woman's childbearing phase.

In the sphere of conception, one looks to the integrity of the process of ovulation and of the ovum itself. First, as just mentioned, menstrual cycles can occur without ovulation, at older ages especially. When ovulation does occur and is followed by conception, fewer of the ova fertilized might be normal and prove viable. If so, the frequency of miscarriages with an abnormal conceptus would be expected to rise with advancing age. In examining these questions, we consider fecundability, miscarriage, and perinatal loss, in turn.

Fecundability

Of all the barriers to reproduction in older women, reduced fecundability is probably the most crucial and the least understood. Ovulation is a minimum condition for conception. Normally, regular menstruation indicating satisfactory endocrine function and a physically intact reproductive system must also be present. Even then, conception may not occur.

As noted previously, one index of fecundability is the monthly probability of conceiving; another is conception delay. Neither index can of itself discriminate between dysfunction related to the ovum (e.g., imperfect ova) and that related to the uterus (e.g., impediments to implantation). In practice, both indices refer to recognizable fecundability; most observations on fecundability in human beings have been confined to clinically recognized pregnancies. One exception is a study that provides data on losses in the early postimplantation stage, beginning about one week after conception (Wilcox et al. 1988).

Other problems of sampling and analysis can also affect interpretation of these indices. When observations begin with women known to have conceived, problems of sampling can lead to overestimates of recognizable fecundability. Infecund women are not included, and those who are slow to conceive may be underrepresented. A potential problem of analysis in samples identified by a recognized pregnancy arises in the designation of the maternal age at which attempts to conceive began. The longer the duration of involuntary infecundability, the older the woman will be when conception ensues. Thus, the relevant age for the prevalence of infecundability is the age at which the attempt to conceive began, and not the age at which a birth or a miscarriage shows that the attempt has succeeded or failed.

In demographic studies, unrefined data may also produce skewed sampling and mistaken estimates of recognizable fecundability. Estimates are likely to disregard the requirement that regular menstruation, which is a surrogate for ovulation, persists throughout the observation period. With the passing of time, as older women near the menopause, the proportion with irregular menstruation and anovular cycles grows. Thus, some women are fecundable at the beginning of the period of observation and infecund at the end. As a result, assessments made at the beginning of an observation period place too many women in the denominator, as candidates for conception, and underestimate average fecundability. The reverse is also true; assessments made at the end of the observation period (among women who are now older by the duration of that period) place too few women in the denominator and overestimate average fecundability. Since anovular cycles are a characteristic of older women, errors will be greatest for women in menopausal transition. Hence, fecundability estimates taken from the end of an observation period, and consequently at older ages, tend to exaggerate the apparent disjunction between fecundability (as manifested in menstrual cycles and the presence of ova) and realized fertility.

With these cautions in mind, we can weigh the available information. In the New York City study of miscarriages, the time taken to conceive did not increase between 20 and 34 years of age, but thereafter a steep upturn occurred. The finding was consistent among public and private patients, in cases of miscarriage and the pregnant controls who did not miscarry, in smokers and nonsmokers, and in primigravidae and multigravidae (Stein 1985). The pattern is also consistent with data on age changes in ovulation, length of menstrual cycles, and fertility (Barrett and Marshall 1969; Leridon 1977; Schwartz et al. 1980), with analyses from the National Fertility Survey (Aral and Cates 1983; Hendershot 1984), and with at least one carefully controlled study of artificial insemination (Federation CECOS 1982).

The decline in fecundability appears in the late 30s and especially in the 40s, ages not related in any obvious way either to opportunities for being impregnated or to a decline in menstrual function and the availability of ova. A healthy woman typically sustains or even increases her sexual activity (Pfeiffer et al. 1968; George and Weiler 1981; Weg 1983); she menstruates and ovulates with fair regularity (Treloar et al. 1967a; Metcalf 1979); and she retains a store of what appear to be normal oocytes in her ovaries (Costoff and Mahesh 1975).

Signs of menstrual decline appear only gradually thereafter. The advent of menstrual bleeding becomes less regular (Treloar et al. 1967a): the interval between bleeding and ovulation (the follicular phase) shortens first (Sherman et al. 1976) and the interval after ovulation (the luteal phase) later. Such menstrual irregularity is not by itself diagnostic of infecundability. Many younger, recognizably fecund women have cycles as irregular as those of older and apparently infecund women (Treloar et al. 1967a).

Although there is thus no patent connection between fecundability and the endocrine functions that regulate menstruation or sustain a pregnancy, localized endocrine dysfunction is not ruled out. If menstruation and ovulation are seemingly normal, the ovaries, ovarian follicles, and the ova themselves remain as possible loci for subfecundity. For instance, in women in their mid-40s endocrine dysfunction might be attributable to a decline in either number or function of the ovarian follicles. Although the follicle-stimulating hormone (FSH) and the luteinizing hormone (LH) produced by the pituitary have been found at expected levels, the estrogen produced by the follicles has been found at reduced levels (Sherman et al. 1976; Wise 1983). The decline in fecundability, it seems fair to conclude, is partly a result of a declining ovarian endocrine system.

MISCARRIAGE

Miscarriage rates begin to rise in women at ages 30 to 35 years (Stevenson et al. 1959; Warburton and Fraser 1964; Pettersson 1968; Taylor 1969; Shapiro et al. 1971; Naylor 1974; Leridon 1976; Harlap et al. 1980a; Stein et al. 1980; Hassold and Chiu 1985). The rise could be the consequence of an excess of chromosomally aberrant losses, chromosomally normal losses, or both. If chromosomally aberrant losses are a factor in the age trend for miscarriage, they raise an underlying question of the quality of the ovum and the viability of the resulting conceptus in the aging women. If chromosomally normal losses are a factor in the age trend, they raise the different underlying question of uterine function and the capacity to sustain the pregnancy in the aging woman.

Trisomy 21 has an undisputed and longstanding connection with maternal age. Trisomies of all chromosomes taken together—whether they are collected at miscarriage, at induced abortion, at prenatal diagnosis, or at birth—are also now known to rise in frequency with maternal age. At birth, besides trisomy 21, only trisomies 13 and 18 and those of the sex chromosomes occur at measurable frequencies. The remaining trisomies do not concentrate anywhere but among miscarriages, so that systematic examination of their maternal age relations had to wait on a sufficiency of karyotyped miscarriages (Hassold et al. 1984b). Full discussion of the role of trisomies, which account for a part of the relations of age with miscarriage, is deferred to the next chapter.

Chromosomally normal miscarriages, like trisomic miscarriages, are associated with increased maternal age (Stein et al. 1980; Hassold and Chiu 1985). It follows that factors other than the chromosomal comple-

Table 17-2 Maternal age and karyotype at miscarriage: odds ratios for chromosomally normal, trisomic, and other chromosomally aberrant miscarriages compared to live births in New York City and Honolulu

Maternal age (in years)	Chromosomally normal	Trisomic	Other chromosomally aberrant
New York City			
15–19	1.0	0.8	1.1
20–24 (reference)	1.0	1.0	1.0
25–29	1.0	1.2	0.9
30–34	1.2	2.1	0.8
35–39	1.7	4.9	1.0
40–44	2.6	15.3	1.4
45–49	1.7	31.3	0.0
Honolulu			
16–19	1.0	0.5	1.0
20–23 (reference)	1.0	1.0	1.0
24–29	0.9	1.4	1.3
30–35	1.2	2.7	1.1
36–39	1.9	6.0	1.7
40–49	2.1	15.6	1.3

Sources: New York City data (with Warburton, unpublished). See Warburton et al. 1986 for a description of the sample. Honolulu data are computed from Hassold and Chiu (1985). Presentation of the data did not permit grouping in the usual 5-year age groups.

ment must be taken into account. The animal experiments discussed earlier provided some clues about such factors: in mice, aging of the dam induced, first, a decline in uterine function and later a deficiency of normal ova. Among women, therefore, one might expect to observe, first, a rise in chromosomally normal miscarriages as uterine function declines and later a rise in trisomic miscarriages as the ova lose their integrity.

The age patterns of miscarriage actually observed in the best available data do not conform with these expectations (Table 17-2). With chromosomally normal miscarriage, no steep rise is seen until the middle and late 30s. With trisomic miscarriages, in contrast, a very gradual but steady rise in frequency begins early; the frequency in each successive age group is greater than in the one before, and the rise becomes much steeper at around 30 years of age. These contrasting age patterns are illustrated for the New York City data in Figure 17-2.

Clearly, chromosomally normal conceptions as well as trisomies contribute to the maternal age effect in miscarriages. The idea that the rise in chromosomally normal miscarriage with age points to uterine dysfunction is also compatible with a shift toward earlier stages of gestation observed in miscarriages at later maternal ages (Warburton et al. 1986). There is nothing to suggest that genetic errors in chromosomally normal

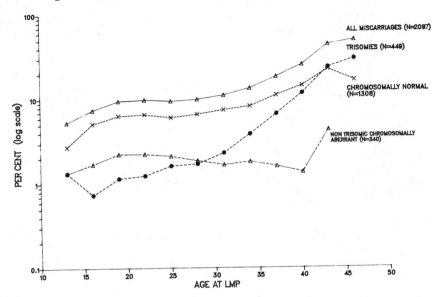

Fig. 17–2 Maternal age and miscarriages: estimated proportions of all recognized pregnancies ending in miscarriage, by karyotype (3-year moving averages).

conceptions relate to maternal age; possible deficiencies in the cytoplasm, which might prejudice early development and relate to maternal age, are purely speculative. The earlier and steeper rise of trisomic as compared to chromosomally normal losses suggests that in humans deterioration of germ cells may precede uterine dysfunction.

In summary, a decline with age in the integrity of the ova, as well as in the ovarian endocrine system and the uterine function that may depend on the system, all appear to contribute to reproductive senescence. The signs of senescence are manifest in functional infertility preceding the menopause on the one hand, and in miscarriage on the other.

CHILDBEARING

First pregnancies deferred to older ages—in so-called elderly primigravida or nullipara—have long been an obstetrical bugbear. It now begins to emerge, in this circumstance as in others, that different risks attach to specific developmental stages (Stein and Susser 1980). Thus, with first pregnancies, the risks may differ by stage, as in the periconception period, before a conception has become viable, and after viability is attained. For instance, in older women, conception delay is a periconceptional outcome no more common with first than with later pregnancies (Stein 1985). For some outcomes of viable pregnancies, however, the combination of a first pregnancy with age does exaggerate risk.

Adverse outcomes after the conceptus becomes viable—namely, stillbirth (or late fetal death), premature delivery, intrauterine growth retardation, perinatal death, and congenital malformation—are the focus of the traditional concerns of obstetricians about the risks of pregnancy in older women. The considerable literature (reviewed by Nortman 1974) sows confusion and reaps confounding. Although the effects of aging on reproduction were remarkable and consistent in the experimental studies reviewed, the effects of gravidity, as tested by the deferral of mating till later ages, were demonstrable in some studies but not in others. In studies of maternal age and gravidity in human beings, confounding of one factor by the other tends to have been insufficiently controlled. Epidemiological studies are generally compatible with experimental ones, however, in that age overshadows gravidity as a factor in reproduction.

Some of the analytic deficiencies have been repaired in more recent epidemiological analyses. At the same time, pregnancy outcome has improved overall as new methods and standards have been adopted in obstetric practice. Findings that depart from past expectations might thus be attributed in part to the sophistication of statistical analysis, in part to the sophistication of obstetric practice, and perhaps to both.

In an analysis of perinatal outcome in all New York City births for the years 1976 to 1978, adjustments were made for several confounding factors such as public or private medical care, ethnicity and race, maternal education, marital state, and previous reproductive loss (Kiely et al. 1986). For low birth weight (<2500 grams), stillbirths, and neonatal mortality, overall results were much as expected: women of 35 years and more had higher risks than younger women, and women bearing their first child were also at higher risk than those who had borne other children. Essentially similar findings for each of these outcomes have been reported for births in Sweden between 1976 and 1980. In addition, in Sweden older women were found to be at greater risk for bearing very large infants (>4500 grams) (Forman et al. 1984). It can be no surprise to obstetricians that the risks of age and parity, being additive, were considerable for a first delivery in an older woman.

More detailed analysis, however, requires some revision of received views. In New York City, age and parity affected outcome differently in the prepartum, intrapartum, and newborn periods. We consider *stillbirths* first. Stillbirths that occurred before the onset of labor (prepartum) were separated from stillbirths that occurred during labor (intrapartum).[1] With prepartum stillbirths, maternal age alone carried an excess risk; parity did not. With intrapartum stillbirths, the risks with age and parity were reversed: maternal age did not add to risk but parity did, especially nulliparity and high parity (≥4 births).

These findings seem open to the eminently reasonable interpretation

[1]Stillbirths included all births after 24 completed weeks of gestation that showed no signs of life at delivery.

that age is a key factor in a woman's capacity to sustain the gestation of the developing organism, as appears to be the case in miscarriages as well. Likewise the experience and trial of previous delivery appear as a key factor in successful parturition. In the past, however, it was an article of faith among obstetricians that older women carried a high risk of intrapartum fetal death because of their age. If that was indeed so, as seems likely, we may infer that the problems specific to older women that caused the high risks have been largely overcome. As yet, no comparable analyses exist that could confirm or disprove the point. At this time, it seems that the raised risks of intrapartum stillbirths inhere in parity alone, and those of prepartum stillbirths inhere in age alone.

Although no other study has reported analyses exactly comparable with this New York City study (types of stillbirths have not generally been separated and analytic control has been less systematic) some supportive results exist. In large-scale Swedish data, antepartum fetal death in particular has been associated with older maternal age in both primigravidae and multigravidae (Forman et al. 1984). In several U.S. studies, undifferentiated late fetal death was also associated with maternal age (Israel and Deutschberger 1964; Kane 1967). Since by far the greater part of late fetal loss in the developed world is now antepartum, these various American results are in general conformity with those in New York City and Sweden.

With *neonatal mortality*, the patterns of risk with age and with parity in New York City are again distinct. The risks with age are of the same general pattern as those for intrapartum stillbirths: older women have no overall excess risk of neonatal deaths, and nulliparity does carry an excess risk. Again, it is reasonable to suppose that previous experience of delivery alleviates risk, but this is probably not the case since low birth weight is a major intervening factor that originates before delivery (Kiely et al. 1986). Another difference from intrapartum deaths is seen here in joint effects of age and parity for neonatal mortality: among nulliparae, older women carry a higher risk than younger women, and the combined risk for older age and nulliparity is greater than their sum. In New York City, the effect of age on neonatal mortality is confined to the first hour of life and mediated almost entirely by low birth weight. The findings in Sweden are again in conformity in that nulliparae have slightly, though not significantly, higher risks at older than at younger ages. It is of interest also that multigravidae had lower risks at older than at younger ages. The Swedish data for nulliparae and multiparae, taken together, suggest favorable circumstances for parturition at older ages consistent with the generally favorable circumstances for health and health care in that society (Forman et al. 1984).

With regard to maternal mortality, this formidable and preventable problem is largely one of the less developed world (Chapter 16). With respect to age, the available data for the less developed world show that the risks are highest for the very young and the very old. In the developed world today, death in childbirth is extremely rare. The small mortality risk that remains relates strongly to maternal age: women of 35 years and older have a risk fourfold higher than that of younger women, and women 40 years and older have a risk that is higher still. Uterine hemorrhage, embolism, and hypertension are the factors most commonly found in maternal deaths.

CONCLUSION: REPRODUCTION AT OLDER AGES

To summarize the findings on reproduction at later maternal ages, the marked changes with age in fertility and miscarriage can be interpreted in terms of at least three separate elements—infecundability, chromosomally normal loss, and trisomies. All of these components become prominent by the late 30s and early 40s, although the steep rise in the frequency of trisomies begins earlier.

In general, the available evidence points to different processes underlying the several outcomes associated with age. It is not entirely out of the question that the processes underlying these outcomes, especially reduced fecundability and chromosomally normal loss, could flow from a single controlling factor. One candidate for the controlling role is follicular endocrine activity. Yet, if endocrine derangement in the follicles does underlie infecundability, the derangement is not accompanied by other unfavorable outcomes that might then be anticipated. For example, if miscarriages and conception delay result from the same process, the association to be expected between them is not apparent. Among women who have either chromosomally normal or aberrant miscarriages, the time to conception is similar to that among age-matched women who have successful pregnancies (Stein 1985). Nor does it appear that pregnancies lost so early that they can be recognized solely by biochemical tests contribute to the appearance of conception delay (Wilcox et al. 1988).

Miscarriage, too, whether chromosomally normal or trisomic, is unlikely to be the controlling factor that limits reproduction at older ages. Although there is no doubt that reproductive loss through miscarriage in the first half of pregnancy contributes substantially to infertility at later ages, infecundability takes on increasing importance until it becomes an insuperable impediment to female reproduction. In the late fetal and perinatal phases, a single pathogenetic mechanism such as uterine dysfunction might perhaps account for the role of maternal age in raising the risk of both prepartum stillbirths and chromosomally normal miscarriages. The same mechanism might also be invoked for neonatal deaths, and for the low birth weight which in turn moderates most neonatal deaths at all maternal ages.

In the intrapartum phase, superior obstetric care may well have suppressed or alleviated the maternal age factor in stillbirths. Comparisons over time and between countries suggest that a substantial reduction in intrapartum stillbirth rates has taken place as obstetrics has become increasingly proficient (Kiely 1983). Presumably obstetricians have dealt less successfully with the risks of nulliparity and grandimultiparity in intrapartum stillbirths. In newborn deaths, the role of parity, like that of maternal age, is largely accounted for by the lower birth weights it engenders (Chapter 14). Few means of remedying deficiencies in birth weight are available, although some preventable factors have been discovered.

Notwithstanding the increased risk, at later ages, for maternal deaths, prepartum stillbirths, and newborn deaths, older women in the developed world can proceed confidently with childbearing. Not only has the excess risk with age for intrapartum stillbirths apparently been eliminated, but virtually all other risks have been sharply reduced. Prenatal screening for karyotype and serum alpha-protein can forewarn and forearm the older woman against the risk of births with Down's syndrome and neural tube defects. Infants of older women, especially at ages over 40 years, remain somewhat more prone to certain anomalies of heart and central nervous system not discussed here (Nortman 1974; National Center for Health Statistics 1978; Goldberg et al. 1979), but these are rare.

PREGNANCY IN YOUTH

Fecundability

The menarche marks the end of puberty in girls. In theory, menstruation signifies fecundability, although the optimal age for reproduction is not yet attained. The mean age of menarche has changed over time and also differs between and within groups. Presumably fecundability varies in the same fashion. In Europe, from the mid-nineteenth century into the mid-twentieth century, the age at menarche decreased by about 4 months for every decade, although recently that trend has halted (Eveleth and Tanner 1976; Helm and Helm 1984; Dann and Roberts 1984). The trend to precocity coincided with improved socioeconomic and nutritional conditions. Geographic variations likewise relate to social conditions. Within populations in which social class differences have been found, the gradients for mean age at menarche are consistent with good or bad conditions for precocity or delay, respectively.

The onset of the menarche relates to individual growth. In line with this, a steady increase in growth (as indicated by height) accompanied the secular trend toward earlier menarche. Some investigators, indeed, hold that the menarche supervenes only when a growth threshold is crossed; this threshold, it has been supposed, relates to stored body fat (Frisch et al. 1973). In any event, childhood nutrition is a plausible factor that might influence the age of onset of the menarche, and current nutrition is certainly a factor in continuing menstruation. Thus, the age of menarche, a biological phenomenon that is the precondition of fecundability, is itself partly conditioned by environmental factors.

Neither in a social nor in a biological sense does the menarche closely predict age at first pregnancy. Fecundability is likely to be at a low level in the immediate postmenarcheal phase. In these early years, menstrual cycles are typically widely spaced or irregular, sparse in flow, and occasionally anovular (Treloar et al. 1967a). Nonetheless, conception is a possibility, and the menarche obviously sets the lower limits for the age at which a child can be conceived.

Births

Over and above the biological age limits of childbearing, the pattern—including age at first pregnancy—always has been profoundly influenced by social and cultural forces. In the developed world today, and often in the less developed world, childbearing at very early ages occurs under adverse social conditions. Social adversity is a complex of elements that can be disentangled, if at all, only by special effort. With youthful childbearing, the unraveling of the biological from the social origins of reproductive outcomes by statistical analysis is a task not yet accomplished. Evidence of adverse effects on pregnancy that can be attributed, in a strictly biological sense, to the youth of the mother is scant, ambiguous and inconsistent. Pregnancies in the very young (below 15 years) seem to be associated with excess perinatal risk mediated through low birth weight and preterm delivery. With regard to intra-uterine growth, the nutrition of the very young woman must provide for the demands of the pregnancy in competition with those of her own growth. Optimal nutrition must satisfy both and enable the woman to gain weight and store nutrients in the form of fat during the first phase of pregnancy. It has been proposed, and some data have supported the proposal, that the demands of the woman are paramount. Unless these dual energy needs are met, the growth of the fetus may suffer. Results for second births to very young women are notably poor; such pregnancies could further accentuate the demands on the young mother. Other hypotheses point to the immaturity of the pelvic outlet as an impediment to parturition.

In regard to reproductive risks for teenagers, several outcomes for which the crude rates are higher in teenagers have been considered separately. They include hypertension of pregnancy, anemia, cephalo-pelvic disproportion, birth weight, gestational age, and perinatal and neonatal mortality. None provides good evidence for biological effects peculiar to youth (Strobino 1987). Indeed, in the later teenage years, such data as permit a biological interpretation generally indicate reproductive performance that matches, and in some countries excels, that at older ages. Residual suspicion falls on only the very youngest ages.

The strongest test so far is provided by an analysis of neonatal mortality, most of which is mediated through low birth weight. To study these outcomes at the earliest ages, large populations are needed. In the United States, for the year 1983, the national data were analyzed for low birth weight (<2500 grams). In a total of nearly 3 million births, girls under 15 years of age who bore children numbered 891 blacks and 428 whites. Thus, despite the large national population, numbers were suitable for finegrained analysis—by single years of age, separately for blacks and whites—only at ages 15 to 19 years (National Center for Health Statistics 1986). In a different analysis (Geronimus 1986), neonatal mortality in three states was combined for the four years 1976 to 1979. For both low birth weight and neonatal mortality among mothers in their teens, the risks improve progressively from the youngest to the oldest. (In Table 17-3, the measure used is the ratio of the rate for a given age to the rate at the optimal ages, around 25 years.) Much of the disadvantage of the young is social. Maternal education and rural/urban residence account for part of the risk. Maternal size also accounts for a substantial part of the risk. Although height and weight are unquestionably biological, the sources of their variation are not. Both genetic and

Table 17–3 Low birth weight[a] and neonatal mortality[b] among teenage mothers: rate ratios[c] (compared to optimal ages) for whites and blacks, separately

Maternal age	Whites		Blacks	
	Low birth weight	Neonatal mortality	Low birth weight	Neonatal mortality
11–13	—	2.5	—	2.0
14	—	3.8	—	1.5
<15	2.2	—	1.3	—
15	1.8	2.0	1.2	1.1
16	1.8	2.3	1.2	1.0
17	1.6	1.6	1.2	0.9
18	1.5	1.4	1.2	0.9
19	1.4	1.2	1.1	0.8

[a]Less than 2500 grams as a percentage of all live births ($n = 2,923,502$) in the United States, 1983. *Source*: National Center for Health Statistics, 1986.

[b]First births, 1976–1979, Louisiana, Washington, and Tennessee ($n = 305,000$ births). *Source*: Geronimus, 1986.

[c]Reference groups: Low birth weight at ages 25 to 29 years (whites, 5 per cent; blacks, 11.7 per cent). Neonatal mortality at ages 24 to 26 years (whites, 6.1 per 1000; blacks 16.5 per 1000).

social factors contribute to variation in maternal size. Inheritance demonstrably affects individual variation; the social conditions of rearing demonstrably affect group variation. In any event, when education, residence, height and weight are controlled, no uniform pattern of risks for youthful childbearing persists (e.g. Geronimus 1986).

Naturally, the absence of a demonstrable effect unique to biological age does not diminish the importance of the social risk for teenage mothers. This social risk differs in character for different social groups. High relative risks and small numbers among white teenagers (compared to their elders) are balanced by lower relative risks and larger numbers among black teenagers. These differences suggest a two-pronged divergence: in the relative terms of risk, the social factors at work depart further from the norm and hence are more adverse for whites than for blacks, but in absolute terms teenage births among blacks outnumber those among whites.

Chromosome Aberrations

Evidence relating young maternal age to chromosome aberrations is sparse and inconsistent. There has been the suggestion of an increase in hydatidiform mole and Down's syndrome in women under 20 years, and monosomy X has been associated with a decrease in mean maternal age in some samples.

The prevalence of complete hydatidiform moles appears to be raised among women under age 20 years, as well as among women 40 years and older (Yen and MacMahon 1968; Hayashi et al. 1982; Matsura et al. 1984). A complete mole seems to result if an egg does not contribute chromosomes to the conceptus when fertilized by a haploid sperm; the chromosomes of the sperm subsequently double to produce a 46 XX karyotype. The prevalence of Down's syndrome births may also be raised, though only slightly, among women under 20 years; findings are inconsistent and samples are often too small to assess the presence of an effect (reviewed in Hook 1981b).

Monosomy X among miscarriages has been strongly associated with younger maternal ages in some settings, but not in others. This inconstancy is not likely to be accounted for by inconsistent or flawed methods. The findings suggest an environmental factor correlated with youth that is active only in some locations. In Geneva and New York City, mean maternal age for monosomy X miscarriages is, on average, 2 to 4 years younger than for live births (Kajii and Ohama 1979; Warburton et al. 1980b, 1986). In those monosomies that survive to birth in the form of Turner's syndrome, maternal age is also somewhat low (Carothers et al. 1980). In Hiroshima and Honolulu, on the other hand, the average maternal age in miscarriages with monosomy X was similar to that in births (Kajii and Omaha 1979; Hassold and Chiu 1985). In other studies

(Lazar et al. 1973; Lauritsen 1976; Creasy et al. 1976), the absence of an association between young maternal age and monosomy X miscarriage is not easy to discount, because chromosomally normal miscarriages were used for comparison. Since the maternal age of chromosomally normal miscarriages is raised, the result should be biased toward enhancing an association with young maternal age.

The inconstancy of the maternal age association may reflect differences between populations in the proportions of cases resulting from the absence of a maternal sex chromosome, on the one hand, and that of a paternal sex chromosome on the other. In Honolulu the parental origin of the X chromosome could be established by molecular analysis in 27 monosomy X miscarriages. In the six cases (22 per cent) in which the X chromosome was paternal in origin, mean maternal age was significantly less than in the 21 cases in which it was maternal. Thus, the association with younger maternal age may be confined to cases with an absent maternal X chromosome (Hassold et al. 1988). If this relation is constant across populations, then the proportion of cases due to an absent maternal X chromosome may be higher in samples in which monosomy X is associated with younger age than in those in which it is not.

Environmental factors might influence the incidence of monosomy X with either an absent maternal or paternal sex chromosome, and so produce variations in relative frequencies and in mean maternal age between populations. Two observations in the New York City miscarriage study are compatible with the notion that environmental factors, rather than young age per se, may underly associations with maternal age. First, the association was not with an absolute measure of youth, but was relative to the mean age for a given social stratum. Thus, the shift toward younger maternal age was of the same size in private and public patients even though the average age of private patients is about 5 years older than that of public patients (Warburton et al. 1986). Second, among miscarriages with monosomy X, paternal age was raised (Hatch 1985). Possibly, therefore, a large difference between maternal and paternal ages is an underlying factor in the monosomy X condition. Whatever the explanation, the strong but inconsistent associations suggest a localized environmental factor.

CONCLUSION

In conclusion, maternal age as a factor in reproduction must be seen in social context to be fully understood. In less developed countries, social disadvantage is widespread, and often concentrated in very young mothers and in older mothers of high parity. In more developed countries, very young mothers are also almost invariably at a social disadvantage.

Older mothers, by contrast—especially those who begin childbearing at a late age—are often relatively privileged. Social advantage and disadvantage are invariably connected with many factors such as diet, work, infections, and access to care.

Hence, social and biological factors are closely interwoven in the reproductive manifestations of both age and parity, and they are not uniform across the world or across any single society. Overall, in the developed world adverse outcomes with youthful pregnancies relate primarily to social rather than biological factors: biological advantage balances social disadvantage. Adverse outcomes in the pregnancies of older women exhibit the converse: social advantage balances biological disadvantage. The fifth decade is a significant transitional phase of life for women. Reproductive senescence is accompanied by other functional changes related to the hypothalamic–pituitary–ovarian axis, such as bone loss and a hormonal balance slowly tilting toward the androgens and virilization. Yet by the standards of a developed society, women in their early 40s are young. It is not impossible that technical and social means can be found to palliate or circumvent the obstacles to reproduction in older women. We have seen that, under good circumstances, the risks of parturition at older ages are largely eliminated. The risk at birth of chromosomal aberrations at older ages can be detected and avoided in a majority of cases. Finally, the postulated connections of endocrine and uterine dysfunction to infecundability and miscarriage point the way to possible interventions in the future.

18 Aging and Reproduction: II. Trisomy

In public health, scientific issues assume significance not only for the degree to which they are fundamental to the prevention and cure of health disorders, but equally for the scale of their impact on people's lives. By both standards, trisomies outweigh other chromosomal aberrations, and the trisomy of chromosome 21 outweighs other trisomies. The supernumerary chromosome that characterizes the trisomic karyotype can originate in any one of the 23 pairs, but in clinically recognized pregnancies it does not do so equally. At birth, trisomies of chromosome 21 and the sex chromosomes are the most frequent and trisomies 13 and 18 appear; all are rare (reviewed by Bond and Chandley 1983). At miscarriage, the five most frequent, in descending order, are trisomies 16, 22, 21, 15 and 13 (Hassold et al. 1984b).

The displacement of the chromosome that produces trisomy can arise, in theory, at any stage of meiosis in the germ cells of either parent. In the maternal germ cell, the extra chromosome could be acquired either before conception, at some time in the extended course of the first chromosomal division (meiosis I), or at the time of conception during the brief course of the second division (meiosis II). In the paternal germ cell, also, the additional chromosome could be acquired at meiosis I or II, but meiosis I is completed over a much shorter period, and meiosis II is completed well before fertilization. The possibility has also been raised that the displacement could arise after conception, with the chromosomal separation occurring during mitosis as the zygote begins to divide (Ford and Roberts 1983).

The phase of meiosis in which the chromosomal displacement occurs can sometimes be determined from the maternal or paternal origin of the extra chromosome. This origin can be inferred from careful study of morphological features of the chromosome specific to some individuals and transmitted from parent to child. Such polymorphisms can be recognized in the karyotypes of dividing somatic cells examined during the metaphase of mitosis. The parental source of a chromosome is marked by visible and distinctive polymorphisms that are shared by the affected offspring and one of the parents.

Assignments of parental origin have depended mainly on judgments about what is observed under the microscope. Experience of observer error in many fields tells us that, among laboratories, judgments differ in reliability and validity. Moreover, the cytogenetic method does not succeed in all cases. More recently cytogenetics has been supplemented by molecular genetics. DNA probes determine the identity in parent and child of the nuclear material of the chromosomes comprising the trisomy. Although not many cases have yet been studied, DNA probes will apparently be able to establish identity in a larger proportion of cases than polymorphisms do. At the time of writing, no series has been large enough to challenge the distribution of the parental origins of trisomies based on cytogenetic study. Combining cytogenetic and molecular techniques is likely to yield virtually complete assignment (Stewart et al. 1988).

The ability to assign a parental origin to the extra chromosome in trisomies has led to the revision of some longstanding assumptions. In particular, the strong association of Down's syndrome with maternal age seemed to exclude a paternal source. Cytogenetic studies (and the few molecular studies)—albeit selectively sampled and with the observer not necessarily blind to which parental karyotype was being examined— indicate that the source of trisomies is certainly not exclusively maternal. In clinically recognized pregnancies, about 80 per cent of the trisomies of chromosome 21 have a maternal source. According to studies of polymorphisms (which may be incompletely informative on this point), some 70 per cent arise at the first maternal meiosis and about 10 per cent at the second maternal meiosis. The 20 per cent with a paternal source seem more evenly divided between first and second meiosis (13 per cent versus 7 per cent, respectively; Hassold et al. 1984a). For other trisomies, to an even greater extent than with trisomy 21, the predominant source is the first maternal meiosis. Although far fewer than for trisomy 21 births, reports from observations at miscarriage exist for trisomies 3, 4, 9, 13–15, 16, 21, and 22 (Hassold et al. 1984a).

Although these direct observations have modified our ideas of parental origin of trisomies (and hence of the etiology), they leave unchallenged the maternal predominance first inferred from the link of trisomy 21 to maternal age. Epidemiological studies of karyotyped miscarriages corroborate this link for several other trisomies, although not for all. The distributions of trisomies by maternal age seen in collections of miscarriages from New York City and Honolulu (Hassold et al. 1984b; Hassold and Chiu 1985; Risch et al. 1986) permit some statements to be made.

First, maternal age effects were not the same for all trisomies: at older ages, the steepness of the rise in frequency varied with the particular

Table 18–1 Maternal age and trisomy: mean maternal age of trisomic and chromosomally normal miscarriages and of live births in New York City and Honolulu

Trisomy	New York City	Honolulu	Combined	Difference compared to births
2	28.3 (24)	28.6 (23)	28.5	2.5
3	23.0 (1)	28.1 (9)	27.6	1.6
4	25.5 (10)	27.0 (24)	26.5	0.5
5	23.0 (2)	25.8 (4)	24.8	−1.2
6	27.0 (1)	25.4 (11)	25.5	−0.5
7	32.4 (18)	28.2 (17)	30.3	4.3
8	25.8 (10)	26.9 (21)	26.6	0.6
9	25.2 (12)	34.1 (17)	30.4	4.4
10	34.5 (6)	29.0 (10)	31.1	5.1
11	———	32.0 (2)	32.0	6.0
12	———	25.9 (7)	25.9	−0.1
13	30.7 (26)	31.6 (26)	31.1	5.1
14	32.1 (16)	30.5 (15)	31.3	5.3
15	31.4 (28)	32.4 (33)	31.9	5.9
16	28.9 (115)	30.0 (184)	29.5	3.5
17	34.0 (2)	29.0 (4)	30.7	4.7
18	32.8 (17)	32.8 (20)	32.3	6.3
20	34.8 (13)	34.0 (14)	34.4	8.4
21	32.9 (37)	29.3 (55)	30.7	4.7
22	34.4 (29)	32.0 (79)	32.7	6.7
Total	30.5 (367)	30.1 (575)	30.3	
Chromosomally normal	27.0 (1307)	27.1 (1134)	27.0	
Live births	26.0 (37,776)	25.9 (15,408)	26.0	

Source: Data from Hassold et al., 1984b.

chromosome or group of chromosomes. It appears that the smaller the chromosome[1] involved in the trisomy, the higher the mean maternal age tends to be (Table 18-1) (Hassold et al. 1984b). The pattern also holds for most of those autosomal trisomies seen only at miscarriage, as well as for the few (13, 18, 21) seen at birth.

Chromosome size can be grouped into three broad classes: small (13–22), intermediate (6–12), and large (2–5). Figure 18-1, based on New York City data (Risch et al. 1986), shows the shape of the frequency curves for the most numerous autosomal trisomies. Among trisomies of the small class (excepting trisomies 13 and 16), the rise in frequency with maternal age tends to be steep after age 30. With trisomy 16, the rise in frequency with age is slow and steady; with trisomy 13 the rise is steady

---

[1]The chromosome numbering system was founded on the ranking of chromosomes according to size. Higher numbers designate smaller chromosomes. As data have accumulated, the fit between designated number and size has not turned out to be quite perfect.

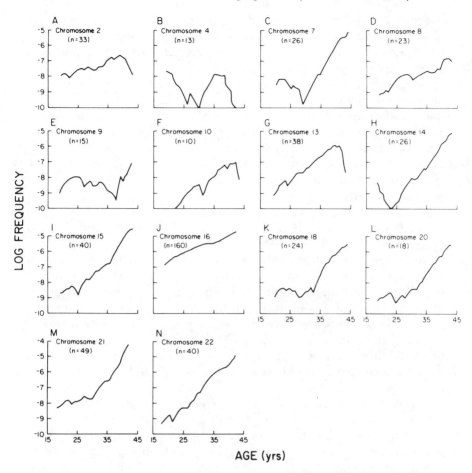

Fig. 18–1 Estimated frequency of trisomic miscarriages and maternal age for several individual chromosomes (log^e frequency smoothed). (From Risch et al. 1986)

until age 40 and then declines. Among trisomies of the intermediate class, the relationships to maternal age are more variable. For most the mean maternal age is raised, and the slope of the increase with age is similar before and after the age of 30 years. Among trisomies of the large class, no relation to maternal age is evident.

It follows from these age relations that chromosome size relates to the distribution of trisomies between younger and older maternal ages (Hassold and Chiu 1985; Risch et al. 1986). In the New York City study, individual trisomies were examined for evidence of discontinuity in the patterns of increase with age. These discontinuities were taken as grounds for the existence of an age-independent class, the size of which could then be estimated. A constant rate of change between successive maternal ages, as in trisomy 16, produces a constant slope; such a curve suggests age-dependence with no suggestion of an age-independent class. A slow or absent rise in frequency at younger maternal ages and a rapid rise at later ages, as in trisomy 21, produces a discontinuous slope; such a curve suggests the existence of an age-independent as well as an age-dependent class. Penrose's postulate of two classes for trisomy 21— frequency being dependent on maternal age in one and age-independent in the other (Penrose 1933)—predated the visualization of karyotypes. From the existence of this age-independent class, he deduced that inherited forms of the syndrome would be found, a deduction since amply confirmed. The known inherited forms, however, are translocations and constitute only a small part of the age-independent class, not all of it as he had surmised.

It is evident that in karyotyped miscarriages, age-independence of trisomies emerges in the same manner as for Down's syndrome at birth (Risch et al. 1986). The size of the postulated class varies with the specific chromosome involved. For 14 trisomies, numbers were sufficient to analyze maternal age relations statistically as well as by inspection of the frequency curves. In a group of six mostly small trisomies (7, 14, 15, 18, 20, 21), the slope of the maternal age curve appeared to be discontinuous above and below 30 years of age; these suggest age-independent classes of substantial size (perhaps 30 to 40 per cent). In another group of six trisomies mixed in size (2, 8, 10, 13, 16, 22), the slope of the maternal age curves appeared to be continuous and increasing above and below 30 years of age: these provide no grounds for the existence of an age-independent class. For the remaining two trisomies (4, 9) the slopes displayed no coherent relationship to maternal age.

The differences between trisomies of different chromosomes in relation to maternal age suggests heterogeneity in the mechanisms of origin. Insofar as maternal age patterns are similar for trisomies of chromosomes when grouped by size, or by the position of the centromere, attention is turned to mechanisms particular to the physical configuration of the individual chromosome affected. Divergences in the patterns of age relations for trisomies of chromosomes within a single group (i.e., they are of similar size and centromere position) may point to even greater heterogeneity in mechanisms. Indeed, the causes of trisomies of an individual chromosome, such as 21, may be heterogeneous. Thus, the data described above indicate that Penrose's postulate for trisomy 21 of an admixture of maternal age-dependent and age-independent classes can reasonably be extended to several other trisomies.

Trisomies of the sex chromosomes behave in a manner distinct from the trisomies of many autosomes, and they also differ among themselves in their frequencies and in the lethality and severity of their effects. Those that survive to birth provide most maternal age data; at miscarriage, the numbers with sex chromosome trisomies are too few to be informative. At birth, sex chromosome trisomies are relatively common and harbinger milder impairments and disabilities than most other trisomies. Trisomies with an extra X chromosome—all 47 XXX and an unknown fraction of 47 XXY—conform with the overall trisomy pattern of raised maternal age (Court-Brown et al. 1969; Carothers et al. 1978). Y chromosomes are the smallest of all, and yet sex chromosome trisomies with an added Y chromosome (47XYY) have not been associated with older maternal age (Court-Brown et al. 1969; Carothers et al. 1978; Robinson et al. 1979).

MOSAICISM

A mosaic trisomy occurs when different cell lines coexist in the same individual. In the usual mosaic form, one line is trisomic and one is normal. It seems likely that mosaicism generally originates as a non-mosaic form of trisomy and that, in the course of development, some trisomic cell lines are shed in favor of normal cell lines.

Mosaicism occurs more often in nonacrocentric[2] trisomies, virtually all of which end in miscarriage, than in acrocentric trisomies, some of which survive to birth. Hence, mosaicism occurs much more frequently among trisomies at miscarriage than at birth. At miscarriage mosaicism is found in 5 to 8 per cent of all trisomies (Creasy et al. 1976; Warburton et al. 1978; Hassold 1982); in Down's syndrome at birth, mosaicism is found in 1 to 2 per cent (Mikkelsen 1977). The frequency of mosaicism is similar among acrocentric trisomies at miscarriage and at birth (Stene and Warburton 1981; Hassold 1982).

As noted, the origin of mosaicism could be either in a primordial trisomic zygote, or in a chromosomally normal zygote later transmuted at mitosis. Mean maternal age in mosaic trisomies at miscarriage, however, resembles mean maternal age in the complete trisomies (Creasy 1977; Warburton et al. 1978; Hassold 1982b). This resemblance between mosaic and complete trisomies, with their common divergence from chromosomally normal losses, points to the origin of mosaicism in a zygote that is initially trisomic. Cytogenetic studies support the notion that mosaics result from postconception changes in complete trisomies: in at least five trisomy mosaics in which the point was explored, it was deduced that the extra chromosome in the trisomic cell lines had arisen during meiosis (Niikawa et al. 1977; Hassold 1982b, 1984a).

PATERNAL AGE

Whether or not paternal age relates to trisomy is a question that has not been finally settled. An association of paternal age with trisomy 21,

---

[2]In an acrocentric chromosome (13–15, 21–22), but not in others, the centromere is located off-center.

strong at first sight, more often than not vanishes with adjustment for the effects of maternal age. Once this was demonstrated in the early 1930s (Penrose 1933; Jenkins 1933), the question was not again seriously considered for almost half a century (Erickson 1978). New interest in a paternal role was provoked by the discovery that in about 20 per cent of instances of Down's syndrome, the additional chromosome 21 was paternal in origin. Material stemming from live births, prenatal diagnostic karyotypes, and miscarriages has become available to pursue this point.

The fact that a minority of trisomies are paternal in origin (reviewed in Juberg and Mowrey 1983; Hassold et al. 1984a) could reflect restricted opportunities for paternal factors to influence the formation of trisomies. In male germ cells, we noted, meiosis does not begin until puberty. Factors that might affect meiotic divisions and produce trisomies through nondisjunction are thus unlikely to be effective before puberty. Thus, other relevant effects of aging in the male, such as less frequent intercourse, might need to be taken into account. Such factors could bear on the theories, discussed later, that relate trisomy formation to the interval between ovulation and fertilization (e.g., German 1968; Jongbloet 1971).

Paternal age in the populations of developed countries and in most monogamous societies, although usually a few years greater than maternal age, is closely bound with it. On statistical analysis, maternal age always has had a distinctly more robust association with Down's syndrome than paternal age. To separate the effects of paternal and maternal age, and thus elucidate the unique role of paternal age, involves logical as well as statistical questions. Maternal age retains the more plausible role in theory, since the extra chromosome appears to be maternal in some 80 per cent of cases. It is therefore logical, in searching for an effect of paternal age over and above that of maternal age, to adjust for the effects of maternal age; the overlap between maternal and paternal effects is thereby allocated to maternal age. In the absence of a residual effect of paternal age, this logic leads to the conclusion that paternal age has no effect independent of maternal age, despite the one case in five with a paternal origin.

Because of the steep rise in trisomy 21 with maternal age beyond the age of 35 years and the strong tie between maternal and paternal age, meticulous analytic control is needed to evaluate paternal age effects. When 5-year maternal age intervals have been used (numbers often being too small to support adjustment in single years) positive associations between trisomy 21 and paternal age have sometimes emerged (Erickson 1978; Lamson et al. 1980). When more refined single-year maternal age intervals have been used, statistically significant associations with paternal age have usually not been found (Sigler et al. 1965b; Cohen et al. 1977; Erickson 1978, 1979; Erickson and Bjerkedal 1981; Regal et al. 1980; Hook et al. 1981; Hook and Cross 1982; Roth et al.

1983; Ferguson-Smith and Yates 1984). With one exception in an amniocentesis study (Stene et al. 1981), null results persist when the focus is on "older" fathers. Most studies leave room for an increase in risk of trisomy 21 of up to 1 per cent for each year of paternal age.

Tests for paternal age effects can be broadened by drawing on the large array of trisomies seen at miscarriage (Lauritsen 1976; Hassold et al. 1980a). Among these, only the New York City study (Hatch 1983) controlled for maternal age. Although in a first phase of that study higher paternal age was associated with trisomy at miscarriage in young women, in the later phases the result was not replicated. It is clear, from all studies taken together, that no substantial effect of paternal age on trisomy should be expected.

THEORIES ABOUT MATERNAL AGE

Several hypotheses have been advanced to explain the maternal age association of trisomies (see Polani 1981; Bond and Chandley 1983; Hassold and Jacobs 1984). The process is often described as nondisjunction: namely, the failure of homologous chromosomes at meiosis to pair or to remain paired. A "weathering" theory postulates structural changes in the chromosomes of the oocyte as it matures, since decades of exposure to life experience pass between the fetal stage of oogenesis, when the first meiotic division begins, and ovulation, when it is completed. Opportunities have been seen by some for the action of such environmental factors as irradiation (Alberman et al. 1972a,b). One postulate (Penrose 1965) was that during this long interval decay might affect the spindle, a key structure in meiosis. Another postulated mechanism for weathering involves the nucleolus of small acrocentric chromosomes (Polani et al. 1960); the findings reported earlier on the maternal age relations of trisomies at miscarriage, not all of which are acrocentric, put this out of court as a general explanation.

Another hypothesis—the "production line" theory—places the original karyotypic error early, in the fetal stage of development when the oocytes are laid down. Those oocytes laid down last, it is suggested, are the most vulnerable to nondisjunction and also the last to be selected for ovulation in the mature female (Henderson and Edwards 1968). The later an oocyte is laid down, so the theory goes, the fewer are the chiasmata that bridge and bind together chromosome pairs, and thus, the greater the likelihood of univalent pairs being formed.

One strut of the theory—last in, last out—proved congruent with recent experiments in mice: the oocytes that were latest to enter meiosis in the female fetus were also latest to ovulate in the mature female (Polani and Crolla 1989). The second strut—that chiasmata are fewer in oocytes laid down late in fetal development—is compatible with some but not all experiments (Speed 1977; Speed and Chandley 1983). An apparent depletion of chiasmata typified oocytes in older mice, as predicted by the theory; also, when chiasmata were fewer, univalent or unpaired chromosomes were more common, especially among the smaller chromosomes (Henderson and Edwards 1968; Polani and Jagiello 1976). It remains to be shown that univalent chromosomes are the predecessors of disomic ova and hence of trisomy in the zygote. Some experiments argue against such a connection (Polani and Jagiello 1976; Speed 1977).

Two mechanisms, asynapsis and desynapsis, have been advanced as the possible basis for the production line theory. With asynapsis, the lack of binding chiasmata might fail to align the homologous pairs. With desynapsis, already paired chromosomes with fewer bonds might be predisposed to precocious separation, displacement, and disomy when the members of each pair draw apart during the first meiotic division. Small chromosomes are supposedly more at risk than large ones, because they have few chiasmata to begin with.

A failure of some kind at the synapsis of chromosome pairs has been reported in Down's syndrome (Warren et al. 1987). In individuals with Down's syndrome, the particular supernumerary chromosome 21 involved had fewer of the recombinations of genetic material that occur during pairing than either of the two members of the chromosome 21 pair that should normally have been present. Recombinations were also fewer than in the members of the chromosome 21 pairs of the mother and unaffected kin of the affected person. The deficiency of recombinations in the supernumerary chromosome, it was suggested, might result from a deficiency of chiasmata and hence of crossovers from one member of a chromosome 21 pair to the other.

Another class of hypotheses postulates that hormonal deficiency induces premature senescence in the reproductive process (e.g., Rundle et al. 1961; Crowley et al. 1979). Here a link between Down's syndrome and Turner's syndrome can be cited in support. Turner's syndrome is the expression of the 45XO monosomy or its mosaic form, and gonadal dysgenesis is a feature of the phenotype. Low fertility and early reproductive senescence are the consequence. A search of world literature yielded a collection of 25 women with the syndrome; between them they had had 58 pregnancies resulting in 35 births (Reyes et al. 1976; King et al. 1978). Although none of the pregnancies was conceived at an age later than 31 years, 3 infants of the 35 had Down's syndrome. In such collected reports of remarkable conjunctions, reporting bias is always an uncomfortable presence. This Down's syndrome frequency is nonetheless high enough to justify a hypothesis.

None of these theories comfortably and generally accommodates recent human data. Figure 18-1 alone is salutary. As discussed previously, different trisomies begin to rise in frequency at different maternal ages;

accordingly no single underlying disorder acting at some modal age can explain all trisomies. Second, the patterns of maternal age relations in trisomies do not accord in any straightforward way with the age effects in the better understood endocrine and physiological functions. With trisomy 21 taken alone, endocrine aging accords somewhat better than for all trisomies together.

Some theories about causes of trisomy lend themselves to testing and representation by epidemiological modeling. One of these (German 1962) is that ova that give rise to trisomy 21 are "overripe," having persisted unfertilized longer than usual, and that such ova are more open to fertilization in older couples. Sexual intercourse, it was supposed, declines in frequency as couples age; attendant on this change in mating behavior, intervals between insemination lengthen, and an ovum remaining in the reproductive tract has a greater chance of becoming overripe before it encounters fertilizing spermatozoa. At the biological level, animal data give some support to the overripe ovum theory, but human data are more recalcitrant (Penrose and Berg 1968; James 1978).

The theory implicates the second meiotic division, which is in process at the moment of fertilization of the ovum; yet at least four out of five human trisomies involve an error at the first meiotic division. From an epidemiological perspective, the theory suggests that the increase in trisomy with maternal age should be concomitant with a decrease in sexual intercourse. Such concordance is not evident for Down's syndrome and cannot underlie all trisomies since different trisomies manifest different patterns of increase with age. Reports of a higher incidence of Down's syndrome in Catholics have been taken as supportive (Jongbloet et al. 1978). The Catholic church recommends family spacing by the "rhythm" method, which defers intercourse to the "safe period" after ovulation; and the risk of inadvertent fertilization of an overripe ovum, it is suggested, might be greater during intercourse insufficiently deferred after ovulation.

The "attrition" theory (Stein et al. 1986) turns attention to the survival of aberrant conceptions in the subclinical phase of pregnancy. This theory takes at face value the poor fit in terms of maternal age between supernumerary chromosomes at their origin and trisomies actually observed. The theory proposes that the maternal age distribution of trisomies is the result, not of the process that generates trisomies, but of a maternal process in the subclinical phase that screens and rejects aberrant conceptions. This explanation is supported by an epidemiological model based on the data in Table 18-2.

It has been commonly, and indeed naturally, supposed that the association of maternal age with trisomies is established at fertilization, and arises because the numbers of disomic ova increase with maternal age and result in the formation of a trisomic zygote. Paternal age, it can be assumed from the preceding discussion, is scarcely related to trisomy.

Table 18–2 Survival of trisomies: for each chromosome, observed frequencies of disomies in sperm; ratio of maternal to paternal origin of trisomies; rate per 1000 among miscarriages of each trisomy, *calculated* and *observed*; and ratio of observed to calculated rates

Chromosome	Disomies per 1000 sperm (D)[a]	Ratio of maternal/ paternal origin (M/P)[b]	Calculated trisomies per 1000 miscarriages (A_c)[c]	Observed trisomies per 1000 miscarriages (A_o)[d]	Ratio of observed to calculated rates (S)[e]
13	1	9/1	167	17.3	0.10
15	1	9/1	167	18.1	0.11
16	1	9/1	167	79.4	0.48
21	3	3/1	200	24.5	0.16
22	1	9/1	167	27.4	0.16

[a]The incidence of a particular disomy per 1000 sperm, a measure of the potential paternal contribution to trisomies.

[b]The ratio of maternal to paternal origin of the trisomies of each chromosome.

[c]The *calculated* maximum proportion possible of trisomies per 1000 miscarriages:

$$A_c = \frac{D(1 + M/P)}{0.4 \times 0.15}$$

[d]The *observed* proportion of trisomies per 1000 miscarriages. The ratio A_o/A_c gives the fraction of all trisomies that have survived to miscarriage.

[e]S = ratio of A_o to A_c.

Source: Adapted from Stein et al. 1986.

Based on these suppositions, maternal age must relate to trisomies of maternal and not of paternal origin. As the woman becomes older, and the proportion of disomic ova increases, the maternal contribution to the frequency of trisomies should increase. This contribution can be measured by the ratio of maternal to paternal origins of trisomies (the M/P ratio). The observed maternal age association with trisomy requires an M/P ratio in women over 40 years of age that is 10 times higher than that in women under 25 years of age.

In fact, up to the time of this writing, the M/P ratio estimated from the available literature shows no appreciable increase with maternal age (Table 18-3; Stein et al. 1986). The absence of a maternal age effect in this ratio, if upheld, rules out an increase with maternal age in ova defective at fertilization. An appreciable maternal age effect is absent also for that majority of trisomies arising at the first maternal meiotic division (MMI). From these observations, the attrition theory holds that the strong maternal age association with trisomies must arise after fertilization.

The theory also holds that the maternal age association must arise before pregnancies are clinically recognized. This modifies a proposal we made some years ago specifically with respect to the phase of pregnancy involved. We proposed that miscarriage might serve as a screening device for chromosome and other anomalies: in older women, who

Table 18-3 Parental origin by maternal age in Down's syndrome: ratios, by maternal age at birth, of i. maternal to paternal origin of the supernumerary chromosome (M/P) and ii. error at first meiotic division (MMI) to all other types of error (*n* = number of informative cases of trisomy)[a]

Maternal age	M/P, rounded	MMI/all other origins
<20	7 (8)	0.6 (8)
20–24	3 (48)	1.6 (46)
25–29	3 (65)	1.5 (61)
30–34	3 (58)	1.6 (52)
35–39	6 (35)	3.1 (33)
40–44	3 (39)	1.6 (37)
45–	∞ (5)	0.7 (5)
Total	258	242

[a]*Sources*: Wagenblicher et al. (1976), Vienna; *n* = 34, M/P = 1.8. Hansson and Mikkelsen (1978), Copenhagen; *n* = 26, M/P = 2.7. Mattei et al. (1980), Marseilles; *n* = 51, M/P = 4.1. Mikkelsen et al. (1980), Funen; *n* = 45, M/P = 8.0; Zealand; *n* = 34, M/P = 3.2. Magenis and Chamberlin (1981), Seattle; *n* = 39, M/P = 4.0. del Mazo et al. (1982), Spain; *n* = 37, M/P = 1.3.

Source: Stein et al. 1986.

are less capable of rejecting aberrant conceptions, more trisomies would survive to later phases of pregnancy (Stein et al. 1975c). This theme has also been discussed in relation to trisomy 21 by others in terms of clinically recognized pregnancies (Ayme and Lippman-Hand 1982; Hook 1983).

Regarding clinically recognized pregnancies, the New York City data on karyotypes from miscarriages now controvert this notion. To serve as an index of attrition in clinically recognized pregnancies, we take the estimated proportion of all trisomies 21 that are lost in miscarriage. This proportion rises from 54 per cent in women under 30 years to 67 per cent in those 30 years and older (Warburton et al. 1986). Such an increase in the estimated proportion of trisomies miscarried is opposite to the expectation that follows from the failure of a postulated screening mechanism; in the clinical phase of pregnancy, a screening failure at later maternal ages should produce a decrease in attrition and a smaller proportion of trisomies lost. Length of gestation, taken as an index of survival of trisomies, also goes against a lowered rate of loss in older women. Their trisomy 21 conceptions (as well as conceptions of some other chromosomally aberrant and normal zygotes) miscarry sooner and survive for a shorter time than those in younger women. Thus, undue survival of trisomies in the clinical phase of pregnancy can be ruled out as a mechanism for the observed maternal age relations of trisomies at birth.

On the basis of these two observations on parental origin and clinically recognized loss, the attrition theory argues, by exclusion, that the maternal age association with trisomy 21 occurs in the subclinical phase of pregnancy. Two corollaries follow: among younger women trisomic conceptions are depleted after the onset of fertilization but before clinical recognition; and any screening mechanism that accomplishes this must be less sensitive as maternal age advances. This loss of sensitivity permits the survival of trisomies and so produces their association with older maternal ages in both clinically recognized losses and births.

Attrition in the subclinical phase of pregnancy has been unmeasurable (although the phase after implantation is now coming within biochemical reach). The model nonetheless rests on observations that can be tested by methods within technical reach of current cytogenetics and molecular biology. As more and better data accrue, therefore, the model is capable of being rejected or verified. In this regard, in accordance with the attrition theory, studies of unfertilized human ova from in vitro fertilization found no relationship between aneuploidy and maternal age (Pellestor and Sele 1988), although this single result is not yet secure (see Chapter 6). It is of note that studies of zygote formation located a mechanism for aneuploidy in very early mitotic divisions after fertilization and found these mitotic errors especially in older women (Ford 1984).

Once sound data become available for the key parameters, the proposed model makes it possible to infer changes with maternal age both in the frequency of trisomic conceptions and in their rates of attrition in the subclinical phase. For the present, the estimates (Table 18-2) are of limited validity and reliability because of the paucity of studies and of numbers, and uncertainties attached to studies of the genetic origin of the error. Hence, a main contribution of the model is that the attrition theory can be tested rigorously as the needed data accumulate.

CONCLUSION

Close to 100 years have gone by since the increasing risk of Down's syndrome with increasing maternal age was described (Shuttleworth 1909). It is now clear that the majority of autosomal trisomies increase in frequency with maternal age, at least among recognized pregnancies. The majority appear, in cytogenetic studies, to arise from a maternal error at meiosis I; it remains for molecular studies to test this result. There are, however, variations between the trisomies in absolute frequency, in the patterns of change with maternal age, in viability, and in the extent to which errors at maternal meiosis I appear to predominate. The differences and similarities between the individual trisomies set guidelines in testing theories about the biologic processes that give rise to them.

19 Pregnancy Number: Problems of Analysis

Some pregnancy outcomes appear to vary in frequency with either gravidity or parity. Gravidity refers to the total number of pregnancies that a woman has had, and parity refers to the total number of births, usually both liveborn and stillborn. The interpretation of such associations can be difficult, because there are many routes through which spurious associations might be produced. Sources of confounding include associations with maternal age, different individual risks among women (or couples) for the outcome under study, selective fertility, and direct causal connections between the outcome of one pregnancy and the next. For example, an immunologic mechanism was postulated to explain the higher average birth weights of second births compared to first births (Warburton and Naylor 1971).[1] With regard to miscarriage as well, an increase in risk with increasing number of pregnancies might implicate immunologic changes, most likely for the chromosomally normal component.

In this chapter we describe some of the methodologic challenges that must be faced in seeking unbiased estimates of associations between pregnancy outcome and pregnancy number. As a specific illustration of the general problem, we take miscarriage as the outcome, and examine the ways in which analyses have been approached and the problems encountered. We use the term "gravidity" to refer only to the total number of pregnancies a woman has experienced, and the terms "pregnancy number" or "rank" to refer to a particular pregnancy within a pregnancy sequence.

PREGNANCY NUMBER AND MISCARRIAGE: METHODOLOGIC ISSUES

A question raised, but not adequately answered, is whether or not an individual woman's risk of miscarriage changes with each additional

[1]This hypothesis has been tested, with conflicting results (Warburton and Naylor 1971; Magnus et al. 1985).

pregnancy beyond that expected on the basis of age alone. Most purported examinations of this question have in fact addressed a question subtly different. They have made estimates for individual women from the changes in the average risk of miscarriage for all women at each pregnancy number. In other words, all pregnancies at a given rank have been the subject of the analysis, with no regard paid to the composition of the sample of women who contribute those pregnancies at each rank. When there is variability in the risk of chromosomally normal miscarriage from woman to woman (heterogeneity), and when the numbers and timing of the pregnancies that they undertake are influenced by the outcomes of previous pregnancies (selective fertility),[2] a comparison of average miscarriage rates at successive pregnancy ranks may be misleading. Variations in the rate of miscarriage with pregnancy number may merely reflect differences in the individual risks typical of women contributing pregnancies at different pregnancy ranks, rather than any biologic effect of pregnancy rank per se. An alternative explanation—that one miscarriage causally affects the next—has received less consideration.

We begin by illustrating how these two phenomena—heterogeneity and selective fertility—can operate together to confound those analytic approaches that have most often been used in relating pregnancy number and miscarriage. We then briefly discuss other methodologic issues that bear on such analyses (for reviews see Leridon 1976; Wilcox and Gladen 1982). We draw especially on one analyst who has provided a framework within which to study the influence of pregnancy order on risk of miscarriage, taking into account the effects of heterogeneity in risk among women, selective fertility, maternal age, and other factors governing current gravidity, such as the spacing between pregnancies (Levin 1986).

Two observations are compatible with the proposition that, at a given age and pregnancy number, heterogeneity exists among women in the risk of miscarriage. One is that women with chromosomally normal losses have increased rates of miscarriage at subsequent pregnancies; another is that chromosomally normal losses tend to recur (Chapter 9). Such associations can be anticipated in the presence of heterogeneity of risk: because women with a history of miscarriage (compared with those without prior loss) tend to overrepresent women at naturally higher risk, as a group they will manifest higher rates of loss in later pregnancies.

The term "stopping rule" (Levin 1986) formalizes the notion that, for a variety of reasons, women differ in the total number of pregnancies they complete. Some of these reasons relate to the outcomes of earlier pregnancies and may affect the distribution of pregnancy sequences

---

[2]An equivalent to selective fertility as a term for describing compensatory reproductive responses to given pregnancy outcomes is "differential continuation rates" (Leridon 1976).

observed. Behavior that governs reproduction might be impelled, for example, by the number of children desired, and by the discouragement or compensation that occurs after repeated pregnancy losses (see Reed and Kelly 1958; Billewicz 1973; Leridon 1976).

To exemplify the various approaches that have been taken in examining the effects of pregnancy number and the pitfalls involved, we have constructed a hypothetical cohort in which only two variables affect outcome: women are heterogeneous for the risk of miscarriage, and each woman follows one of two stopping rules that govern her reproductive behavior. Table 19-1 sets out the distribution of outcomes for the first two pregnancies from this cohort; L indicates a live birth and A a miscarriage. Ordinarily, the investigator can observe only the sequences from the total sample, that is, the cell in the lower right corner.

The cohort includes two types of women: women at a low (10 per cent) risk of miscarriage in every pregnancy, comprising 90 per cent of the cohort; and women at a high (50 per cent) risk of miscarriage in every pregnancy, comprising 10 per cent of the cohort. The distribution of stopping rules is as follows: 50 per cent of women stop reproduction after having their first birth and 50 per cent stop after having their first two pregnancies. For each woman the risk of miscarriage (p) is taken to be a fixed characteristic that does not vary with age or pregnancy number. The "choice" of stopping rule is assumed to be independent of the woman's underlying risk of miscarriage. In this cohort, 14 per cent of first pregnancies miscarry.

When neither the risk status of each woman nor the stopping rule is known, one approach to analyzing data of this kind is to contrast the proportions of pregnancies ending in miscarriage at pregnancy ranks 1 and 2. We refer to this as the *marginal association* between pregnancy rank and miscarriage. This tabulation (Table 19-1, I) suggests that the rate of miscarriage is 0.14 in pregnancy 1 and then increases to 0.153 in pregnancy 2.

The inference that the risk of miscarriage increases with pregnancy number would be in error, however. The error is produced because this analytic approach does not take into account the fact that the rule "stop after first live birth" has the effect of removing a greater proportion of low-risk women than of high-risk women from pregnancy rank 2. (In Table 19-1, high-risk women comprise 10 per cent of first pregnancies and 13.2 per cent of second pregnancies.) Analyses of this type have been used, albeit with analytic adjustment for the effects of maternal age, to support the conclusion that the rate of miscarriage increases with pregnancy number (Stevenson et al. 1959; Warburton and Fraser 1964; Shapiro et al. 1971; Naylor 1974). In two samples in which the likelihood of continuing reproduction was greater after a live birth than after a miscarriage, the rate of miscarriage did not vary with pregnancy number within age strata (Leridon 1976).

Table 19–1 Reproductive histories in a hypothetical population: expected distribution of pregnancy outcomes in a population composed of women at low and high risk of miscarriage and following two stopping rules[a]

Stopping rule (% of population)	Pregnancy sequences	90% Low risk women ($p = .10$)	10% High risk women ($p = .50$)	Total population (100%)
Stop after first live-birth (0.50)	L	0.4050	0.0250	0.4300
	LL	0	0	0
	LA	0	0	0
	AL	0.0405	0.0125	0.0530
	AA	0.0045	0.0125	0.0170
Stop after second pregnancy (0.50)	L	0	0	0
	LL	0.3645	0.0125	0.3770
	LA	0.0405	0.0125	0.0530
	AL	0.0405	0.0125	0.0530
	AA	0.0045	0.0125	0.0170
Total	L	0.4050	0.0250	0.4300
	LL	0.3645	0.0125	0.3770
	LA	0.0405	0.0125	0.0530
	AL	0.0810	0.0250	0.1060
	AA	0.0090	0.0250	0.0340

[a] Key to abbreviations: L = live birth, A = miscarriage (spontaneous abortion); p = rate of miscarriage in each pregnancy.

[b] Investigator can only observe the distribution of sequences in the total population.

I. Marginal rates of miscarriage:

Pregnancy	Rate
1	0.140 [AL + AA]/Total
2	0.153 [LA + AA]/[LL + LA + AL + AA]

II. Analysis of sequences:

Among sequences of two pregnancies, each with one miscarriage, the proportion with the sequence LA is 0.053 and that with the sequence AL is 0.106. The dearth of sequences with LA compared to AL has been misinterpreted to suggest that the risk of miscarriage decreases with increasing pregnancy number.

III. Among sequences with two pregnancies, the rates of miscarriage at pregnancies 1 and 2 are as follows:

Pregnancy	Rate
1	0.246 [AL + AA]/[LL + LA + AL + AA]
2	0.153 [LA + AA]/[LL + LA + AL + AA]

IV. Estimate of the odds at miscarriage of pregnancy 2 compared to those of pregnancy 1, taking into account the likelihoods of continuing reproduction after a live birth and after a miscarriage on the first pregnancy are as follows:

Observed odds on miscarriage in second pregnancy versus odds in first pregnancy among those with one miscarriage: LA/AL = 0.053/0.106 = 0.5.

Proportion continuing reproduction after live birth: 0.43/0.86 = 5.

Proportion continuing reproduction after miscarriage: 0.14/0.14 = 1.

Likelihood ratio for continuing reproduction after live birth compared to after miscarriage: (0.43/0.86)/(0.14/0.14) = 0.5.

Estimated odds on miscarriage in second pregnancy versus miscarriage in first pregnancy = observed odds ratio LA/AL divided by the likelihood ratio for continuing reproduction: 0.5/0.5 = 1.

Another approach to assessing the effects of gravidity is to study the distribution of pregnancy sequences of the same length and same number of miscarriages (Naylor 1974; Naylor and Warburton 1979). Within sequences of the same length and number of miscarriages, an imbalance in the number of sequences in which the miscarriage occurs in the last pregnancy as opposed to the first has been interpreted as supporting an effect of pregnancy number. The principle is analogous to the estimation of association in matched pairs studies; here the matched pairs are the first two pregnancy outcomes. In theory, if the risk is constant between pregnancies, the proportion of pairs AL should equal the proportion of pairs LA, simply because $pq = qp$.

However, in our example (Table 19-1, II), among sequences of two pregnancies with one birth and one miscarriage, the proportion of sequences with a birth followed by a miscarriage (LA) is less than the proportion with a miscarriage followed by a birth (AL). This inequality arises because the rule "stop after first live birth" depletes the two-pregnancy sample of a greater proportion of low-risk women than of high-risk women. The inference that the risk of miscarriage is lower in the second pregnancy than in the first is incorrect.

A third approach (Roman et al. 1978; Bakketeig and Hoffman 1979; Naylor and Warburton 1979) is to stratify the sample by gravidity at the time of observation and to contrast the proportion of pregnancies ending in miscarriage (or perinatal death) at each pregnancy rank. For example, among women with two pregnancies, the rate of miscarriage is 0.246 in the first pregnancy and 0.153 in the second (Table 19-1, III). As before, both rates are higher than the 0.14 rate at first pregnancy in the entire cohort because women with two pregnancies overrepresent high-risk women. The apparent decrease in risk from pregnancy 1 to 2 arises as before because the rule "stop after first live birth" biases the sample of women with two pregnancies. Trends of this sort have been erroneously interpreted as suggesting that risk decreases with increasing pregnancy number (Roman et al. 1978; Bakketeig and Hoffman 1979) as has before been noted (Mantel 1979; Golding et al. 1983).

From the examples set out here, it is clear that if women (or couples) are heterogeneous in the risk of miscarriage, selective fertility may produce spurious associations with pregnancy number. Spurious associations will not arise in the presence of only one of these two phenomena. Thus, in the presence of heterogeneity of risk, a promising approach to estimating changes in the odds of miscarriage with pregnancy number takes account of selective fertility (Levin 1986). Estimated odds are adjusted for variation in the observed rates of undertaking additional pregnancies, given previous pregnancy outcomes, as well as for other characteristics such as maternal age and spacing between pregnancies. The approach is robust in the presence of heterogeneity of risk.

For example, in the hypothetical cohort, consider the estimation of changed risk between first and second pregnancy among women with two or more pregnancies. As in the analysis of sequences already set out, the analysis begins by contrasting the numbers of two sets of pairs, namely, pairs in which a live birth is followed by a miscarriage (LA), and pairs in which a miscarriage is followed by a live birth (AL). In our example the proportion of women with LA is 0.053 and the proportion with AL is 0.106—an odds ratio of 0.5. This estimate must be adjusted for the likelihood of continuing to pregnancy 2 depending on the outcome of pregnancy 1. That is, the odds must be divided by the ratio of the likelihood that women who had a live birth in the first pregnancy continue to a subsequent pregnancy to the likelihood that women who had a miscarriage in the first pregnancy will likewise continue: $(0.43/0.86)/(0.14/0.14) = 0.5$. The resulting estimate of the odds ratio is unity $(0.5/0.5)$, indicating correctly that the risk of miscarriage does not change between pregnancies 1 and 2 (see Table 19-1, IV).

ESTIMATES OF THE LIKELIHOOD OF STOPPING REPRODUCTION

Stopping rules can be observed directly only in samples composed of women who have completed reproduction. None of the data that have been used to search for the effects of pregnancy number on miscarriage are of this type, although one investigator attempted to limit analyses to complete sibships (James 1974). Two alternate sources of data are the reproductive histories of women identified at an index pregnancy, and the reproductive histories of women identified for reasons other than pregnancy.

The majority of analyses to assess the effects of pregnancy number on miscarriage have used the first sampling strategy. By the nature of the strategy, all reproductive histories are incomplete. One assumption, usually implicit, is that the factors that influence a woman to stop reproducing are stable over time (Leridon 1976; Levin 1986). Even if this assumption is roughly correct, it can be shown that the probabilities of continuing reproduction cannot be consistently estimated from a sample of this type, and thus the relation of miscarriage risk to pregnancy number cannot be assessed (Levin 1986).

The alternative strategy uses the reproductive histories of women ascertained for reasons other than pregnancy, for example, an occupational cohort or a representative sample of women of reproductive age (Leridon 1977). In samples of this type it is possible to obtain a consistent estimate of the probabilities of stopping reproduction given previous outcomes, age, and other factors. In a representative sample of women of childbearing age of this kind, in Martinique, the overall probability of stopping reproduction was found to be greater after miscarriage than after birth (Leridon 1977). Although the analysis did not take into account the differential likelihoods of continuing reproduction, an analysis of the published data that does so supports the original conclusion that pregnancy number effects were absent (Levin, personal communication).

Other phenomena too can produce misleading marginal associations between pregnancy rank and miscarriage rate. These include maternal age—since the risk of miscarriage increases with age and a woman is older at each successive pregnancy—recall of the outcomes of pregnancy that differ for recent pregnancies and those long past, and spacing between pregnancies that differs with the outcome of the earlier pregnancy. Several such factors, as well as differential stopping rules in the presence of heterogeneity of risk, could act together to produce a spurious marginal association between pregnancy rank and miscarriage. Computer analyses that model changes in risk with several of these factors have simulated associations similar to those reported in the literature (Wilcox and Gladen 1982). For all this, the demonstration that spurious results may emerge from an incorrect analytic strategy does not provide an answer to the question of interest. Thus, although no result shows that the risk of miscarriage changes with pregnancy number, neither does any result demonstrate conclusively that it does not. Future research will need to address this open question in a manner that guards against the biases outlined in this chapter.

V The Physical Environment, Reproduction and Surveillance

20 Surveillance of Reproductive Outcomes: I. Keeping Watch

Dangers to health in the physical environment have been envisaged ever since the Hippocratic writers related health disorders to "airs, waters, and places." Epidemiologists aiming to control environmental dangers engage in two main kinds of public health activity. One kind of activity is surveillance—simply to keep watch in a systematic way. Warning signals come from various observation points, sometimes from routine data collection systems, at other times from systems custom-built to meet a particular need for surveillance. The epidemiological function is to set up or devise observation points and to interpret the signals.

The second kind of activity is to pursue such leads as come to attention. Epidemiologists can be moved to act by signals from surveillance systems, clinicians, affected individuals, or the public. They can be impelled by the cogency of collateral scientific evidence or scientific intuition about the existence of danger in the environment; or they may be merely the servants of public authorities, or of the public at large in whom a sense of danger has been aroused with more or less justification. Epidemiologists are called on to demonstrate or refute the existence of danger.

What steps can and should be taken to ensure prompt recognition of hazards to reproduction that newly enter the physical environment? An epidemic intelligence system must early arouse suspicion that something may be amiss. After such an alert, further study must be undertaken to fortify or dismiss suspicion, and means of intervention must be weighed. Calls to action do not always wait on these props to prudence. Even before a judgment can be reached that an association is causal or that an intervention will be effective, something may have to be done.

With teratogens and physical and toxic hazards generally, the successes and failures of the past in discovering and preventing their effects may instruct us. In this chapter we first consider the grounds for undertaking surveillance of reproductive outcomes in light of the past discoveries of environmental teratogens. We ask ourselves what might be learned and applied from that experience. We go on to describe approaches to monitoring, the problems that are encountered, the statistical techniques that have been used, and the factors that influence the yield of these approaches. In the next chapter we consider the problems of following leads. These involve designing and mounting tests to demonstrate the effects of potential dangers or, failing that, to draw the limits around what the effects might be.

TERMS AND DEFINITIONS

Before we proceed to the substance of this chapter, readers may be aided by a note on the terminology we have arrived at in considering these matters. Although both in technical and lay writings surveillance is often used as a synonym for monitoring, we think it worthwhile to separate the two terms as others have attempted to do (Weatherall and Haskey 1976). We treat surveillance as an umbrella term, and monitoring as one element of surveillance.

Surveillance, in our usage, describes a general, continuing and purposeful system for following frequencies of potentially adverse exposures or outcomes, or both, through time. The system may employ an array of means and encompass an array of exposures and outcomes. Surveillance systems are exemplified by the continued sampling of air, soil and water for pollution and of food for contamination, by the tracking of sales of drugs, and by routine scrutiny of reproductive outcomes in vital statistics or registries. Surveillance is likely to involve a combination of routine procedures. Thus, surveillance encompasses the whole set of activities deployed to detect untoward environmental exposures and the unexpected variation or emergence of health outcomes, whether increments and decrements in common disorders or the appearance of new and strange ones. In an optimal system, baselines refer to the *population at large.* Surveillance of given exposures generally aims to work from a baseline determined from a safety threshold or a norm for the population at large. Surveillance of given outcomes aims to work from a baseline of rates in the population at large.

Monitoring, in our usage, describes the watch, by means of a single system that collects data, for particular signals of either exposure or effect. The implied purpose of this well-tried approach to prevention is to initiate action, although whether action follows or not is a matter of judgment, will and resources. *Outcome monitoring* is the continuing enumeration of specified events (here, reproductive events) in a manner that allows potentially adverse departures from baseline values to be detected and acted on. *Exposure monitoring* is the continuing measurement of indices of potentially hazardous exposures. For example, levels of radiation in the working environment and some pollutants in the ambient air are continuously sampled; bacterial and chemical contaminants in water, soil and food are periodically sampled. Monitoring commonly works from data self-contained within the system, without reference to the population at large.

Outcomes tend to yield discrete variables that are compared with expected numbers; exposures more often yield continuous variables that are compared with a threshold for safety. Thus, outcome monitoring is usually based on numerator data and expressed in terms of events (say, low-birth-weight births), occasionally in terms of an index on a continuous measurement scale (say, mean birth weight). Comparisons are with expected values, usually derived from the same self-contained data source as counts or means averaged over preceding "nonepidemic" time intervals. Exposure monitoring is usually based on sampling by time and location and expressed in terms of continuous measurement scales (say, carbon monoxide levels), occasionally in terms of counts (say, numbers of bacteria seen in a microscopic field in a sample of specimens). Comparisons are usually made with safety thresholds derived from antecedent experience or some best estimate. Meaningful interpretation of such self-contained monitoring results requires certain assumptions. With outcomes, for example, numerator counts require the tacit assumption of an unchanging denominator in the population at large. For exposures, assumptions are made about what levels are unsafe or otherwise undesirable, as well as about average levels experienced by the population at large.

In this chapter, we deal first with the overall question of surveillance—its rationale and approach to problems. Discussion of monitoring approaches follows.

THE GROUNDS FOR SURVEILLANCE

Epidemiology, with its origins in medicine, leans naturally toward health outcomes rather than exposures as a beginning point for study. Systematic and continuing measurement has been devoted to the surveillance of health disorders. The monitoring of environmental exposures—in water, air, factory and farm—has been the public health task of sanitary and environmental engineers. What follows here respects this traditional division of tasks; our main concern is with the surveillance and monitoring of reproductive health disorders.

The use of already existing surveillance systems and the creation of special systems for the purposes of monitoring changes in reproductive outcomes, particularly malformations, is relatively recent public health practice. Because formal monitoring systems rest on assumptions about their relations with the experience of the population at large, they operate most comfortably where knowledge is sufficient to establish sound population norms, and where departures from those norms give good grounds for responding to them. In the field of prenatal development, population norms are far from established, and surveillance is still in a phase of exploration, testing and hoped-for discovery. Formal surveillance systems do not exclude discoveries through other routes. It is through these other routes that past discoveries have been made. We examine some of these for their possible relevance to discovery through formal approaches.

The overall success of any approach to surveillance or monitoring might be assessed in terms of the lapse of time between the appearance of a new environmental hazard and the recognition of its adverse effects. A review of past discoveries by this criterion might hold some lessons for those undertaking surveillance. How long did it take to identify the connection between hazard and effect and by what means was it accomplished? Naturally, in using examples from the past, allowance must be made for the technical advantages of the present as well as for the public health and clinical alertness aroused by the discoveries themselves. We shall consider, in turn, knowledge engendered by clinical insight into the disease process, by epidemiological insight into disease occurrence, by systematic research, and by stimulus from the lay public.

Clinical Insight

The earliest route to the discovery of connections between exposure and birth outcome depended on the synthesis of clinical observations about pathogenesis. The route is not necessarily straightforward and simple. In the absence of an appropriate conceptual framework, clinical skill and technique alone may not lead to appropriate answers. A prototype is provided by teratogenic effects that give rise to congenital syphilis. The definitive descriptions of congenital syphilis, in the 1850s (Fournier 1886, Hutchinson 1887), preceded by half a century the discovery of the spirochete *Treponema pallidum* (Schaudinn and Hoffmann 1905). In truth, the story of the idea of syphilis as a teratogen took much longer to evolve than a mere half-century. We begin with this story to illustrate the governing role that concepts and paradigms can play in discovery.

Paracelsus recognized the common source of congenital and adult syphilis in the sixteenth century. This came about, we surmise, because features of the disease in the newborn, such as those localized in skin and mucous membranes, resemble those of secondary syphilis in the adult. Paracelsus lived at the time when syphilis presented as a new disease. At the very end of the fifteenth century, it had begun to spread across Europe in epidemic force. The manifestations of secondary syphilis in the mother would often have been present at the birth of an affected child. Sharp observation could connect them unaided.

Nonetheless, centuries passed before the observation of Paracelsus took on general significance for teratogenesis in biomedical thinking.

His dynamic concept of epidemic disease governed by stellar motion (King 1963), one may argue, was a hindrance. Perhaps one may remind the reader of the famous aphorism of Claude Bernard (1865) that discoveries come to the prepared mind. The preparation Bernard advocated was the steadfast and imaginative pursuit, in depth, of an area of study. Social context also prepares the mind. A century and more after Bernard, Thomas Kuhn (1970) clarified the role of conceptual paradigms in limiting the questions posed and the answers offered. A new paradigm was needed before syphilis would be properly understood as a teratogen.

In the very instance in question, Ludwik Fleck—a predecessor of Kuhn by some decades in the sociology of scientific ideas—took the history of syphilis over four centuries for his case study of the "genesis and development of a scientific fact" (Fleck 1935). In this work, Fleck traced the twists and turns in concepts of syphilis—the shifts in the disorders, signs and symptoms that were included and those that were excluded—until, finally, the modern concept was reached. This now familiar multicausal model attributes the disease to a single organism, but one that impinges on the different susceptibilities of individuals under varying environmental conditions of transmission.

Once a new overriding paradigm guides the thought and concepts of a science, information from many different sources contributes to new discoveries. The teratogenic link between mother and infant that had been recognized with syphilitic infection lay dormant and without further application in teratology until the link was again recognized with the discovery of rubella and malformations in 1941. Historical analysis teaches us that such delays are to be anticipated until a new paradigm emerges that can accommodate new ideas and formulations. The moral for the epidemiologist is that effective surveillance, like effective research, must assimilate and apply current understanding as well as knowledge. Surveillance can probe more deeply for disorder as it mobilizes new and refined techniques for capturing change at the physiological, cellular and molecular levels, as well as at the clinical level.

Epidemiological Insight

An astute clinician opened the route to the discovery of the teratogenic effects of rubella. This discovery anticipated by decades the isolation of the organism. The discovery depended on a sense of population frequencies and rare events combined with insight into the distribution of the shared experience of a cohort. As we saw in Chapter 2, the immediate antecedent of recognition was appreciation of an epidemic of an apparently noninfectious disorder—namely, a cluster of cataracts in very young children. The new insight was the common membership in a birth cohort of children whose mothers had been pregnant at the time of a recent rubella epidemic and gave a history of infection (Gregg 1941). With rubella, unlike syphilis, the effects in infants offered no manifest clue that they shared a common origin with the effects of the virus in postnatal life.

A similar history of discovery attaches to the teratogenic effects of diethylstibestrol (DES) on the reproductive tract of those exposed to it in utero. Adenocarcinoma of the vagina, an extremely rare cancer in young women, was the signal for the discovery. Over a short period in Boston, a gynecologist observed several of these cancers in young women (Herbst and Scully 1970). The link with prenatal diethylstibestrol is a salient demonstration, we noted in Chapter 3, of the utility of case-control studies in addressing new and mysterious diseases.

In the previous decade, consciousness of the teratogenic potential of therapeutic drugs had been roused by the discovery of the effects of thalidomide when used as an antiemetic in pregnant women. In October 1960 two cases of a new limb reduction deformity were reported at a meeting in Germany (Kosenow and Pfeiffer 1960); other reports from German physicians followed (Wiedemann 1961). Two investigators, one in Australia and one in Germany, suggested a link with thalidomide (McBride 1961; Lenz 1962). Later, corroboration of the uniqueness of the malformations observed was aided by the availability of data on which to base expectations of frequency. These were derived retrospectively from a coincidental study of 37 years of records of birth defects in Hamburg (Lenz and Knapp 1962; Lenz 1965) and, also, from a congenital malformation registry in Liverpool (Smithells 1962). As time went on, the causal connection of thalidomide with limb reduction deformities was reinforced by the decline in frequency as the drug was withdrawn from the market (Frantz 1963; Smithells and Leck 1963; Lenz 1965).

The discovery of this therapeutic hazard and the felt need for monitoring gave a fillip to the 1950s notion of maintaining systematic registries of congenital anomalies (Newcombe et al. 1959; McKeown and Record 1960; Smithells 1962). Indeed, had the present Swedish monitoring system been in place, according to one estimate the epidemic would have been signaled after the birth of only seven affected infants in a 4-month period (Kallen and Winberg 1968). In fact, before the epidemic was discovered nearly a year and a half had passed, in the course of which at least 153 affected births occurred (Holtzman and Khoury 1986).

In each of these modern examples, the avenue to discovery was an epidemic, which is a frequency of any condition excessive for a given time, place and population. The characteristics of the epidemic alone were sufficient to lead to the indictment of the causal factors. Change in frequency was rapid and sharp, occurring over a short period of time. In each instance, awareness was heightened by a relatively high degree of specificity-in-the-effect. It was, of course, also necessary that these epidemics of normally rare events impinge on the awareness of keen observers. A general approach to improve discovery through surveillance, however, must reduce reliance on clinical insight. Surveillance systems should be able to capture small silent epidemics, or large ones early in their course, because of their capacity for continuous quantitative assessments. Thus, effective surveillance should ensure that no real changes in disease pattern are missed even if they are subtle and entirely undramatic.

Systematic Research

Besides clinical and epidemiological insight, systematic research—biological, experimental, clinical and, not least, epidemiological—is an avenue to discovery of ever-growing importance. Thus, clinical observation has benefitted from reinforcement by biological and epidemiological knowledge in yielding discoveries. The discoveries of the teratogenic effects of androgenic hormones and of isotretinoin (Chapter 3) can each be attributed to clinical observation combined with broad biological knowledge. These drugs were given under the supervision of physicians. Anticipations of the activity of each—masculinization with androgens (Jost 1955) and specific malformations with isotretinoin (Lammer et al. 1985)—existed in experimental work and, for androgens, also in clinical observations in children and adults. With such forewarnings, untoward effects would not be expected to escape the prepared mind for long.

Laboratory investigation of the properties of chemicals and drugs, and animal experiments to test their effects in a variety of species, may point to their potential as human teratogens and narrow the search. The capacity of a substance to bring about mutagenesis in laboratory cell preparations is an initial indicator that a substance may have the potential for harm. Experimental studies in animals can then test the teratogenic potential of the suspect substance and serve as the basis for guidelines in human pregnancy.

Conversely, the plausibility of a positive finding in human beings is enhanced by a positive finding in any one species of animal. So far, all teratogens found to affect human beings are said to be also teratogenic in at least one animal. In the corollary, if an agent has no adverse effect in many species of animals—say, seven or more—doubt is cast on a positive association in human beings. Only consistency of a positive association on replication in human beings rebuts the null results of such experiments (see Chapter 1).

In the domain of epidemiology, the ultimate confirmation of suppositions of risk founded on animal or laboratory studies is in human populations. Research pursued in a systematic manner is often essential to such confirmation. For some agents, the lead for investigations of their teratogenic potential came, not from clinical, epidemiological or experimental insight, but from systematic epidemiologic research. In matters of public health, systematic epidemiological research may draw on sources developed specifically for surveillance, or on secondary analyses of data collected for other purposes.

The idea of using registries for epidemiological description and explanation is not a new one, especially for secondary analysis. Historians have assigned the very beginnings of quantitative epidemiology to John Graunt's secondary analysis in the seventeenth century of the London Bills of Mortality (these weekly reports were an early monitoring device, kept to give warning of any rise in mortality that could signal the onset of a plague epidemic). Later, beginning in the late nineteenth century, registries of psychiatric disorders (Jarvis 1855; see Grob 1978) and of mental deficiency (Kanner 1964) were used in similar fashion for secondary analysis. The motives for the initiation of registries of mental deficiency in particular were not free of political intent; "mainline" eugenics aimed to remove persons of low intelligence from society, in which they were perceived as a danger (Gould 1981; Kevles 1985). Nonetheless, secondary analysis of the registers did much to forward epidemiological understanding (Susser 1968, 1976).

Vital statistics, the routine collection by political jurisdictions of health and demographic data, provide existing registration systems that can be put to good use in surveillance. From the time William Farr took up his appointment as Compiler of Medical Statistics in the General Register Office in 1839, he promoted the use of vital registration systems of births, marriages and deaths for secondary analyses. In his hands, this approach became standard and continues in use. For example, in Britain in the 1960s, deferred mortality from neural tube defects signaled the increase in both survival and disability produced by surgical ventricular shunts in the newborn with hydrocephalus (Adelstein 1974). In New York City, the frequencies and types of malformations registered at birth have been related to the frequencies of an array of notifiable diseases (Siegel and Greenberg 1959, 1960). Other attempts to use vital statistics have proved more frustrating. In British Columbia a linked system was developed from the registries of births and deaths in the late 1950s precisely for the purpose of monitoring congenital defects (Newcombe et al. 1959). This system produced many interesting data but few signals of untoward clusters. Possibly ascertainment was deficient, or possibly no substantial epidemics occurred during a surveillance period that continued for several years.

In summary, systematic laboratory and animal research can inform or be informed by research in human beings. In the systematic collection of quantitative data on disease in populations we can perceive both antecedents and resources for surveillance. These forerunners include the secondary analysis of vital statistics, the linking of different vital statistics systems or data sets in the same system, and the evolution from public health notification of infectious disease to registers of noninfectious disease maintained continuously and enumerated periodically.

The Lay Public

Concerns of the lay public have been an added stimulus to the instigation of teratogenic research in recent years, although as yet they have led to few discoveries. The public has become watchful of the hazards of drugs, food additives, environmental toxins, and irradiation. It was the public, moved by the potential victims, who most insistently posed the questions about the teratogenicity of caffeine, heavy metals, powerlines, and Agent Orange, to name only a few examples. In some of these instances, the scientific grounds for the questions have been slender. Such tenuous suspicions present a special class of social and political problems. For scientists, to substantiate or falsify them requires intense and, not infrequently, diversionary attention. At the same time, the public stimulus has undoubtedly invigorated and sometimes enriched the study of a number of health problems.

MONITORING REPRODUCTIVE OUTCOMES

Procedures for monitoring that are sensitive enough to assess changes in the incidence of adverse outcomes of pregnancy over time are much needed. Subtle but real effects do not quickly impinge on clinical perception and much less on the public consciousness. Thus, in Australia, although deafness was on record for decades, epidemics of congenital rubella that went unremarked were eventually discovered only when reconstructed by hindsight (Lancaster 1951). Systematic surveillance might have identified the epidemics at the time they occurred.

The diagnosis of birth defects continues to be the task of individual physicians. In the United States and other countries today, however, the clinical observer need not be the sole repository of the experience and memory by means of which changes in frequency are quickly brought to light. Computerized notification systems can now absorb the reports of many physicians continuously and assemble them for display at any time.

Several malformation registries now monitor changes in prevalence— the Centers for Disease Control Metropolitan Atlanta Congenital Defects Program and the Birth Defects Monitoring Program (Edmonds et al. 1981), the International Clearing House for Birth Defects (Flynt and Hay 1979), and its offshoot, the EUROCAT project (Lechat et al. 1985). Such systems have the capacity to register the points in time at which reports of malformations exceed an "expected" baseline rate. The investigator specifies beforehand the level at which an "excess" is signaled, taking into consideration the probabilities of false alerts (errors of commission) and missed alerts (errors of omission).

Existing systems for monitoring congenital defects have in common the aim of examining changes over time or between regions. Some of the large systems have joined in an association that provides quarterly reports (International Clearing House for Birth Defects Monitoring Systems 1982). Similarities in trends between regions can thus be noted. The more sophisticated systems also provide a sampling frame on which to mount case-control studies or, through record linkage, to relate exposure to outcomes. Groups can be selected for study from registry or vital statistics systems to the extent that appropriate variables can be derived from the information entered—for example, occupation, place of residence, and demographic characteristics.

The utility of a reporting or registration system for the prompt detection of changes in frequency and their causes is affected by several issues that vary with local circumstances and practice; we discuss a few of the more general of these. Issues of *case definition and ascertainment* involve the range of outcomes coded, and the degree of diagnostic refinement with which they are specified. In addition, the extent of collected data bears on the degree to which analyses can be refined. Issues of *population and measures of change* include the size of the population, the measures of frequencies, and the baseline rate of the outcome. Issues of *monitoring technique* arise because choices among more or less elaborate or sophisticated methods must be made.

Case Definition and Ascertainment

The range and specificity of coding has immediate consequences. The range of outcomes recorded sets an absolute limit on what effects can be detected by surveillance. A system cannot detect differences in the frequency of outcomes that were not specified beforehand as within its purview, nor of those for which ascertainment is very incomplete. The endpoints that can be included with profit in birth defect notifications do not represent all the outcomes that could result from teratogens. Any system of registration has practical limits. Those who record are usually physicians, nurses or other designated hospital personnel. The choice of outcomes is limited by their capacity to record completely and accurately and by the lack of standard procedures among them. A classification system for recording outcomes may prove too spare to prove useful, or too complex and cumbersome to operate.

Completeness of ascertainment is also affected by how wide and systematic a net is cast. Results differ according to whether all or some hospitals are included, or whether institutions for chronic care, diagnostic screening clinics, office practitioners, and voluntary agencies participate (McKeown and Record, 1960). Notifications made at birth do not net defects that emerge later in life. Notifications made at later ages do not net defects in children who do not survive to those ages (Susser 1968). With all these limitations, notification systems do tend to cover handicaps that impose the gravest burden on survivors and their families.

Vital statistics can be expected to extend the population range of ascertainment and the power of surveillance that employs other data sources such as those from hospitals, physicians, and notification systems. Vital statistics encompass all births, and at least some of the outcomes recorded might be affected by maternal exposures during pregnancy. Many public health authorities routinely collect population statistics on infants born alive, which include, at a minimum, sex, birth weight, duration of gestation, and neonatal and postneonatal mortality; some also attempt to record, with varying levels of success, early as well as intermediate and late fetal deaths (National Center for Health Statistics 1980).

In practice these outcomes, excepting perinatal mortality, have seldom been monitored for changes over time. More often, data already collected have been used for a retrospective search for adverse effects of environmental toxins on reproduction. In the notorious area of the chemical dump in the Love Canal, New York, effects of exposure on birth weight, but not on malformations, could be sought and putatively shown in vital records of an earlier period (Vianna 1980; Vianna and Polan 1984). Knowledge of the frequency of malformations was to be had only by resorting to a purposive survey.

The constraint of the narrow requirements for information in vital statistics and the often low ascertainment levels cannot be ignored. Even within the range of conditions that can be captured at birth by the monitoring system, the degree of diagnostic specification sets limits. As we argued in the chapters on teratogenesis, a disadvantage of grouping diagnostic entities is the possible masking of change. When a constituent diagnosis comprises a small proportion of a grouped category, even a steep rise may be overwhelmed by the lack of change in the large proportion of the group as a whole. Whether a new hazard will cause a single or many malformations is quite uncertain beforehand.

Prudence dictates the collection of detailed information, so that the analyst may have the best of both worlds. Computers facilitate recording; today the main impediments to a satisfactory system are likely to be the maintenance of standardized and reliable procedures for diagnosis and coding, and the interval between events and reports of events. Data collateral to a given outcome are important to interpretations of frequency changes and hypotheses about their causes. Thus, registration systems—whether for vital statistics generally or malformations only—will yield collateral data. They usually include items on maternal age and such other characteristics as ethnicity, obstetric history and place of birth. In some systems selected information such as medication use is recorded; in others census information on occupation and other variables can be linked to registries (see Kallen et al. 1984 for review).

When recorded or linked data are sufficient, they can be used to generate hypotheses about the likely causal agent. An early step is to analyze background data to indicate whether a change in prevalence might be a result merely of demographic change in the population at risk, or whether a change affects a subgroup that can be defined in terms of recorded characteristics. When changes are confined to one or two medical facilities, a change in methods of ascertainment is the first hypothesis to be tested.

Populations and Measures of Change

Population rates of incidence at inception or prevalence at birth reflect most closely the underlying truth the monitor aims to discover, but they are seldom accessible. Cumulative incidence—a measure of the cumulative rate of events in a cohort at selected points in the life course or in calendar time—except by good fortune is unlikely to be available for reproductive outcomes with the continuity that surveillance or monitoring require. Period incidence—the traditional measure, approximating incidence density, of the average rate of events over a specified period in a dynamic population—requires the continuous maintenance of knowledge about the source and completeness of ascertainment of cases for the numerator and periodic knowledge about the population from which these cases are drawn for the denominator. Thus, for practicability, in a monitoring system outcomes are typically measured in terms of numerators. For rare, discrete outcomes, monitoring usually relies on counts (e.g., number of malformations per month). With other more common outcomes, the monitoring index may be cast in the form of proportions (e.g., percentage of trisomies among miscarriages) and, with quantitative characteristics, in the form of means (e.g., birth weight).

For discrete events, to depend on numerator data is to place the indices of change at a further remove from the true variation in the population at large than incidence or prevalence rates.[1] In the absence of population denominators, data restricted to numerators require some internally generated baseline against which to measure departures from expected values. These expectations must be created by statistical techniques. To generate baseline expectations, most monitoring techniques resort to average numbers of events over time; the averages are derived

---

[1]In the discussion of monitoring, we restrict the term "rates" to data that relate the number of events to the denominator population or sample from which the numerator events are drawn.

from stretches of time, generally preceding the monitoring phase, for which requisite data are available. In the "sets" technique, the time interval between events, and not the number of events over time, provides the monitoring index.

Several conditions—besides the quality, scope, and reliability of ascertainment already discussed—affect the speed with which one can recognize change in the occurrence of an outcome and also the likelihood that an alarm is false. We consider first the statistic used to measure change and to serve as a signal or alert that something may be amiss. In a monitoring system, change in the baseline parameters for outcomes of interest has three ready measures: relative risks for counts, odds ratios for proportions, and differences in means for continuous variables. In each case the use of these proportionate measures of association is suggested by standard statistical analyses for prototypical distributions such as the Poisson for counts, binomial for proportions, and Gaussian for continuous variables.

These rules are not inviolable, nor are the choices unalterable, and specific goals may be better served by variants. For example, when monitoring is used to plan resource allocations, an additive measure of change in expected counts may yield information more relevant to the purpose than the proportionate or multiplicative measure of relative risk. The following generalizations, as with most malformation monitoring, relate to changes in the number of outcomes counted, and to natural or canonical measures of the change. (The canonical measure of change with a Poisson distribution is the log relative risk; with a binomial distribution, it is the log odds ratio.)

In general, the likelihood of detecting a change in the frequency of any given outcome increases as the size of the population under surveillance increases, with the proviso that prevalence rates and ascertainment rates are fixed. If either of these rates in the comparison populations under surveillance are not the same, exceptions to the rule can occur. For example, ascertainment of cases may be more complete in smaller than in larger monitoring systems; the increase in the numbers of cases observed might then compensate for the smaller size of the denominator population (Kallen et al. 1984).

The advantages of a larger population are illustrated by example. In a setting with roughly 1000 births per month, consider a monthly count of neural tube defects with a baseline expectation of one case per month and with an assumed Poisson distribution (as the approximation to the binomial distribution for rare outcomes). Under these assumptions, doubling to two or more cases in one month would occur with probability 0.26, or about once in 4 months on average. In a population 10 times larger, with 10,000 births per month and a monthly expectation of 10 cases, doubling to 20 or more cases in one month would occur with a probability of less than 0.001, or once in a thousand months. The doubling in counts would, by convention, be judged insignificant in the smaller population and highly significant in the larger.

These considerations bear on how quickly a monitoring scheme can signal an alert. To achieve an acceptable rate for false alarms, a monitoring scheme must not be sensitive to random fluctuations that occur with a likelihood as high as 0.26, as in the preceding example. In general, with a fixed false alert rate (or alpha level) a monitoring system will signal the same true multiplicative change or relative risk more rapidly in the larger population than in the smaller.

Detectability is also affected by the baseline rate of the outcome in a given population, but to different effect for multiplicative versus absolute or additive change. When the baseline rate, and consequently the expected count, is high (and population sizes and ascertainment rates are equal), a given *multiplicative change* will be judged statistically significant more quickly than when the baseline rate is less. The numbers set out in the previous example can be used to illustrate this point if the expectations of 1 and 10 cases per month in the two settings are taken to pertain to two different malformations. Note that for additive change, however, the opposite obtains: a given *additive change* is less likely to lead to prompt detection when the baseline rate is high than when it is low. This is because—when the rate is high—in Poisson distributions a given mean shift entails both a smaller relative risk and a smaller shift in standard deviation terms.

This rule is relevant to the day-to-day clinical situation: change ordinarily impinges on an individual observer dealing with individual cases in absolute and not multiplicative terms. Hence with phocomelia and with vaginal adenocarcinoma in young women, their very rarity made more probable the recognition of change and the consequent discovery of the new teratogens thalidomide and diethylstilbestrol, respectively. Changes in the absolute numbers of cases were noticed because they deviated from previous experience. Of course, in population terms, such additive changes correspond to large relative risks.

The monitoring situation differs from the clinical situation, however, and for monitoring under ordinary conditions the rule for additive change and population size is less relevant. Relative risk is what impinges on a monitoring system. In monitoring, therefore, the first rule ordinarily applies: given a particular population size and outcome, the greater the rise in the underlying baseline rate of the outcome (and hence the greater the relative risk) the more readily the change will be detected. The size of the increase reflects both the strength of association between the causal factor and outcome, and the proportion of the population exposed to the causal factor. Thus, with the strength of association between factor and outcome held constant, the larger the proportion of the population exposed, the more ready detection is.

Should a population be highly saturated by a suspect causal factor—

for instance, tea or coffee in many developed countries—the small proportion who remain unexposed might present the same problems of detecting an effect on outcomes as a rare exposure might do. Requirements for numbers or statistical power might have to be met by purposeful design. In other words, monitoring is not usually an appropriate technique for discovering the effects of widespread and habitual exposures. The technique might be productive in the special circumstance when there is a decline in a common exposure that is or is not accompanied by a decline in a given outcome.

Statistical significance rests on the probability that an observation is incompatible with the null hypothesis of no association; the test is designed to guard against giving undue weight to a chance association (type I error). Statistical power is the probability that a true association of a given size can be found statistically significant; tests of power guard against falsely interpreting a failure to find a significant association as indicative of a true absence of association (type II error). For the efficient operation of a monitoring system, the calculation of similar kinds of probabilities is desirable. On the one hand, the type I error probability serves as a guide to the average time between false alerts; on the other hand, power (1 minus type II error probability) serves as a guide to how quickly, if at all, a true epidemic of a particular magnitude might be detected.

As in studies with fixed sample sizes, in monitoring the probabilities of type I and type II errors are usually inversely related: the more stringent the requirement to avoid false alerts, the longer the lag time is before an alert is signaled, and the lower the power to detect a true epidemic. The likelihood of detecting an epidemic, it will by now be evident, is influenced by the size of the population monitored, the baseline rate of the outcome, and the magnitude of the increase in underlying rates (which itself depends on three factors: the strength of the association between the causal factor and the outcome, the proportion of the population that is exposed, and the duration of the increase).

In the computation of power, magnitude is a preset value against which the probability of detection is estimated. In monitoring, magnitude must be conceived differently from what is usual in studies of fixed sample size. When the size of the sample is fixed, magnitude is ordinarily measured by the single dimension of the level of the increase in the rates under study. The fact that monitoring is an open-ended process through time adds a new dimension. The magnitude of an epidemic can be defined as the number of excess cases above baseline. This excess is the product of the level of the increase in baseline rates (e.g., the ratio of p_1, the new rate during the epidemic, to p_0, the baseline rate) and the duration of this increase.

Thus, in order to represent epidemic change of a particular magnitude, one must reckon in the time over which the increase persists. The same number of total excess cases might be produced in a variety of ways, for example, by large increases in baseline rates of short duration, or by modest increases of longer duration. The manner in which these two dimensions are subsumed in the concept of magnitude will influence (sometimes implicitly, sometimes explicitly) the criteria used to define an alert in monitoring systems using different statistical techniques.

In the same vein, monitoring systems differ from studies of fixed sample size in that investigators proceed by collecting and evaluating data over variable and often unspecified time periods. To apply the concepts of type I errors and type II errors to monitoring, therefore, the time period over which monitoring is to be carried out must be specified in advance. No doubt, if monitoring continued indefinitely, ultimately an epidemic that resulted from a new and persisting exposure would be detected. At the same time, if monitoring were to extend indefinitely, chance fluctuations in frequency inherent in the underlying variability of the outcome are likely to be encountered.

Hence the investigator needs to specify the maximum tolerable frequency of false alerts over a specified period of monitoring and, also, what size of effect is worthy of an alert and subsequent follow-up. How quickly the monitoring system detects such changes for given baseline rates in the population at large can then be determined. The capacity to detect small-scale change must be balanced against the capacity to avoid false alerts; these capacities are complementary and tied to each other. As we said earlier, the size of effects to which the system is sensitive should not be so small that many changes, insignificant in a practical sense, become grounds for an alert. The opposite danger is that the system may be too insensitive to signal an alert for quite large increases. The frequency with which false alerts can be tolerated is governed in part by the effort required to respond to them, for example, in follow-up research.

Monitoring Techniques and Analysis

Once the intended duration of monitoring and the size of effects to which the system will be sensitive have been decided, several analytic techniques are available to evaluate changes in frequencies over time. Monitoring programs for outcomes, we have emphasized, are ordinarily self-contained with respect to the data collected—for example, counts of malformations but not of the total cohort of births in the population at large that give rise to them. Unless the data refer to the population at large, therefore, monitoring requires methods that assume a stable population or adjust for population change. The speed with which a true increase can be detected varies somewhat between techniques; it varies also with such characteristics of the epidemic as the size of the increase in underlying baseline rates, duration, and periodicity.

A commonly used method tests whether the observed number of malformations differs from that expected by more than a prespecified number of standard deviations (e.g., Shewhart 1931; Van Dobben de Bruyn 1968). The baseline expectations are computed from a nonepidemic period that precedes monitoring. Since most malformations are rare, in a homogeneous and stable population the assumption that frequencies are distributed as a Poisson variable is often appropriate. For some outcomes, the distribution of counts is better described by the negative binomial distribution (Weatherall and Haskey 1976).

The method is easy to apply. For each time interval, observed numbers of each outcome need only be compared with a threshold preset to signal an excess. A disadvantage is that in testing observations from single time intervals, evidence accumulated over consecutive time intervals is ignored. Thus, epidemics that persist over adjacent intervals may be missed if, in any one time interval, the number of events falls short of the threshold chosen to signal a significant increase.

Another approach is the "sets" technique (Chen 1978, 1979; Gallus et al. 1986). In monitoring rare malformations, it is convenient to switch from the rate measure (malformations per unit time) to the reciprocal measure of interarrival times (time between successive malformations). In the sets procedure, a threshold interarrival time is prespecified, and an "event" is declared when an interarrival time falls below the threshold. When a run of N consecutive "events" occurs, where N is a small integer such as 1, 2, or 3, the system signals an alert. The threshold value and N are design parameters. The procedure is simple to implement, but efficiency is lost by dichotomizing "events" as above or below threshold. Hence, the sets procedure is not optimal for monitoring, although for very rare outcomes the inefficiency may not be substantial.[2]

A third approach, the cumulative summation (cusum) technique, takes account of persistent change by combining evidence sequentially over time. Consecutive excesses of counts above a reference value are accumulated until their cumulative sum crosses a prespecified level above the running minimum of cumulative sums, which then constitutes the signal of change in the mean number of events. The reference value is chosen so that the cumulative sums have a net downward drift under the baseline rate or count, but a net upward drift with an elevated rate or count worthy of detection. The cusum technique was introduced (Page 1954) for industrial quality control, and has been intensively studied.

---

[2]Published comparisons with the cusum technique (see later) have sometimes been misleading because the comparisons were not based on like distributional assumptions (e.g., the cusum technique designed for Poisson counts rather than geometric interarrival counts has been compared to the sets procedure, which is based on interarrival counts). It can be shown that the sets procedure is a nonoptimal special case of a cusum procedure appropriately adapted to geometric data (Levin, personal communication). Similar observations have been made by others (Kennett and Pollack 1983; Chen 1979).

The method has been applied to a monitoring system for malformations (Weatherall and Haskey 1976) and also in a retrospective evaluation of changes over time in karyotypes among miscarriages (Levin and Kline 1985). Figure 20-1 illustrates the latter.

When the cusum technique is applied in prospective monitoring, the design criteria are most often expressed in terms of average run length (ARL). The reference value and alert level are chosen to achieve certain values of ARL under the null and epidemic conditions. The cusum procedure is designed to ensure that, in the absence of change, the average waiting time before a false alarm (the "false alert waiting time") is sufficiently large. Subject to this condition, the procedure seeks to minimize the average waiting time between the change in the mean frequency of an event and the signal of this change (the "true alert waiting time").

The *false alert waiting time* is analogous to statistical significance and the avoidance of type I error. For example, the false alert waiting time speaks to the following question: if the underlying baseline rate of spina bifida is constant, how long will it take, on average, for the system to signal a false increase in the rate of spina bifida? The *true alert waiting time* is analogous to statistical power and the avoidance of type II error. The true alert waiting time speaks to the question: if the underlying baseline rate of spina bifida were to increase fivefold, how long would it take, on average, for this increase to be judged statistically significant in the monitoring system? The cusum procedure possesses certain optimality properties with respect to its stated goals. To wit, as the false-alert waiting time criterion is set larger and larger, the procedure approaches (and asymptotically attains) the theoretical lower limit for the true alert waiting time in any surveillance system (Lorden 1971). Other types of optimality have been discussed (Moustakides 1986).

Effectiveness and Efficiency of Monitoring

The degree to which surveillance or monitoring is successful can be considered in terms of both effectiveness and efficiency (Cochrane 1972). *Effectiveness* is simply a measure of effect, the degree to which the intended objective is met. With monitoring, the broad question posed is how quickly alerts to change in the baseline rates of the population under study were discovered. To arrive at a quantitative assessment, the question must be given more specific form. Some commonsense level of change needs to be agreed on as constituting an appropriate signal for a "lead," in much the same way as appropriate levels for statistical significance depend on convention. In a monitoring system, as noted above, the change is best specified as the scale of an epidemic or cluster; scale would be measured in terms of the increase in baseline rates and the duration of the increase. As with all such conventions, the monitoring

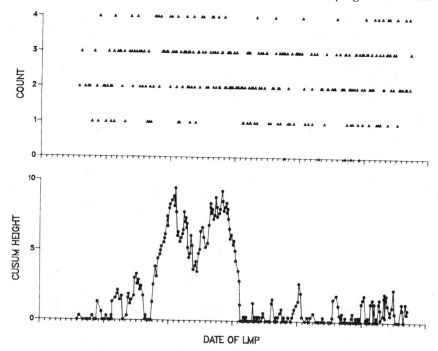

Fig. 20–1 Chromosomally normal miscarriages in one New York City hospital for 5 years from August 1, 1976 (dated by LMP). Top: Numbers of chromosomally normal losses (counts of 0, 1, 2, 3 or 4 per unit of 4 karyotypes). Bottom: Cumulative sum (cusum) chart shows a five-month epidemic ending early in 1978. Data were analyzed in units of 4 karyotypes with an expected mean of 2.4 chromosomally normal per unit; reference value for the cusum was 2.71; the conditional significance level of the maximum cusum was 0.02. (Adapted from Levin and Kline 1985.)

net will capture some chance fluctuations larger than the specified level and it will miss small-scale epidemics that do not break through the undifferentiated surface below the statistical threshold.

In a monitoring system for exposure, an index of effectiveness is its capacity to detect quickly true changes in the underlying level of exposure. Similarly, for outcomes, an index of effectiveness is its capacity to detect quickly changes in the underlying baseline rate. Hence effectiveness can be measured in terms of the lapse of time between a change in the underlying baseline rate of an outcome and the recognition of this change. Thus, a usual measure of effectiveness is simply the true alert waiting time: the average time interval between a change of specified scale in the baseline level and the signal of this change. The shorter the true alert waiting time, the more effective the system is.

Efficiency is a measure of the economy of means. Two systems with the same average true waiting times may not be equally efficient. Given equal true alert waiting times, the longer the time interval between false alerts, the more efficient the system is. An overall index of efficiency would best combine the true and false alert waiting time measures. Different monitoring techniques can thus be compared for the speed with which they signal increases of a particular size and duration, while holding constant the rate of false alerts.

A monitoring system that samples from a larger population, or deals only with numerator data, can be viewed as a screen to detect changes in the underlying baseline level of exposure or rate of outcome. In this context, we can ask whether some of the more familiar indices of effectiveness and efficiency for screening tests can be applied to monitoring systems. With screening tests for disease, one index of effectiveness is the *sensitivity* of the test, that is, the probability that persons with the disease (as judged by a more valid criterion) will screen positive. Indices of efficiency are the predictive values of the test. These indices combine information on sensitivity, specificity, and the prevalence of disease in the population being tested. With screening tests for disease, *positive predictive value* is the proportion of persons with a positive test who do in fact have the disease; *negative predictive value* is the proportion of persons with a negative test who in fact do not have the disease.

The measures of sensitivity, specificity and predictive values in screening for diseases are analogous in broad concept but not easily extended in practice to monitoring systems. In some part, this is because monitoring is a process that takes place over time, and the goal is not simply the detection of changes in baseline rates (analogous to the detection of disease), but also the *rapid* detection of these changes. The difficulties that arise are illustrated by attempting to define these indices for monitoring.

Sensitivity might be defined as the probability that an increase of a particular magnitude in the underlying baseline rate will be signaled within a specified time interval of its occurrence (say, one year). Conversely, if the baseline rate is unchanged, specificity might be defined as the probability that no alert is signaled over the time period. Definitions of this sort have the weakness that they require specification of the duration of the epidemic and the introduction of an arbitrary time interval within which it must be signaled.

We might ask in what way the true alert waiting time, a less arbitrary and more usual measure of effectiveness, relates to the definition of sensitivity given here. In comparing two monitoring systems, if the sensitivity of one system exceeds that of the other for all time intervals, then the true alert waiting time of the system with greater sensitivity will be shorter than that of the system with lower sensitivity. The converse is true only in special cases: with an exponentially distributed waiting time, the average waiting time is inversely related to sensitivity; that is, the shorter the true alert waiting time, the greater the sensitivity of a monitoring system. Similarly, in comparing different monitoring systems, the false alert waiting time will be longer in the system with greater specificity for all time intervals.

To extend the concept of predictive values to monitoring poses yet another problem. In screening tests, the computation of predictive values requires knowledge of the prevalence of disease. In monitoring, the analogous rate would be the frequency of epidemics of particular magnitudes. For example, we might consider the observation period to be a sequence of one-month intervals, and the frequency of epidemics would be the fraction of these intervals in which an increase in baseline rate of specified size occurred. The positive predictive value of an alert would be greater for exposures and outcomes with more frequent increases in baseline rates. Conversely, when no alert is signaled, the negative predictive value will be greater with lower frequencies of epidemics.

Monitoring is a device to alert us to possible changes in baseline rates that cannot be predicted in advance. Thus, it is rarely possible to specify the expected frequency distribution of epidemics. If the experience of monitoring systems thus far is any guide in the absence of requisite data, the frequency of epidemics of malformations may be low. This suggests that the positive predictive value of alerts in malformation monitoring systems may also be low.

The concept of predictive value serves to remind us that not all alerts signal changes in the underlying baseline rates, nor does the absence of alerts ensure that underlying baseline rates are unchanged. It appears, however, that the more conventional definitions of sensitivity, specificity, and predictive value have limited utility in defining the effectiveness and efficiency of monitoring systems, even though the systems themselves can be viewed as screens for changes in a larger population or, when counts are monitored, in baseline rates.

The evaluation of alerts signaled rests in surveillance. Surveillance goes beyond monitoring; it addresses the reality and scale of epidemic change in the population at large by gathering all available kinds of relevant data. It asks whether the monitoring system has in fact reflected a change in baseline rates. If so, it seeks the source. Ideally, it first asks whether the increase derives from changes in ascertainment or diagnosis or the frequency of known risk factors. If not, new causes of the disorder are sought. The next chapter thus explores the ways in which leads from monitoring systems, and from other sources, are followed.

21 Surveillance of Reproductive Outcomes II. Following Leads

The physical environment may arouse public health vigilance. Suspicion rises either with an undue frequency of some adverse outcome, or with an undue exposure to a possible hazard. In response, the search for causes of the excess cases, or for the effects of the suspect exposure, is a major commitment and a late rather than initial step. Untoward outcomes require confirmation. Spurious increases resulting from changes in ascertainment procedures or diagnosis need to be ruled out. In the face of uncertainty, action might be deferred until surveillance has demonstrated persistence of the excess. Untoward exposures are sometimes dramatic, as with large-scale nuclear or chemical accidents, but more often insidious and chronic. With large-scale environmental disaster, delay in assessing effects is, of course, inappropriate and not to be tolerated. With either form of exposure, nonetheless, an important and frequently neglected step is to seek out and measure or, at the least, estimate the accretion of physical constituents that are suspect.

With the change in outcome confirmed, an appropriate undertaking might be a case-control study. Comparisons of affected and unaffected pregnancies might discover exposures that could have led to the adverse outcome, or confirm the occurrence of a suspect exposure more often in cases than in controls. The data for such studies could come from those available in a monitoring system, or from special surveys. Where the alarm is set off by a major accident, prospective cohort studies might be called for at the outset. With exposures such as radiation, long-term monitoring might be appropriate. These approaches are not a first recourse. The particular circumstances, the level of suspicion, feasibility and economy dictate the choice. In what follows, we outline various grounds for choosing one or another approach to investigating a presenting problem (Report of Panel II 1981).

The aim of an epidemiological investigation is to elicit relationships between exposure and outcome that cannot be accounted for by differences between comparison groups extraneous to the relationships. To accomplish this aim, sources of extraneous variation need to be controlled. Characteristics of the comparison groups may differ in factors that affect the frequency of both exposure and outcome. Aside from the inherent character of the comparison groups, they may differ artifactually simply because modes of ascertainment or of data collection were not the same for each group.

The degree to which rigor can be achieved depends largely on the research strategy chosen, which in turn is limited by the resources and the effort to be deployed. The gravity of the outcome in terms of severity and the possible numbers involved are a first consideration in this deployment. A rational choice of strategy is governed by the strength of the suspicion that justifies the research. Low levels of suspicion, when no more than hints and intimations point to risk, can justify ventures only if they can be mounted with ease, speed and economy. Such facility usually sacrifices precision and detail. High levels of suspicion may be created or reinforced by these "quick and dirty" studies. The more intense the suspicion, which is to say the stronger the hypothesis or the intuition, the greater the effort called for. Here we classify study designs by the levels of effort required to mount them (Susser 1968; Stein et al. 1981a).

Level I.   These studies draw on existing and accessible data. They usually provide the least precision in definition of exposure, the smallest range and the least detailed description of outcomes, and the fewest data for safeguarding the comparability of study groups. Estimations of exposure must usually depend on the averages for a population, as when they are based on the proximity of homes to a toxic waste site, or on knowledge that water sources are contaminated. Rarely is it possible to distinguish the exact exposure of either parent or the duration of exposure. Indeed, even the fact of exposure may be in doubt.

With respect to outcome, Level I studies may draw on vital certificate data or special registries of malformations; thus, in most circumstances the range of outcomes is limited to birth weight, perinatal mortality, sex of offspring, and possibly malformations among births. In most places, birth certificates provide data on a few potentially confounding variables such as maternal age, but records of personal habits such as cigarette smoking or alcohol drinking are not to be expected. Causal inferences are likely to be weak. Both positive and negative findings may need a second level of study.

Despite all these limitations, such studies are efficient; they reward the level of effort involved in a first search by providing leads to possible environmental influences. The potential of such studies should not be underrated when secondary analyses can be carried out on archived research data (Hyman 1972). One example was the search in the National Collaborative Perinatal Project data set for the consequences of maternal alcohol abuse after the fetal alcohol syndrome was described (Jones et al. 1974). No systematic histories of maternal alcohol use or of alcoholism were taken. Nonetheless records in which there was a mention of alcoholism were pulled and reviewed and culled to define a small group that probably was alcoholic during pregnancy. Under these circumstances, the identification of some children with features compatible with the syndrome added substantially to the evidence available up to that time.

Another example was a large Australian case-control study of 8517 infants with congenital malformations and 8517 without such anomalies, matched for maternal age and time of birth (Donovan et al. 1983). This study was designed to test the suggestion that the offspring of men who had served in the Vietnam War were at raised risk for some or all birth defects. A defoliant, Agent Orange, had been used to clear large tracts of jungle and was the suspected agent. Vietnam army service was established through linking birth record data on fathers with military records. Large-scale, economical, anonymous and expeditious, this study was able to set the worst fears of the servicemen at rest. At the same time, such a study could in no way address or resolve all the major issues.

Level II. These studies extend beyond the reach of routinely available or already collected data: they engage the researchers in field surveys, the data from which can be cast in cross-sectional or case-control forms. Field surveys permit the collection of data that gain in information and precision because of specified hypotheses. Questions can focus both on the exposure of individuals and on potentially confounding variables, and they enable outcome variables to be refined by means of detailed histories and direct examination.

Thus, the range of outcomes can go beyond what is readily obtained through routine sources, and includes others obtainable on interview (e.g., early fetal deaths or sexual dysfunction) or else on special examination (e.g., the quality of semen, or the level of particular hormones or particular antibodies). Precision in the definition of exposure gained through personal interviews can be further improved by examining homes and domestic animals, as well as water, vegetation, topography, and weather.

Contact with the people under study to obtain such data requires tact and care, and benefits from the support of local community and political organizations. When properly carried out, many Level II studies provide information on exposure and outcome that can be analyzed at the individual level.

An example is a study in the United States of the same Agent Orange problem investigated at Level I in Australia. The Centers for Disease Control undertook to test the possible connections between army service in Vietnam and fathering a child with birth defects (Erickson et al. 1984). A case-control design was adopted, with nearly 5000 cases and 3000 controls. This investigation was much more costly than the Australian study, because all the individual parents of cases and controls were interviewed at length on the telephone. Data on location and duration of service were obtained by interview and also from the military record. With detailed data available, the analysis could be more sophisticated, especially regarding the control of potential confounding variables. The results for this Level II study were, like those of the Level I study, essentially negative.

The scientific basis for the hypothesis under test in this study was somewhat tenuous; strong grounds for suspecting a male exposure, at times often well before insemination, are hard to find. The rationale was rather social and political. This is not necessarily to say that the study was without justification. A large number of men had been exposed; high degrees of individual anxiety were attached to the question, and national concern was stimulated by attention from the media and congressional representatives.

Level III. These studies are longitudinal. Like those of Level II, they usually involve the collection of field survey data. The increment in cross-sectional information from the survey is enhanced by the follow-up of cohorts of exposed and unexposed individuals. With this prospective element, Level III studies add an important dimension; events are observed as they unfold over time.

In some circumstances follow-up can be achieved without contact with study subjects. In Finland, occupations of parents are registered and can be linked with hospital discharge registries as well as malformation registries (Hemminki et al. 1983a). In Sweden and Norway, census data can be linked to birth registry data that include information on malformations (see Kallen et al. 1984 for review). In Canada, cohorts with particular occupational and other exposures, or with particular medical conditions, can be followed by linkage with data bases for mortality and cancer incidence (Smith and Newcombe 1980). In England and Wales, longitudinal follow-up has been effected by creating cohorts from a 1 per cent random sample of the national census and following them through the national vital registration systems and through death and cancer registries (Adelstein 1974).

In the United States, with its 50 states and many independent sources of data, such linkages between data systems have been more difficult. Hence, Level III studies must usually be effected, after the exposed and unexposed subjects are assembled at the start of the study, by individual follow-up to ascertain outcome. Special populations do exist, however, from which historical cohorts can be constructed, as has been done with studies of asbestos from union records (Selikoff 1968), and with studies of multiple outcomes from military records (Beebe 1960, 1962; Kurtzke et al. 1979). In all such ventures that aim to study the relations of a particular exposure and outcome, ingenuity and luck play a large part.

When an entire cohort can be followed without severe losses to follow-up, Level III studies are likely to provide the strongest evidence for causal inference. Exposure is defined before the outcome occurs and to that degree is unbiased. Participation involves self- and social selection; bias from that source is controlled by complete follow-up of the cohort. On the other hand, such studies, laborious and difficult to carry out, require both diligence and patience. Years may pass before a study is completed and decisions consequent on the findings can be made.

As an example of a Level III study, we again draw on a study of the exposure of servicemen to defoliants in Vietnam in relation to birth defects in their offspring. A cohort of men was identified who, having served in the Air Force squadron that sprayed the defoliant, had been in close proximity to the suspected agent. The reproductive experiences of these men and their spouses were compared with those of a cohort who had served in another squadron not connected with the defoliant. This study shared with other cohort studies the advantage that a wide range of reproductive outcomes could be examined, for example, fertility, miscarriage, birth weight, malformations, and learning defects. On the other hand, it also shared the typical disadvantages of limited numbers with regard to outcome. Again, the results have not supported the suspicion of adverse effects on reproduction (Lathrop et al. 1984).

To conclude this brief consideration of these three levels of effort, we note first that the discussion of strategies is by no means exhaustive. Many ingenious approaches have been devised by enterprising researchers, and many more will be. Among the innovations not discussed here are efforts that heavily involve the members of a community in studying their own environmental problems, with all the hazards of bias and the rewards of incentive entailed (Lagakos et al. 1986). Although studies of exposures and effects at the individual level are nearly always more cogent and to be preferred to study at the ecological level, some problems have lent themselves well to this approach. Indeed, some problems can be addressed only at the ecological level. Properly approached, areas become the unit for estimating sample size and for analysis. Thus, for example, randomization and analysis at the level of groups was the approach taken in an evaluation of the effects of vitamin A on child mortality in Indonesia (Sommer et al. 1983; National Research Council 1986). Such large-scale undertakings are the exception. The group approach used to evaluate the Women Infants and Children (WIC) food and nutrition program in the United States (Rush 1988), for example, used a nonrandomized quasi-experimental design, in which areas penetrated more or less fully were compared.

For reasons of practicability and cost, in research on the physical environment designs of choice are the exception. Researchers must make do with a variety of devices and a weaker level of inference. In the main, we have emphasized the characteristics of studies that aid interpretability. The refinement achieved by classifying exposure from the experiences of individuals rather than of groups brings power with the refinement. Further refinement is gained by specifying the duration, timing, dose, and route of exposure.

The predictive power of hypotheses is sharpened when adverse outcomes are selected because they are the most likely to occur and not merely because they are available in routine records. Limits are placed on the degree of confounding when data can be acquired with which to test the comparability of study groups. Finally, bias is removed and the stringency of the test of a hypothesis is enhanced by the independent ascertainment of exposure and outcome. Level III studies can meet nearly all of these desiderata; Level II studies can meet many; Level I studies can meet few. Level II studies are perhaps most vulnerable in their capacity to maintain independence between exposure and outcome status: interviews with affected and unaffected individuals often provide the only data on exposure or outcomes, which raises the potential for differential recall and bias. Level I studies tend to fall short in many areas, although they offer the most economical and least intrusive means of examining the research question.

OUTCOMES

The possible adverse outcomes of reproduction affected by environmental exposures are many. Any or several of the endpoints listed in Table 21-1 can be examined. The inclusions and exclusions in the list are both pragmatic (the endpoints are capable of being measured in an epidemiologic study) and theoretical (the endpoints have been shown to vary in frequency).

No one has used all the outcomes listed to test for effects on reproduction. Choices made among them have often seemed arbitrary or ill-considered. Yet the selection of appropriate endpoints for study may be the most crucial scientific decision made. The issues to be weighed in such a choice are many: biological coherence; the frequency of the outcome in the unexposed; accessibility of data; the statistical costs of interpreting associations with single or multiple endpoints; and the financial costs and technical problems of data-gathering. For purposes of surveillance, monitoring and analysis, each outcome variable must be approached with due respect for epidemiological pitfalls.

Table 21-2 shows crude frequencies for indices of reproductive outcome in unexposed populations. It should be borne in mind that two- and threefold differences can be found between groups defined by such factors as age, social class and race.

Table 21–1 Potential sentinels of prenatal environmental exposure: reproductive and developmental disorders

Sexual dysfunction
   decreased libido
   impotence

Sperm abnormalities
   decreased number
   decreased motility
   abnormal morphology

Subfecundity
   abnormal gonads, ducts, or external genitalia
   abnormal pubertal development
   infertility (of male or female origin)
   amenorrhea
   anovulatory cycles
   time to conception

Complications of pregnancy and parturition
   toxemia
   hemorrhage

Chromosomally normal loss
   subclinical
   miscarriage
   intermediate and late fetal death
   intrapartum fetal death
   death in the first week

Chromosomal aberration
   subclinical
   miscarriage
   intermediate and late fetal death
   births (or detected at induced abortion or prenatal diagnosis)

Birth weight
   decreased (without distinction of preterm or growth retardation)
   growth retarded

Gestational age at delivery
   premature
   postmature

Altered sex ratio

Multiple births

Birth defects
   major
   minor
   specific types

Infant mortality

Childhood malignancies

Childhood morbidity

Childhood mortality

Age at menopause

Table 21–2 Expected frequencies of some potential sentinels of environmental exposure

Event	Frequency (%)	Denominator
Azoospermia	1	Men
Birth weight <2500 grams[a]	5–15	Live births
Failure to conceive after one year of unprotected intercourse	10–15	Couples
Miscarriage	10–20	Pregnancies
Chromosome aberration at miscarriage	40–50	Miscarriages
Chromosome aberration at amniocentesis (women ≥35 years)	2	Amniocentesis specimens
Late fetal deaths (≥28 weeks)	1–4	Late fetal deaths + live births
Birth defects	2–3	Live births
Chromosome aberration at birth	0.6	Live births
Neural tube defects	.005–1.0	Late fetal deaths + live births
Severe mental retardation[b]	.4	Children to age 15

[a]Also, birth weight can be analyzed as a continuous variable.

[b]Includes children with chromosomal aberrations (primarily trisomy 21).

EXPOSURES

In recent years, it is not uncommon that the call for public health action comes from community residents who suspect chemical or physical pollution of the environment is causing adverse effects. When the starting point is the exposure, the requirements for the choice and construction of outcome variables differ from those when studies begin with effects. Whether laboratory or clinical knowledge is available to guide us to likely effects is a matter of chance and history.

The exposure, physical or chemical, may be difficult to specify in terms of both constituents and quantity. An accident in a nuclear plant, as at Three Mile Island in 1979, emits radiation for which monitors provide measures of some kind, even if they are suspected of covering an incomplete spectrum of radiation. But such an accident may well cause chemical interactions with emissions of which there are no measures. Chemical waste sites, too, commonly defy precise description of constituents, and hence the identification of relevant exposures. Contaminants may be multiple and several of them equally suspect. The responsible agents may be neither one or many of these individual contaminants, but new products formed through their interaction.

Besides knowledge of the nature of the exposure, the timing of exposure is crucial to causal inference, as we illustrated for teratogenesis in Part I. Frequently both the time of onset and duration of relevant exposure are inexactly known, or not known at all. With an acute exposure, as in a nuclear accident or a breakdown in a chemical plant, measures of contaminants at the time of the accident give investigators valuable if partial information for following up consequences. The measures can be complemented and refined by the tracing and testing of likely routes of exposure. The inhalation of polluted air, drinking of contaminated water, eating of contaminated vegetables, and direct contact with contaminated materials in homes or schoolyards all could have a part.

With past or chronic exposures, estimates are less likely to be obtainable. Estimates of past exposure may be needed to provide a baseline against which to compare acute exposure, or to weigh the contribution of past exposure to current effects that follow a presumed latent period. In most circumstances, epidemiologists must be content with descriptions of exposure based on the sampling, more or less adequate, of the current environment. Information on the stability of concentrations over time, or on the by-products that may have been formed, is seldom if ever recoverable. Sometimes, by good fortune, routine data from environmental monitoring in previous years are available.

Even if the nature, concentration, timing, and route of exposure are known, these descriptors are frequently ecological, in that they relate only to a site and to a population at that site. Data for each individual on the probable dose, time, and duration of exposure are difficult to obtain, except for some special hazardous occupations and special exposures. In the absence of such data, individuals must usually be allocated to an exposure class on the basis of an average exposure at a site. In the investigation of hazards to reproduction, such allocations are a blunt probe in most cases.

Some exposures can be measured from deposits or residues in the tissues of exposed individuals. DDT, polychlorbiphenyl and some other exposures can be inferred from serum or from biopsies of fat tissue. For instance, measurements of blood specimens taken from the umbilical cord were used to test the effect of polychlorbiphenyl on birth weight (Fein et al. 1984). Plutonium exposure has been estimated, after many years in the body, from the elimination patterns of this radioactive substance. With this element, precise estimates of dose have been obtained from measurements of urine (Lawrence 1962). In men exposed during World War II, ostensibly accurate dosage has been calculated from successive measurements over 20 years (Hempelmann et al. 1973).

The problems of measuring exposures are well illustrated by studies of pollution of the ambient air (Holland et al. 1979; Shy 1979). Air pollution was the subject of more sustained research over the first three post-World War II decades than was any other form of chemical and physical exposure except radiation. Yet even with an automated monitoring system, as in New York City in the 1960s, uncertainties abound about the nature and levels of exposure (Goldstein and Landowitz 1977).

The several pollutants measured constituted a relatively small number of all the contaminants suspected of polluting the ambient air of the city, and of these not all were efficiently monitored. Quite probably many contaminants emitted by various manufacturing plants were not even suspected. For pollutants such as smoke and sulfur dioxide that could be monitored, measurements carried out at the same time but at different sites in the city correlated only modestly, if at all, with each other. Thus, if the measures were accurate, which is not certain, exposures were local and varied substantially from place to place. This is not to say that measurement of ambient and indoor air, and of other sources of pollutants in water, soil and workplace, cannot be greatly improved by technical advances. Improvements now underway include estimates that take account of topography, wind direction, and meteorological conditions.

Changing estimates of radiation effects tell another cautionary tale. The dosimetry of the atomic bombs at Hiroshima and Nagasaki is the foundation for official views about the effects of radiation on cancer, including the particular effects of prenatal exposures. Exposure levels were estimated from what is known about the bombs and the bomb sites; effects were estimated from the cohorts of survivors now followed for more than 40 years. With later study, it has become evident that the neutron dose ascribed to the one-of-a-kind Hiroshima bomb was probably too high by a factor of 10. The main exposures were to gamma rays, much less carcinogenic than beta rays. Hence the observed effects must be attributed to lesser doses than was previously thought and the risks attached to those doses revised upward accordingly. In addition, as the exposed cohorts age, the range of effects has expanded, and effects have grown larger in those exposed prenatally relative to those exposed as adults. Estimates of relative risks for cancers overall have increased twofold to threefold; for those exposed young five- to sixfold; and for childhood leukemia about tenfold. A quadratic dose–response model has been used, with an assumed threshold before any dose has an effect. If the more likely linear model is assumed as the basis for estimates instead, the overall risk of various outcomes is doubled again (Roberts 1987; Radiation Effects Research Foundation 1987; Lambert 1988).

Epidemiologists must be content with indices of exposure that are less than perfect. In the usual way, and in the absence of detailed information of the movements of individuals from place to place, misclassification of the exposure status of the individual is virtually certain to occur, with a consequent reduction in the statistical power to detect associations between specific exposures and given outcomes. Under these conditions, the discovery of any relationship of an exposure to an outcome must usually be considered an impressive feat and a matter of good fortune.

Finally, in dealing with exposures as in other matters, rational public health action relates to populations and is necessarily founded on statistics. Some statistics have been created specifically for the purpose of estimating the potential mass effect of an exposure that has a known or putative risk for specified outcomes. These *attributable risk* statistics have widespread application in public health. In matters of planning, policy and evaluation, the statistics are germane for estimating population burden. Attributable risk statistics require comparison data—exposed versus unexposed compared in terms of outcome, or cases versus controls compared in terms of exposure. They also require estimates for the population affected of the frequencies of both exposure and outcome, or of both exposure and relative risk. With monitoring that produces self-contained numerator data only, albeit continuously over time, the necessary comparisons are often lacking. By contrast, a fully deployed surveillance system can be expected to produce population rates as opportunity arises.

Attributable risk bears on the weighing and the burden of a particular outcome in the population at large. We noted that the magnitude of an epidemic can be described in terms of the number of cases that occurred in excess of expectation over a given period among those who dwell in the location under surveillance. If a known or putative causal factor or a risk factor has been identified, attributable risk gives a sense of the importance of the factor to the occurrence of a disorder in such a population. The statistic indicates the proportion or amount of all cases attributable to the particular factor under study. It depends jointly on the strength of association between exposure and outcome (risk ratio) and the frequency of exposure among the total number of cases in the designated study population. The statistic can be stated either as that fraction of all cases that can be attributed to the factor (*attributable fraction* or *etiologic fraction*) or as the arithmetic excess of cases (*excess risk*). Since two terms contribute to the attributable risk—the risk ratio and the frequency of exposure in the population—if one is large and the other trivial, the attributable fraction is small. Thus, even when a factor has a very strong association with an outcome, unless or until a sufficient proportion of the population has been exposed, the proportion of cases attributable to the factor (or the number of excess cases) may be low (reviewed in Susser et al. 1985a; Khoury and Holtzman 1987).

SOCIAL AND POLITICAL QUESTIONS

Investigators of environmental effects must expect to encounter human problems as well as technical problems. Studies of the effects of chemical dump sites on the health of those who dwell nearby are illustrative. Sites for dumps are likely to be chosen precisely because the surrounding populations are small and dispersed. The range of outcomes represented will in consequence be limited. Lack of statistical power may forbid interpretation of the variety of effects of interest, even in large populations.

Social, political and economic questions obtrude on these technical questions and impede investigation. Once the alarm has been sounded, a highly charged atmosphere quickly develops (Levine 1982). Whole communities, and the sense of identity and security of residents, have been undermined by a preventible industrial disaster (Erikson 1976). Anger and fear pervade communities when a serious health hazard is suspected. The situation is likely to be shot through with conflict. In the affected communities, mistrust of authority tends to accompany suspicion. Local bureaucrats, on their side, tend to respond defensively in attempts to circumscribe legal responsibility for the emerging situation (Freudenberg 1984). Government authorities want to avoid the political consequences. Companies, corporations, or entrepreneurs want to avoid the economic consequences.

The hostilities of an adversarial atmosphere make it difficult or impossible to learn from disaster or potential disaster. Access to plants, records, and exposed people may be blocked (Paigen 1981). Data obtained by personal interview, especially in the aftermath of an acute event or in the persisting turmoil of public concern, are subject to unconscious or even conscious bias. The person interviewed may be an interested party or a victim with a corresponding state of mind. Critical reviewers, parties at risk of litigation because of their responsibilities in relation to the exposure, and paid "expert" witnesses from whatever side, can be expected uniformly to cast doubt on all available data.

In recent years we have learned that even supposedly open democratic governments are not always to be trusted in such matters. After the nuclear plant accident at Windscale in 1957, the British government is reported to have suppressed knowledge of its large scale for the next 30 years (Dickson 1988). In the U.S., the Army is likewise reported to have suppressed information of the radiation risks of nuclear weapons testing in Colorado and Utah in the 1950s. The fact of contamination over several decades from the plants controlled by the Department of Energy is becoming known only as this book goes to press, and its extent is still to be fully established. Whenever possible, the prudent investigator seeks validation in other evidence of the information purveyed by government, industry and interested parties.

These real-life problems influence both the design of a study and the inferences that can be drawn from it when completed. The first question likely to be raised by a community concerned about potential exposure is whether exposure is associated with ill health. The question involves statistical significance. In the event of a negative result, a second question likely to be raised is the likelihood that a particular investigation could have failed to detect health effects that were in fact present. This question involves statistical power.

The epidemiologist increasingly plays two roles: as researcher into the causes and consequences of health disorders and as counselor on public health issues. The two roles are not always in harmony. The researcher may be restrained by rigorous judgment from inferring that a factor is harmful. At the same time, the counselor may be constrained by prudence to advise regulation or withdrawal of the factor because of a reasonable possibility that it could be hazardous. The role of the counselor is generally the more pressing. Many public health questions demand immediate responses and quick decisions. By contrast, causal inference is usually a long-drawn-out process that depends on repeated tests and the gradual evolution of knowledge. The researcher must nonetheless guard jealously the right to insist on unbiased observations, sound design, logical constructs, and careful analyses. In the absence of laboratory experiments on human beings, these are the foundations for sound inference in human reproduction.

Bibliography

Abbott A., Siebert J.R., and Weaver J.B. 1977 Chondrodysplasia punctata and maternal warfarin treatment *Br Med J* 1:1639–1640.

Abel E.L. 1980 Smoking during pregnancy: A review of effects on growth and development of offspring *Hum Biol* 52:593–625.

Abel E.L. 1984 *Fetal Alcohol Syndrome and Fetal Alcohol Effects* Plenum Press, New York.

Abel E.L. 1985 Fetal alcohol effects: Advice to the advisors *Alcohol Alcoholism* 20:189–93.

Adelstein A.M. 1972 The Medical Division of the Office of Population Censuses and Surveys. I. Objectives and Methods *Health Trends* 4:2.

Adelstein A.M. 1974 National statistics In D. Barltrop, ed. *Paediatrics and the Environment* Fellowship of Postgraduate Medicine, London, pp. 57–67.

Ainsworth M. 1967 *Infancy in Uganda* Johns Hopkins University Press, Baltimore.

Alberman E. 1973 The epidemiology of spontaneous abortions and their chromosome constitution In A. Boué and C. Thibault, eds. *Les accidents chromosomiques de la reproduction* Institute National de la Sante et de la Recherche Medicale, pp 305–316.

Alberman E. 1981a The abortus as a predictor of future trisomy 21 pregnancies In F. de la Cruz and P. Gerald, eds. *Trisomy 21 (Down syndrome) Research Perspectives* University Park Press, Baltimore, pp 69–76.

Alberman E. 1981b The scope of perinatal statistics and the usefulness of comparisons In R. Chester, P. Diggory, and M. Sutherland, eds. *Changing Patterns of Childbearing and Child Rearing* Academic Press, London.

Alberman E., and Peckham C.S. 1977 Infections and pregnancy In C.R. Coid, ed. *Long-Term Effects Following Infections in Pregnancy* Academic Press, London, pp 489–514.

Alberman E., Polani P.E., Fraser Roberts J.A., Spicer C.C., Elliott M., and Armstrong E. 1972a Parental exposure to X-irradiation and Down's syndrome *Ann Hum Genet Lond* 36:195–208.

Alberman E., Polani P.E., Fraser Roberts J.A. et al. 1972b Parental X-irradiation and chromosome constitution in their spontaneously aborted foetuses *Ann Hum Genet Lond* 36:185–194.

Alberman E., Creasy M., and Polani P.E. 1973 Spontaneous abortion and neural-tube defects *Br Med J* 4:230–231.

Alberman E., Elliott M., Creasy M., and Dhadial, R. 1975 Previous reproductive history in mothers presenting with spontaneous abortions *Br J Obstet Gynaecol* 82:366–373.

Alberman E., Creasy M., Elliott M., and Spicer C. 1976 Maternal factors associated with fetal chromosomal anomalies in spontaneous abortions *Br J Obstet Gynaecol* 83:621–627.

Alberman E., Roman E., Pharoah P.O., and Chamberlain G. 1980 Birth weight before and after a spontaneous abortion *Br J Obstet Gynaecol* 87:275–280.

Albert R. E. and Oman A. R. 1968 Follow-up study of patients treated by x-ray epilation for tinea capitis I. Population characteristics, posttreatment illnesses, and mortality experience *Arch Env Hlth* 17:899–918.

Alexander G.R., Tompkins M.E., Altekruse J.M., and Hornung C.A. 1985 Racial differences in the relation of birth weight and gestational age to neonatal mortality *Publ Health Rep* 100:539–547.

Alfi O.S., Chan R., and Azen S.P. 1980 Evidence for genetic control of nondisjunction in man *Am J Hum Genet* 32:477–483.

American Academy of Pediatrics 1967 Committee on fetus and newborn: Nomenclature for duration of gestation, birth weight and intra-uterine growth *Pediatrics* 39:935–939.

American College of Obstetricians and Gynecologists 1977 *Guidelines on Pregnancy and Work.* National Institute of Occupational Safety and Health, Rockville, MD.

American Society of Anesthesiologists 1974 Occupational disease among operating room personnel: A national study *Anesthesiology* 4:321–340.

Amin-Zaki L., Majeed M.A., Elhassani S.B., Clarkson T.W., Greenwood M.R., and Doherty R.A. 1979 Prenatal methylmercury poisoning. Clinical observations over five years *Am J Dis Child* 133:172–177.

Anctil A., Joshi B.J., Lucas W.E., Little W.A., and Callagan D.A. 1964 Prematurity: A more precise approach to identification *Obstet Gynecol* 24:716–721.

Andersen F., Johnson T.R.B., Flora J.D., and Barclay M.L. 1981a Gestational age assessment. I. Analysis of individual clinical observations *Am J Obstet Gynecol* 139:173–177.

Andersen F., Johnson T.R.B., Flora J.D., and Barclay M.L. 1981b Gestational age assessment. II. Prediction from combined clinical observations *Am J Obstet Gynecol* 140:770–774.

Anderson G.D., Blidner I.N., McClemont S., and Sinclair J.C. 1984 Determinants of size at birth in a Canadian population *Am J Obstet Gynecol* 150:236–244.

Andre-Thomas M., Chesni Y., and St. Anne-Dargassies S. 1960 The neurological examination of the infant (Little Club Clinics in Developmental Medicine, No. 1) National Spastics Society, London.

Andrews J. and McGarry J.M. 1972 A community study of smoking in pregnancy *J Obstet Gynecol* 79:1057–1073.

Angell R.R., Templeton A.A., and Aitken R.J. 1986 Chromosome studies in human in vitro fertilization *Hum Genet* 72:333–339.

Annegers J.F., Elveback L.R., Hauser W.A., and Kurland L.T. 1974 Do anticonvulsants have a teratogenic effect? *Arch Neurol* 31:364–373.

Antonov A.N. 1947 Children born during siege of Leningrad in 1942 *J Pediatr* 30:250–259.

Aral S.O. and Cates W. 1983 The increasing concern with infertility. Why now? *JAMA* 250:2327–2331.

Armstrong E.G., Ehrlich P.H., Birken S., Schlatterer J.P., Siris E., Hembree W.C., and Canfield R.E. 1984 Use of a highly sensitive and specific immunoradiometric assay for detection of human chorionic gonadotropin in urine of normal, nonpregnant, and pregnant individuals *J Clin Endocrin Metab* 59:867–874.

Armstrong E.G., Birken S., Moyle W.R., and Canfield R.E. 1986 Immunochemistry of Human Chorionic Gonadotropin In *Biochemical Actions of Hormones*, Vol XIII, Academic Press, pp 91–127.

Arthur R.K. Jr. and Kaltreider D.F. 1956 The elderly nullipara: An analysis of the hazards of late first viable pregnancy, with especial reference to caesarean section *Obstet Gynecol* 8:215–222.

Aschheim S. 1930 Die Schwangershcaftsdiagnose aus dem Harne In: A. Martin, A. Doderlein, L. Seitz, H. Sellheim, and G.A. Wagner, eds. *Abhandlungen Aus der Geburtshilfe und Gynakologie und ihren Grenzgebieten*, Vol 3, Verlag Von S. Kaerger, Berlin.

Ashford J.R., Fryer J.G., and Brimblecombe F.S.W. 1969 Secular trends in late foetal deaths, neonatal mortality, and birth weight in England and Wales 1956–1965 *Br J Prev Soc Med* 23:154–162.

Ashford J.R., Read K.L.Q., and Riley V.C. 1973 An analysis of variations in perinatal mortality amongst local authorities in England and Wales *Int J Epidemiol* 2:31–46.

Askrog V. and Harvald B. 1970 Teratogen effekt af inhalationsanaestetika *Nordisk Med* 83:498–500.

Aurelius G., Radestad A., Nylander I., and Zetterstrom R. 1987 Psychosocial factors and pregnancy outcome *Scand J Soc Med* 15:79–85.

Australian In Vitro Fertilization Collaborative Group 1985 High incidence of preterm births and early losses in pregnancy after in vitro fertilization *Br Med J* 291:1160–1163.

Avery, G.B., Monif G.G.R., Sever J.L., and Leikin S.L. 1965 Rubella syndrome after inapparent maternal illness *Am J Dis Child* 110:444–446.

Axelson O., Edling C., and Andersson L. 1983 Pregnancy outcome among women in a Swedish rubber plant *Scand J Work Environ Health* 9 (suppl 2):79–83.

Axelsson G. and Rylander R. 1982 Exposure to anaesthetic gases and spontaneous abortion: Response bias in a postal questionnaire study *Int J Epid* 11:250–256

Axelsson G. and Rylander R. 1984 Validation of questionnaire-reported miscarriage, malformation and birth weight *Int J Epid* 13:94–98.

Axelsson G., Jeansson S., Rylander R., and Unander M. 1980 Pregnancy abnormalities among personnel at a virological laboratory *Am J Ind Med* 1:129–137.

Axelsson G., Lutz C., and Rylander R. 1984 Exposure to solvents and outcome of pregnancy in university laboratory employees *Br J Ind Med* 41:305–312.

Aylward G.P., Hatcher R.P., Leavitt L.A., Rao V., Bauer C.R., Brennan M.J., and Gustafson N.F. 1984 Factors affecting neurobehavioral responses of preterm infants at term conceptional age *Child Dev* 55:1155–1165.

Ayme S. and Lippman-Hand A. 1982 Maternal-age effect in aneuploidy: Does altered embryonic selection play a role? *Am J Hum Genet* 34:558–565.

Ayme S. and Lippman-Hand A. 1983 Maternal age and altered embryonic selection: A reply to Carothers and to Warburton, Stein and Kline *Am J Hum Genet* 35:1064–1066.

Bachrach C.A. and Horn M.C. 1988 Sexual activity among US women of reproductive age *AJPH* 78:320–321.

Baillie M., Allen E.D., and Elkington A.R. 1980 The congenital warfarin syndrome: A case report *Br J Ophthal* 64:633–635.

Baird D. 1977 Epidemiology patterns over time In D. Reed and F.J. Stanley, eds. *The Epidemiology of Prematurity* Urban & Schwarzenberg, Baltimore, pp 5–15.

Baird D. 1980 Environment and reproduction *Br J Obstet Gynaecol* 87:1057–1067.

Baird D. and Thomson A.M. 1969 In N.R. Butler and E. Alberman *Perinatal Problems.* Livingstone, London.

Baird D., Baumgartner L., Chaudhuri K.C., Gomez F., Lelong M., and Lesinski J. 1961 Expert Committee on Maternal and Child Health in Geneva, 1960 *WHO Hlth Org Tech Rep Ser* 217:1–116.

Baird D.D. and Wilcox A.J. 1985 Cigarette smoking associated with delayed conception *JAMA* 253:2979–2983.

Baird D.D., Wilcox A.J., and Weinberg C.R. 1986 Use of time to pregnancy to study environmental exposures *Am J Epidemiol* 124:470–480.

Baker G. 1785 An essay concerning the cause of the Endemial Colic of Devonshire (1767), 3rd Ed. *Med Tr Lond* 1:175–256, Delta Omega Soc. 1958, Baltimore.

Baker-Faulkner E. 1925 Protective Labor Legislation with Special Reference to Women in the State of New York Vol 116, Columbia University Studies in History, Economics, and Public Law; reprinted 1976 ed., AMS Press, New York.

Bakketeig L.S. 1977 The risk of repeated preterm or low birth weight delivery In D.M. Reed and F. Stanley, eds. *The Epidemiology of Prematurity* Urban & Schwarzenberg, Baltimore, pp 231–241.

Bakketeig L. S. and Hoffman H. J. 1979 Perinatal mortality by birth order within cohorts based on sibship size *Br Med J* 3:693–696.

Bakketeig L.S. and Hoffman H.J. 1981 The epidemiology of preterm birth: Results from a longitudinal study of births in Norway In M.G. Elder and C.H. Hendricks, eds. *Preterm Labor*, Butterworths International Medical Reviews, London, pp 17–46.

Bakketeig L.S. and Hoffman H.J. 1983 The tendency to repeat gestational age and birth weight in successive births, related to perinatal survival *Acta Obstet Gynaecol Scand* 62:385–392.

Bakketeig L.S., Hoffman H.J., and Harley E.E. 1979 The tendency to repeat gestational age and birth weight in successive births *Am J Obstet Gynecol* 135:1086–1103.

Bakketeig L.S., Bjerkedal T., and Hoffman H. 1986 Small-for-gestational age births in successive pregnancy outcomes: Results from a longitudinal study of births in Norway *Early Hum Develop* 14:187–200.

Ballantyne J.W. 1902 The problem of the premature infant *Br Med J* 1196–1200.

Baltzar B., Ericson A., and Kallen B. 1979 Delivery outcome in women employed in medical occupations in Sweden *J Occup Med* 2(8):543–543.

Barnes A.B., Colton T., Gundersen J., Noller K.L., Tilley B.C., Strama T., Townsend D.E., Hatab P., and O'Brien P.C. 1980 Fertility and outcome of pregnancy in women exposed in utero to diethylstilbestrol *N Engl J Med* 302:609–613.

Baron J.A. 1984 Smoking and estrogen-related disease *Am J Epid* 119:9–22.

Barrett J. and Marshall J. 1969 The risk of conception on different days of the menstrual cycle *Pop Studies* 23:455–461.

Barron S.L. and Thomson A.M. 1983 Epidemiology of pregnancy In S.L. Barron, A.M. Thomson eds. *Obstetrical Epidemiology* Academic Press, London, pp 1–24.

Battaglia F.C. and Lubchenco L.O. 1967 A practical classification of newborn infants by weight and gestational age *Pediatrics* 71:159–163.

Baumgartner L., Pessin V, Wegman ME and Parker S. L. 1950 Weight in relation to fetal and newborn mortality; influence of sex and color *Pediatrics* 6:329–342.

Beall C.M. 1981 Optimal birthweights in Peruvian populations at high and low altitudes *Am J Phys Anthropol* 56:209–216.

Beard R.W. and Sharp F., eds. 1985 Preterm labor and its consequences Proceeding of 13th Study group of Royal College of Obstet and Gyn, London, pp 15–20.

Beasley R.P., Lin C.C., Hwang L.Y., and Chien C.S. 1981 Hepatocellular carcinoma and hepatitis B virus *Lancet* ii:1129–1133.

Becker M.H., Genieser N.B., Finegold M., Miranda D., and Spackman T. 1975 Chondrodysplasia punctata. Is maternal warfarin therapy a factor? *Am J Dis Child* 129:356–359.

Beebe G.W. 1960 Lung cancer in World War I veterans: Possible relation to mustard gas injury and the influenza epidemic *JNCI* 25:1231–1252.

Beebe G.W., Ishida M., and Jablon S. 1962 Studies of the mortality of the A-bomb survivors: Panel study of the mortality in the medical sample *Radiat Res* 16:253–280.

Beer A.E., Semprini A.E., Xiaoyu Z., and Quebbeman J.F. 1985 Pregnancy outcome in human couples with recurrent spontaneous abortions: HLA antigen profiles, HLA antigen sharing, female serum MLR blocking factors, and paternal leukocyte immunization *Expl Clin Immunogenet* 2:137–153.

Beer A.E., Quebbeman J.F., and Semprini A.E. 1987 Immunopathological factors contributing to recurrent spontaneous abortion in humans In M.J. Bennett and D.K. Edmonds, eds. *Spontaneous and Recurrent Abortion* Blackwell Scientific Publication, Oxford, pp 90–108.

Benenson A.S., ed. 1975 *Control of Communicable Diseases in Man* 12th Ed. American Public Health Association, Washington D.C., pp 272–276.

Bennett P.H., Webner C., and Miller M. 1979 Congenital anomalies and the diabetic and prediabetic pregnancy *Pregnancy Metabolism, Diabetes and the Fetus* Elsevier/North-Holland, pp 207–225.

Beral V. and Colwell L. 1981 Randomised trial of high doses of stilboestrol and ethisterone therapy in pregnancy: Long-term follow-up of the children *J Epidemiol Comm Health* 35:155–160.

Beral V., Grisso J.A., and Roman E. 1985 Is paid employment during pregnancy detrimental to the offspring? In *Prevention of Physical and Mental Congenital Defects* Alan R. Liss, New York, pp 261–264.

Bergman A.B. and Wiesner L.A. 1976 Relationship of passive cigarette smoking to sudden infant death syndrome *Pediatrics* 58:665–668.

Bergner L. and Susser M.W. 1970 Low birthweight and prenatal nutrition: An interpretive review *Pediatrics* 46:946–966.

Bergsma D., ed. 1979 *Birth Defects Compendium* Alan R. Liss, New York.

Berkowitz G.S. 1981 An epidemiologic study of preterm delivery *Am J Epidemiol* 113:81–92.

Berkowitz G.S. and Kasl S.V. 1983 The role of psychosocial factors in spontaneous preterm delivery *J Psychosom Res* 27:283–290.

Berkowitz G.S., Harlap S., Beck G.J., Freeman D.H., and Baras M. 1983 Early gestational bleeding and pregnancy outcome: A multivariable analysis *Int J Epidemiol* 12:165–173.

Berkowitz G.S., Kelsey J.L., Holford T.R., and Berkowitz R.L. 1983 Physical activity and the risk of spontaneous preterm delivery *J Reprod Med* 28:581–588.

Berman S.M., Binkin N.J., and Hogue C.J.R. 1987a Assessing sex differences in neonatal survival: A study of discordant twins *Int J Epidemiol* 16:436–440.

Bern H.A., Jones L.A., Mills K.T., Kohrman A., and Mori T. 1976 Use of the neonatal mouse in studying long-term effects of early exposure to hormones and other agents *J Tox Environ Health Suppl* 1:103–116.

Bernard C. 1865 *An Introduction to the Study of Experimental Medicine* Trans. Green H.C. (1957) Dover Publications, New York.

Bernard R.P. and Sastrawinata S. 1985 Infant outcome, fetal growth, and pregnancy care: Relationships in Indonesian university obstetrics *Acta Pediatr Scand* 319 (suppl):111–119.

Bernard R.P., Sastrawinata S, and Högberg V. 1984 Risk of maternal death in Indonesia and Sweden. Patterns and trends in 3D display in teaching. *Praventivmed* 29:172–73.

Bertin J.E. 1986 Reproduction, women, and the workplace: Legal issues In Z.A. Stein and M.C. Hatch, eds. *Reproductive Problems in the Workplace* Hanley & Belfus, Philadelphia *Occupational Medicine* 1:497–507.

Bibbo M., Gill W.B., Azizi F. et al. 1977 Follow-up study of male and female offspring of DES-exposed mothers *Obstet Gynecol* 49:1–8.

Bierman-Van Eendenburg M.E.C., Jurgens-Van der Zee A.D., Olinga A.A., Huisjes H.H., and Touwen B.C.L. 1981 Predictive value of neonatal neurological examination: A follow-up study at 18 months *Dev Med Child Neurol* 23:296–305.

Biggers J.D. 1969 Problems concerning the uterine causes of embryonic death, with special reference to the effects of aging of the uterus *J Reprod Fertil* 8 (suppl):27–43.

Biggers J.D., Finn C.A., and McLaren A. 1962a Long-term reproductive performance of female mice. I. Effect of removing one ovary *J Reprod Fertil* 3:303–312.

Biggers J.D., Finn C.A., and McLaren A. 1962b Long-term reproductive performance of female mice. II. Variation of litter size with parity *J Reprod Fertil* 3:313–330.

Billewicz W.Z. 1972 A note on birth weight correlation in full sibs *J Biosoc Sci* 4:455–460.

Billewicz W.Z. 1973 Some implications of self-selection for pregnancy *Br J Prev Soc Med* 27:49–52.

Billingham R.E. 1964 Transplantation immunity and the maternal fetal relationship *N Eng J Med* 270:667–672, 720–725.

Binkin N.J., Williams R.L., Hogue C.J.R., and Chen P.M. 1985 Reducing black neonatal mortality: Will improvement in birth weight be enough? *JAMA* 253:372–375.

Birkbeck J.A. 1976 Metrical growth and skeletal development of the human fetus In D.F. Roberts and A.M. Thomson, eds. *The Biology of Human Fetal Growth* Halsted Press, New York, pp 39–68.

Birkbeck J.A., Billewicz W.Z., and Thomson A.M. 1975 Foetal growth from 50 to 150 days of gestation *Ann Hum Biol* 2:319–326.

Birch H.G. and Gussow J.D. 1970 *Disadvantaged Children* Grune & Stratton, Orlando, Fl.

Bithell J.F. and Stiller C.A. 1988 A new calculation of the carcinogenic risk of obstetric X-raying *Statistics Med* 7:857–864.

Bjerkedal T., Czeizel A., Goujard J. et al. 1982 Valproic acid and spina bifida *Lancet* ii:1096.

Bjerre I. and Varendh G. 1975 A study of some biological and socioeconomic factors in low birth weight *Acta Paediatr Scand* 64:605–612.

Blackwell R.Q., Chow B.F., Chin K.S.K., Blackwell B.N., and Hsu S.C. 1973 Prospective maternal nutrition study in Taiwan: Rationale, study design, feasibility, and preliminary findings *Nutr Rep Int* 7:517–532.

Blalock H.M. 1964 *Causal Inference in Non-experimental Research* University of North Carolina Press, Chapel Hill.

Bland P.B. 1919 Influenza in its relation to pregnancy and labor *Am J Obstet* 79:184–197.

Blomquist U., Ericson A., Kallen B., and Westerholm P. 1981 Delivery outcome for women working in the pulp and paper industry *Scand J Work Environ Health* 7:14–118.

Blondel B., Kaminski M., Saurel-Cubizólles M., and Breart G. 1987 *Int J Epidemiol* 16:425–430.

Blum M. 1979 Is the elderly primipara really at high risk? *J Perinat* 7:108–112.

Boldman R. and Reed D.M. 1977 In *The Epidemiology of Prematurity* D. Reed and F. Stanley, eds. Urban & Schwarzenberg, Baltimore pp 39–52.

Bond D.J. and Chandley A.C. 1983 *Aneuploidy* Oxford University Press, Oxford.

Bongaarts J.A. 1975 Method for the estimation of fecundability *Demography* 12:645–660.

Bongaarts J. 1982 Not so unresolved: A reply *Fam Plan Perspect* 14:288–289.

Bongiovanni A.M. and McPadden A.J. 1960 Steroids during pregnancy and possible fetal consequences *Fertil Steril* 11:181–186.

Boué J. and Boué A. 1970 Les aberrations chromosomiques dans les avortements spontanes humains *Presse Medical* 78:635–641.

Boué J. and Boué A. 1973a Chromosomal analysis of two consecutive abortuses in each of 43 women *Humangenetik* 19:275–280.

Boué J. and Boué A. 1973b Anomalies chromosomiques dans les avortements spontanes In A. Boué, C. Thibault, eds. Les Accidentes Chromosomiques de la Reproduction INSERM, Paris, pp 29–56.

Boué J., Boué A., and Lazar P. 1975 Retrospective and prospective epidemiological studies of 1500 karyotyped spontaneous human abortions *Teratology* 12:11–26.

Boué J., Philippe E., Giroud A., and Boué A. 1976 Phenotypic expression of lethal chromosomal anomalies in human abortuses *Teratology* 14:3–19.

Boué A., Boué J., and Gropp A. 1985 Cytogenetics of pregnancy wastage *Adv Hum Genet* 14:1–57.

Bouyer J., Dreyfus J., Lazar P., Collin D., Winisdoerffer G., and Papiernik E. 1988 Prevention of preterm births: Haguenau perinatal study, 1971–1985 *Rev Epidemiol et Sante Publique* 36(2):83–88.

Boyers S.P., Diamond M.P., Lavy G., Russell J.B., and DeCherney A.H. 1987 The effect of polyploidy on embryo cleavage after in vitro fertilization in humans *Fertil Steril* 48:624–727.

Bracken M.B. 1984 Methodologic issues in epidemiologic investigation of drug-induced congenital malformations In M.B. Bracken, ed. *Perinatal Epidemiology* Oxford University Press, Oxford, pp 423–449.

Bracken M.B. and Vita K. 1983 Frequency of non-hormonal contraception around conception and association with congenital malformations in offspring *Am J Epid* 117:281–291.

Brandeis L.D. and Goldmark J. 1908 Brief for the State of Oregon National Consumers' League, New York p 62.

Brandt-Rauf P.W. and Brandt-Rauf S.I. 1986 Ethical aspects of reproductive health in the workplace In Z.A. Stein and M.C. Hatch, eds. *Reproductive Problems in the Workplace* Hanley & Belfus, Philadelphia *Occupational Medicine,* Vol 1, pp 509–515.

Brandriff B., Gordon L., Ashworth L., Watchmaker G., Moore D., Wyrobek A.J., and Carrano A.V. 1985 Chromosomes of human sperm: Variability among normal individuals *Hum Genet* 70:18–24.

Brawner D.L. 1955 Maternal rubella: Results following an epidemic *J Med Assn Georgia* 44:451–454.

Brazelton T.B. 1973 Neonatal behavioral assessment scale *Clinics in Developmental Medicine,* No. 50, Lippincott, Philadelphia.

Brenner W.E., Edelman D.A., and Hendricks C.H. 1976 A standard of fetal growth for the United States of America *Am J Obstet Gynecol* 126:555–564.

Brent R.L. 1977 Radiations and other physical agents In J.G. Wilson and F.C. Fraser, eds. *Handbook of Teratology* Plenum Press, New York, Vol 1, pp 153–223.

Breslow N.E. and Day N.E. 1980 *Statistical Methods in Cancer Research* Vol I International Agency for Research on Cancer, Lyon, France.

Brezowsky V.H. and Dietel H. 1967 Der Einflus von Wetter und Jahreszeit auf Wehenbeginn, Wehendauer, vorzeitigen Blasensprung und Fruhgeburt *Z Geburtshilfe Perinatol* 166:244–270.

Briend A. 1980 Maternal physical activity, birth weight, and perinatal mortality *Med Hypotheses* 6:1157–1170.

Br Med J 1978 Is hyperthermia a teratogen? Editorial 2:1586–1587.

Brody J.A. 1966 The infectiousness of rubella and the possibility of reinfection *Am J Pub Health* 56:1082–1087.

Brook J.D., Gosden R.G., and Chandley A.C. 1984 Maternal aging and aneuploid embryos: Evidence from the mouse that biological and not chronological age is the important influence *Hum Genet* 66:41–45.

Bross O. 1954 Misclassification 2 × 2 tables *Biometrics* 10:478–486.

Brown N.A. and Fabro S. 1983 The value of animal teratogenicity testing for predicting human risk *Clin Obstet Gynecol* 26:467–477.

Brown I., Elbourne D., and Mutch L.K.M.M. 1981 Standard national perinatal data: A suggested minimum data set *Comm Med* 3:298–306.

Brueton M.J., Palit A., and Prosser R. 1973 Gestational age assessment in Nigerian newborn infants *Arch Dis Child* 48:318–320.

Budin P. 1902 Les enfants debiles *Presse Med* 10:1155–1157.

Buehler J.W., Kaunitz A.N., Hogue C., Hughes J.M., Smith J.C., and Rochat R.W. 1986 Maternal mortality in women aged 35 years or older: United States *JAMA* 255:53–57.

Bulmash J.M. 1978 Systemic lupus erythematosus and pregnancy *Obstet Gynecol* 7:153–194.

Bulmer M.G. 1970 *The Biology of Twinning in Man* Oxford University Press, London.

Buncher C.R. 1969 Cigarette smoking and duration of pregnancy *Am J Obst Gynecol* 103:942–946.

Butcher R.L. and Page R.D. 1981 Role of the aging ovary in cessation of reproduction In N.B. Schwartz and M. Hunzicker-Dunn, eds. *Dynamics of Ovarian Function* Raven Press, New York, pp 253–271.

Butler N.R. and Bonham D.G. 1963 *Perinatal Mortality: The First Report of the 1958 British Perinatal Mortality Survey*, Livingstone, Edinburgh.

Butler N.R., Goldstein H., and Ross E.M. 1972 Cigarette smoking in pregnancy: Its influence on birth weight and perinatal mortality. *Br Med J* 2:127–130.

Byrne J. 1981 *Morphologic characteristics of miscarriage: An epidemiologic approach* PhD Dissertation, Columbia University, New York.

Byrne J. and Warburton D. 1979 Some pathological observations in spontaneous abortion *Birth Defects Original Article Series*, Vol XV:137–147.

Byrne J. and Warburton D. 1986 Neural tube defects in spontaneous abortions *Am J Med Genet* 25:327–333.

Byrne J., Blanc W.A., Warburton D., and Wigger J. 1984 The significance of cystic hygroma in fetuses *Human Pathology* 15:61–67.

Byrne J., Warburton D., Kline J., Blanc W., and Stein Z. 1985 Morphology of early fetal deaths and their chromosomal characteristics *Teratology* 32:297–315.

Camacho I. 1950 Expert group on prematurity final report *Wld Hlth Org Tech Rep Ser* 27:1–11.

Campbell S. 1976 The antenatal assessment of fetal growth and development: The contribution of ultrasonic measurement In D.F. Roberts and A.M. Thomson, eds. *The Biology of Human Fetal Growth* Halsted Press, New York pp 15–38.

Carothers A.D. 1983 Evidence that altered embryonic selection contributes to maternal-age effect in aneuploidy: A spurious conclusion attributable to pooling of heterogeneous data? *Am J Hum Genet* 35:1057–1059.

Carothers A.D. 1987 Down syndrome and maternal age: The effect of erroneous assignment of parental origin *Am J Hum Genet* 40:147–150.

Carothers A.D., Collier S., De Mey R., and Frackiewicz A. 1978 Parental age and birth order in the aetiology of some sex chromosome aneuploidies *Ann Hum Genet London* 41:277–287.

Carothers A.D., Frackiewicz A., DeMay R., Collyer S., Polani P.E., Osztovics M., Horvath K., Papp Z., May H.M., and Ferguson-Smith M.A. 1980 A collaborative study of the aetiology of Turner syndrome *Ann Hum Genet London* 43:355–368.

Carr D.H. 1965 Chromosome studies in spontaneous abortions *Obstet Gynecol* 26:308–326.

Carr D.H. 1967 Chromosome anomalies as a cause of spontaneous abortion *Am J Obstet Gynecol* 97:283–293.

Carr D.H. 1970 Chromosome studies in selected spontaneous abortions: 1. Conception after oral contraceptives *C.M.A.J.* 103:343–348.

Carr D.H. 1971 Chromosome and abortion In H. Harris and K. Hirschhorn, eds. *Advances in Human Genetics* 2:201–257, Plenum Press, New York.

Carr-Hill R., Campbell D.M., Hall M.H., and Meredith A. 1987 Is birth weight determined genetically? *Br Med J* 295:687–689.

Carter C.O. 1958 A life-table for mongols with causes of death *J Ment Defic Res* 2:64–74.

Carter C.O. and MacCarthy D. 1951 Incidence of mongolism and its diagnosis in the newborn *Br J Soc Med* 5:83–90.

Carter C.O. and Evans K.S. 1961 Risk of parents who have had one child with Down's syndrome (Mongolism) having another child similarly affected *Lancet* 2:785–788.

Carter C.O. and Evans K.S. 1973 Spina bifida and anencephalus in greater London *J Med Genet* 10:209–234.

Carter C.O. and Marshall W.A. 1978 The genetics of adult stature *Hum Growth* 1:299–305.

Carter C.O., Evans K.A., and Stewart A.M. 1961 Maternal radiation and Down's syndrome (Mongolism) *Lancet* ii:1042.

Cashner K.A., Christopher C.R., and Dysert G.A. 1987 Spontaneous fetal loss after demonstration of a live fetus in the first trimester *Obstet Gynecol* 70:827–830.

Castilla E. 1983 Valproic acid and spina bifida *Lancet* ii:683.

Cawley R.H., McKeown T., and Record R.G. 1954 Parental stature and birth weight *Am J Hum Genet* 6:448–456.

Chalmers B. 1984 A conceptualization of psycho-social obstetric research *J Psychosomat Obstet Gynaecol* 3:17–26.

Chance P.F. and Smith D.W. 1978 Hyperthermia and meningomyelocele and anencephaly *Lancet* i:769–770.

Charlton V. 1984 Fetal nutritional supplementation *Semin Perinatol* 8:25–30.

Chase H.C. 1972 *Comparison of Neonatal Mortality from Two Cohort Studies.* USDHEW 72-1056, Rockville, MD.

Chase H.C. 1977 Time trends in low birth weight in the United States, 1950–1974 In D. Reed and F.J. Stanley, eds. *The Epidemiology of Prematurity* Urban & Schwarzenberg, Baltimore, pp 17–38.

Chavkin W., ed. 1984 *Double Exposure: Women's Health Hazards on the Job and at Home* Monthly Review Press, New York.

Cheek D.B. 1968 Body composition, cell growth, energy, and intelligence *Human Growth* Lea & Febiger, Philadelphia.

Chen R. 1979 Statistical techniques in birth defects surveillance systems In M.A. Klingberg and J.A.C. Weatherall eds. *Epidemiologic Methods for Detection of Teratogens*, (Contributions to Epidemiology and Biostatistics, Vol 1) Karger, New York, pp 184–189.

Christenson P.E., Schmidt H., Jensen O., Bang, H.O., Andersen V., Jordal B. 1953 An epidemic of measles in southern Greenland 1951. Measles in virgin soil *Acta Med Scand* 144:313–322.

Christianson R.E. and Torfs C. 1988 Maternal smoking and Down syndrome. *Am J Hum Genet* 43:545–546.

Christie A.U., Dunham E.C., Jenss R.M., and Dippel A.L. 1941 Development of the center for the cuboid bone in newborn infants *Am J Dis Child* 61:471–482.

Chung C.S. and Myrianthopoulos N.C. 1975 Factors affecting risks of congenital malformations. II. Effect of maternal diabetes on congenital malformatons *Birth Defects* 11:23–38.

Chung C.S., Smith R.G., Steinhoff P.G., and Mi M.P. 1982 Induced abortion and spontaneous fetal loss in subsequent pregnancies *Am J Publ Health* 72:548–554.

Clapp J.F. and Dickstein S. 1984 Endurance exercise and pregnancy outcome *Med Sci Sports Exer* 16:556–562.

Clarke C.A., Donohoe W.T.A., Mc Connell R.B., Woodrow J.C., Finn R., Krevans J.R., Kulke W., Lehane D., and Sheppard P.M. 1963 Further experimental studies on the prevention of Rh hemolytic disease *Brit Med J* i:979–984.

Clarren S.K., Smith D.W., Harvey M.A.S. et al. 1979 Hyperthermia: A prospective evaluation of a possible teratogenic agent in man *J Pediatr* 95:81–83.

Clifford S.J. 1934 Reduction of premature infant mortality through determinants of fetal size in utero *JAMA* 103:1117–1121.

Cochrane A.L. 1972 *Effectiveness and Efficiency* Nuffield Provincial Hospitals Trust London.

Cohen B.H. and Lilienfeld A.M. 1970 The epidemiological study of Mongolism in Baltimore *Ann NY Acad Sci* 171:320–327.

Cohen B.H., Lilienfeld A.M., Kramer, S., and Hyman L.C. 1977 Parental factors in Down's syndrome: Results of the second Baltimore case-control study In E.D. Hook and I.H. Porter, eds. *Population Cytogenetics* Academic Press, New York, pp 301–352.

Cohen E.N., Bellville J.W., and Brown B.W. 1971 Anesthesia, pregnancy and miscarriage: A study of operating room nurses and anesthetists *Anesthesiology* 35:343–347.

Cohen E.N., Brown B.W., Wu M.L., Whitcher C.E., Brodsky J.B., Gift H.C., Greenfield W., Jones T.W., and Driscoll E.J. 1980 Occupational disease in dentistry and chronic exposure to trace anesthetic gases *JADA* 101:21–31.

Collings C.A., Curet L.B., and Mullin J.P. 1983 Maternal and fetal responses to a maternal aerobic exercise program *Am J Obstet Gynecol* 145:702–707.

Comess L.J., Bennett P.H., Man M.B., Burch T.A., and Miller M. 1969 Congenital anomalies and diabetes in the Pima Indians of Arizona *Diabetes* 18:471–477.

Commission on Life Sciences 1986 Methodologies for conducting field trials of vitamin A supplementation National Research Council, Washington, D.C.

Cone T.E. 1961 De Pondere Infantum Recens Natorum *Pediatrics* 28:490–498.

Copeland K.T., Checkoway H., McMichael A.J., and Holbrook R.H. 1977 Bias due to misclassification in the estimation of relative risk *Am J Epidemiol* 105:488–495.

Cooper D.W. and Aitken R.J. 1981 Failure to detect altered rosette inhibition titres in human pregnancy serum *J Reprod Fert* 61:241–245.

Cooper L.Z. 1968 Rubella: A preventable cause of birth defects In *Birth Defects: Original Article Series*, Vol IV, pp 23–35.

Cooperstock M. and Wolfe R.A. 1986 Seasonality of preterm birth in the Collaborative Perinatal Project: Demographic factors *Am J Epidemiol* 124:234–240.

Corbett T.H., Cornell R.G., Endres J.L., and Lieding K. 1974 Birth defects among children of nurse-anesthetists *Anesthesiology* 4:341–344.

Cordero J.F. and Layde P.M. 1983 Vaginal spermicides, chromosomal abnormalities and limb reduction defects *Fam Plan Perspect* 15:16–18.

Correa P., Pickle L.W., Fontham E., Lin Y., and Haenszel W. 1983 Passive smoking and lung cancer *Lancet* ii:595–597.

Costoff A. and Mahesh V.B. 1975 Primordial follicles with normal oocytes in the ovaries of postmenopausal women *J Am Geriatr Soc* 23:193–196.

Coulam C.B., Moore S.B., and O'Fallon W.M. 1987 Association between major histocompatability antigen and reproductive performance *Am J Reprod Immunol* 12:10–12.

Coulam C.B., McIntyre J.A., and Faulk W.P. 1986 Reproductive performance in women with repeated pregnancy losses and multiple partners *Am J Reprod Immunol* 12:54–58.

Court-Brown W.M. and Doll R. 1957 Leukemia and aplastic anaemia in patients irradiated for ankylosing spondylitis *Spec Rep Ser Med Res Counc* No. 295, H.M.S.O., London.

Court-Brown W.M., Law P., and Smith P.G. 1969 Sex chromosome aneuploidy and parental age *Ann Hum Genet* 33:1–14.

Covell G. 1950 Congenital malaria *Trop Dis Bull* 47:1147–1167.

Cradock-Watson J.E., Ridehalgh M.K.S., Anderson M.J., and Pattison J.R. 1981 Outcome of asymptomatic infection with rubella virus during pregnancy *J Hyg Cambridge* 87:147–154.

Cramer D.W., Schiff I., Schoenbaum S.C., Gibson M., Belisle S., Albrecht B., Stillman R.J., Berger M.J., Wilson E., Stadel B.V., and Seibel M. 1985 Tubal infertility and the intrauterine device *N Engl J Med* 312:941–947.

Creasy M. 1977 *The Cytogenetics of Early Human Fetuses* Doctoral Dissertation, University of London.

Creasy M.R. and Alberman E.D. 1976 Congenital malformations of the central nervous system in spontaneous abortions *J Med Genet* 13:9–16.

Creasy M.R., Crolla J.A., and Alberman E.D. 1976 A cytogenetic study of human spontaneous abortions using banding techniques *Hum Genet* 31:177–196.

Cross P.K. and Hook E.B. 1984 Down syndrome and maternal smoking: A negative association *Am J Hum Genet* 36A:905 (Abstract).

Crowley P.H., Gulati D.K., Hayden T.L., Lopez P., and Dyer R. 1979 A chiasma-hormonal hypothesis relating Down's syndrome and maternal age *Nature* 280:417–419.

Cullingworth C.J. 1878 Case Illustrating the Viability of Extremely Small Children, with brief reference to several analogous examples *Obstet J* 6:163.

Czeizel A. and Rode K. 1984 Trial to prevent first occurrence of neural tube defects by periconceptional multivitamin supplementation *Lancet* ii:40.

Dale, E., Mullinax K.M., and Bryan D.H. 1982 Exercise during pregnancy: effects on the fetus *Can J Appl Spt Sci* 7:98–103.

Daling J.R. and Emanuel I. 1977 Induced abortion and subsequent outcome of pregnancy in a series of American women *N Engl J Med* 297:1241–1245.

Daling J.R., Weiss N.S., Metch B.J., Chow W.H., Soderstrom R.M., Moore D.E., Spadoni L.R., and Stadel B.V. 1985 Primary tubal infertility in relation to the use of an intrauterine device *N Engl J Med* 312:937–941.

Dann T.C. and Roberts D.F. 1984 Menarcheal age in University of Warwick students *J Biosoc Sci* 16:511–519.

Davies A.M. and Dunlop W. 1983 Hypertension in pregnancy In S.L. Barron, A.M. Thomson, eds. *Obstetrical Epidemiology* Academic Press, London, pp 167–208.

Davies K.E., Harper K., Bonthron D., Krumlauf R., Polkey A., Pembrey M.E., and Williamson R. 1984 Use of a chromosome 21 cloned DNA probe for the analysis of non-disjunction in Down syndrome *Hum Genet* 66:54–56.

Davies D.P., Gray O.P., Ellwood P.C. et al. 1976 Cigarette smoking in pregnancy: Association with maternal weight gain and fetal growth *Lancet* i:385–387.

Davis P.J.M., Partridge J.W., and Storrs C.N. 1982 Alcohol consumption in pregnancy. How much is safe? *Arch Dis Child* 57:940–943.

Delgado H., Martorell R., Brineman E., and Klein R.E. 1982 Nutrition and length of gestation *Nutr Res* 2:117–216.

Delhanty D.A., Ellis J.R., and Rowley P.T. 1961 Triploid cells in a human embryo *Lancet* 1:1286.

de la Cruz F.F. and Gerald P.S., eds. 1981 *Trisomy 21 (Down syndrome): Research Perspectives* University Park Press, Baltimore.

del Mazo J., Castillo A.M., and Abrisqueta J.A. 1982 Trisomy 21: Origin of non-disjunction *Hum Genet* 62:316–320.

Demakis J.G. and Rahimtoola S.H. 1971 Peripartum cardiomyopathy *Circulation* 44:964–968.

DePorte J.V., Parker S.L., and Parkhurst E. 1943 Statistical aspects of coding and tabulating medical data on birth and stillbirth certificates *Am J Publ Health* 33:651–658.

Dewees W.P. 1836 *Treatise on the Physical and Medical Treatment of Children*, L.A. May, ed. 1977 Dabor Science Publications, Oceanside, NY, p. 30.

Dhadial R.K., Machin A.M., and Tait S.M. 1970 Chromosomal anomalies in spontaneously aborted human fetuses *Lancet* ii:20–21.

Diamond E.L. and Lilienfeld A.M. 1962 Effects of errors in classification and diagnosis in various types of epidemiological studies *Am J Pub Health* 52:137–144.

Dick-Read G. 1942 *Revelation of Childbirth* Heinemann, London.

Dickson D. 1988 Doctored report revives debate on 1957 mishap (news) *Science* 239:556–557.

DiSaia, P.J. 1966 Pregnancy and delivery of a patient with a Starr-Edwards mitral valve prosthesis. Report of a case *Obstet Gynecol* 28:469–472.

Dobson R.L. and Felton J.S. 1983 Female germ cell loss from radiation and chemical exposure *Am J Ind Med* 4:175–190.

Dobson R.L., Koehler C.G., Felton J.S., Kwan T.C.W., and Jones D.C.L. 1978

Vulnerability of female germ cells in developing mice and monkeys to tritium, gamma rays and polycyclic aromatic hydrocarbons. In D.D. Mahlum, M.R. Sikov, P.L. Machett, and F.D. Andrews, eds. *Developmental Toxicology of Energy Related Pollutants* Department of Energy Symposium Series 47.

Dohrenwend B.S. and Dohrenwend B.P. 1969 Social Status and Psychological Disorder Wiley-Interscience, New York.

Donald H.P. 1939 Sources of variation in human birth weight *Proc R Soc Edin* 59:91–108.

Donovan J.W., Adena M.A., Rose G., and Batistutta D. 1983 Case-control study of congenital anomalies and Vietnam service Canberra, Australian Government Publishing Services.

Doring G.K. 1969 The incidence of anovular cycles in women. *J Reprod Fertil* (Suppl 6):77–81.

Dorland's Illustrated Medical Dictionary 26th Ed. 1981 W.B. Saunders, Philadelphia, p. 1317.

Douglas A.C. 1963 The deposition of tetracycline in human nails and teeth: A complication of long term treatment *Br J Dis Chest* 57:44–47.

Doyle L.W. and Kitchen W.H.J. 1987 Prognosis for infants born at 23 to 28 weeks' gestation *Br Med J* 294:55–56.

Drillien C.M. 1957 The social and economic factors affecting the incidence of premature birth *J Obstet Gynaecol Br Emp* 64:161–184.

Dubowitz L.M.S. and Dubowitz V. 1981 The neurological assessment of the preterm and full term newborn infant *Clin Develop Med* No 79, Heineman, London.

Dunn T.B. and Green A.W. 1963 Cysts of the epididymis, cancer of the cervix, glandular cell myoblastoma, and other lesions after estrogen injection in newborn mice *J Nat Cancer Inst* 31:425–438.

Eccles A. 1977 Obstetrics in the 17th and 18th centuries and its implications for maternal and infant mortality *Bull Soc Social Hist Med* 20:8–11.

Eccles A. 1982 *Obstetrics and Gynaecology in Tudor and Stuart England* Kent State University Press, OH.

Ederer F., Myers M.H., and Mantel N. 1964 A statistical problem in space and time: Do leukemia cases come in clusters? *Biometrics* 20:626–638.

Edmonds D.K., Lindsay K.S., Miller J.F., Williamson E., and Wood P.J. 1982 Early embryonic mortality in women *Fertil Steril* 38:447–453.

Edmonds L.D., Falk H., and Nissim J.E. 1975 Congenital malformations and vinyl chloride *Lancet* ii:1098.

Edmonds L.D., Anderson L.E., Flynt J.W., and James L.M. 1978 Congenital central nervous system malformations and vinyl chloride monomer exposure: A community study *Teratology* 17:137–142.

Edmonds L.D., Layde P.M., Flynt J.W., Erickson J.D., and Oakley G.P. 1981 Congenital malformations surveillance: Two American systems *Int J Epidemiol* 10:247–252.

Edwards L.E., Alton I.R., Barrada M.I., and Hakanson E.Y. 1979 Pregnancy in the underweight woman: Course outcome and growth patterns of the infant *Am J Obstet Gynecol* 135:297–302.

Edwards M.J. 1967 Congenital defects in guinea pigs following induced hyperthermia during gestation *Arch Path* 84:42–48.

Edwards M.J. 1968 Congenital malformations in the rat following induced hyperthermia during gestation *Teratology* 1:173–175.

Edwards M.J. 1969a Congenital defects in guinea pigs: Fetal resorptions, abortions, and malformations following induced hyperthermia during early gestation *Teratology* 2:313–328.

Edwards M.J. 1969b Congenital defects in guinea pigs: Prenatal retardation of brain growth of guinea pigs following hyperthermia during gestation *Teratology* 2:329–336.

Edwards M.J. 1981 Clinical disorders of fetal brain development: Defects due to hyperthermia In B.S. Hetzel and R.M. Smith, eds. *Fetal Brain Disorders* Elsevier/North-Holland Biomedical Press, Berlin, pp 335–364.

Edwards R.G. 1980 *Conception in the Human Female* Academic Press, London.

Edwards R.G., Fishel S.B., and Purdy J.M. 1983 *In vitro* fertilization of human eggs: Analysis of follicular growth, ovulation and fertilization In H.M. Beier and H.R. Lindner, eds. *Fertilization of the Human Egg In Vitro* Springer-Verlag, Berlin, pp 169–188.

Edwards R.G., Fishel S.B., Cohen J., Fehilly C.B., Purdy J.M., Slater J.M., Steptoe P.C., and Webster J.M. 1984 Factors influencing the success of in vitro fertilization for alleviating human infertility *J Vitro Fertiliz Embryo Transfer* 1:3–23.

Eichenwald H.F. 1959 A study of congenital toxoplasmosis with particular emphasis on clinical manifestations, sequelae, and therapy. In J.C. Siim, ed. *Human Toxoplasmosis* Vol 2, Munksgaard, Copenhagen.

Elder H.A., Santamarina B.A.G., Smith S., and Kass E.H. 1971 The natural history of asymptomatic bacteriuria during pregnancy: The effect of tetracycline on the clinical course and the outcome of pregnancy *Am J Obstet Gynecol* 111:441–462.

Ellis N.J., Chen H.-C., Jason J., and Janerich D.T. 1986 Pilot study to detect early pregnancy and early fetal loss *J Occup Med* 28:1069–1073.

Elster A.B., Lamb M.E., Tavare J., and Ralston C.W. 1987 The medical and psychosocial impact of comprehensive care on adolescent pregnancy and parenthood *JAMA* 258:1187–1192.

Elwood J.M. 1983 Can vitamins prevent neural tube defects? *Can Med Assoc J* 129:1088–1092.

Elwood J.M. and Elwood J.H. 1980 *Epidemiology of Anencephalus and Spina Bifida* Oxford University Press, New York.

Endo Laboratories, Inc. 1975 Revised Full Prescribing Information for Coumadin, Garden City, NY.

Erhardt C.L. 1963 Pregnancy losses in New York City, 1960 *Am J Publ Health* 53:1337–1357.

Erhardt C. and Nelson F.G. 1964 Reported congenital malformations in New York City, 1958–1959 *Am J Publ Health* 54:1489–1506.

Erhardt C.L., Joshi G.B., Nelson F.G. et al. 1964 Influence of weight and gestation on perinatal and neonatal mortality by ethnic group *Am J Publ Health* 54:1841–1855.

Erickson J.D. 1978 Down syndrome, paternal age, maternal age and birth order *Ann Hum Genet* 41:289–298.

Erickson J.D. 1979 Paternal age and Down syndrome *Am J Hum Genet* 31:489–497.

Erickson J.D. and Bjerkedal T. 1981 Down syndrome associated with father's age in Norway *J Med Genet* 18:22–28.

Erickson J.D., Cochran W.M., and Anderson C.E. 1978 Birth defects and printing *Lancet* i:385.

Erickson J.D., Mulinare J., McClain P.W., Fitch, T.G., James L.M., McLearn A.B., Adams M.J. 1984 Vietnam veterans' risks for fathering babies with birth defects *JAMA* 252:903–912.

Ericson A. and Kallen B. 1979 Survey of infants born in 1973 or 1975 to Swedish women working in operating rooms during their pregnancies *Anesthesia Analgesia* 58:302–305.

Ericson A. and Kallen B. 1986 An epidemiological study of work with video screens and pregnancy outcome: I. A registry study *Am J Indust Med* 9:447–457.

Ericson A., Kallen B., and Westerholm P. 1979 Cigarette smoking as an etiologic factor in cleft lip and palate *Am J Obstet Gynecol* 135:348–351.

Ericson A., Kallen B., Meirik O., and Westerholm P. 1982 Gastrointestinal atresia and maternal occupation during pregnancy *J Occup Med* 24:515–518.

Erikson K.T. 1976 *Everything in Its Path: Destruction of Community in the Buffalo Creek Flood* Simon & Schuster, New York.

Erkkola R. 1976 The physical work capacity of the expectant mother and its effect on pregnancy, labor and the newborn *Int J Gynaecol Obstet* 14:153–159.

Ernhart C.B., Wolf A.W., Linn P.L., Sokol R.J., Kennard M.J., and Filipovich H.F. 1985 Alcohol-related birth defects: Syndromal anomalies, intrauterine growth retardation, and neonatal behavioral assessment *Alcoholism* 9:447–453.

Estryn M., Kaminski M., Franc M., Fernand S., and Gerstle F. 1978 Grossesse et conditions de travail en milieu hospitalier *Rev Franc Gynec* 73:625–631.

Evans D.R., Newcombe R.G., and Campbell H. 1979 Maternal smoking habits and congenital malformations: A population study *Br Med J* 2:171–173.

Evans T.N. and Riley G.M. 1953 Pseudohermaphroditism. A clinical problem *Obstet Gynecol* 2:363–378.

Eveleth P.B. and Tanner J.M. 1976 *Worldwide Variation in Human Growth* Cambridge University Press, London.

Everson R.B., Randerath E., Santella R.M., Cefalo R.C., Avitts T.A., and Randerath K. 1986 Detection of smoking-related covalent DNA adducts in human placenta *Science* 231:54–56.

Faulk W.P., Coulam C.B., and McIntyre J.A. 1987 Reproductive immunology: Biomarkers of compromised pregnancies *Environ Health Persp* 74:119–127.

Federation CECOS, Schwartz D., Mayaux M.J. 1982 Female fecundity as a function of age *N Engl J Med* 306:404–406.

Fedrick J. and Adelstein P. 1978 Factors associated with low birth weight of infants delivered at term *Br J Obstet Gynaecol* 85:1–7.

Fedrick J. and Anderson A.B.M. 1976 Factors associated with spontaneous preterm birth *Br J Obstet Gynaecol* 83:342–350.

Fedrick J., Alberman E.D., and Goldstein H. 1971 Possible teratogenic effect of cigarette smoking *Nature* 231:529–530.

Fein G.G., Jacobson J.L., Jacobson S.W., Schwartz P.M., and Dowler J.K. 1984 Prenatal exposure to polychlorinated biphenyls: Effects on birth size and gestational age *J Pediatr* 105:315–320.

Ferguson-Smith M.A. and Yates J.R.W. 1984 Maternal age specific rates for chromosome aberrations and factors influencing them: Report of a collaborative European study on 52,965 amniocenteses *Prenat Diag* 4:5–44.

FIGO 1976 Lists of gynecologic and obstetrical terms and definitions *Int J Gynaecol Obstet* 14:570–576.

Finch C.E. 1978 Reproductive senescence in rodents: Factors in decline of fertility and loss of regular estrous cycles In E.L. Schneider, ed. *The aging reproductive system* Raven Press, New York, pp 193–212.

Finn C.A. 1962 Embryonic death in aged mice *Nature* 194:499–500.

Finn C.A. 1963a Reproductive capacity and litter size in mice: Effect of age and environment *J Reprod Fertil* 6:205–214.

Finn C.A. 1963b Collagen content of barren and previously pregnant uterine horns in old mice *J Reprod Fertil* 6:405–407.

Finn C.A. 1966 The initiation of the decidual cell reaction in the uterus of the aged mouse *J Reprod Fertil* 11:423–428.

Fisher N.L. and Smith D.W. 1981 Occipital encephalocele and early gestational hyperthermia *Pediatrics* 68:480–483.

FitzSimmons J., Jackson D., Wapner R., and Jackson L. 1983 Subsequent reproductive outcome in couples with repeated pregnancy loss *Am J Med Genet* 16:583–587.

Fleck L. 1935 Genesis and development of a scientific fact In T.J. Trenn and R.K. Merton, eds. (trans. 1979) University of Chicago Press.

Flynt J.W. and Hay S. 1979 International clearinghouse for birth defects monitoring systems. *Contr Epidemiol Biostat* 1:44–52.

Ford C.E. and Evans E.P. 1973 Non-expression of genome imbalance in haplophase and early diplophase of the mouse and incidence of karyotype abnormality in post-implantation embryos In A. Boué and C. Thibault, eds. *Les Accidents Chromosomiques de la Reproduction* INSERM, Paris, pp 271–285.

Ford C.E., Jones K.W., Polani P.E., De Almeida J.C., and Briggs J.H. 1959 A sex-chromosome anomaly in a case of gonadal dysgenesis (Turner's syndrome) *Lancet* i:711–713.

Ford J.H. 1984 Spindle microtubular dysfunction in mothers of Down syndrome children *Hum Genet* 295–298.

Ford J.H. and Lester P. 1982 Factors affecting the displacement of human chromosomes from the metaphase plate *Cytogen Cell Genet* 33:327–332.

Ford J.H. and Roberts C. 1983 Displacement of chromosomes in mitosis: A technique for assessing differential chromosome error *Cytogen Cell Genet* 36:537–541.

Ford J.H. and Russell J.A. 1985 Differences in the error mechanisms affecting sex and autosomal chromosomes in women of different ages within the reproductive age group *Am J Hum Genet* 37:973–983.

Forman M.R., Meirik O., and Berendes H.W. 1984 Delayed childbearing in Sweden *JAMA* 252:3135–3139.

Fourie D.T. and Hay I.T. 1975 Warfarin as a possible teratogen *S Afr Med J* 49:2081–2083.

Fournier J.A. 1886 *La Syphilis Hereditaire Tardive* G. Massor, Paris.

Fraga A., Mintz G., Orozco J., and Orozco J.H. 1974 Sterility and fertility rates, fetal wastage and maternal morbidity in systemic lupus erythematosus *J Rheumatol* 1:293–298.

Frank J.P. 1790 *The People's Misery—Mother of Disease* Trans. (1941) Sigerist H. *Bull Hist Med* 9:81–100.

Frantz C.H. 1963 Increased incidence of malformed infants in West Germany during 1959–1962 *Ill Med J* 123:27–39.

Fraser F.C. 1980 Animal models for craniofacial disorders In M. Melnick, D. Bixler, and E.D. Shields, eds. *Etiology of Cleft Lip and Cleft Palate* Alan R. Liss, New York, pp 1–23.

Fraser F.C. and Biddle C.J. 1976 Estimating the risks for offspring of first cousin matings. An approach *Am J Hum Genet* 28(5):522–526.

Fraser F.C. and Scriver J.B. 1954 A hereditary factor in chondrodystrophia calcificans congenita *N Engl J Med* 250:272–277.

Fraser F.C. and Skelton J. 1978 Possible teratogenicity of maternal fever *Lancet* ii:634.

Fraser F.C., Czeizel A., and Hanson C. 1982 Increased frequency of neural tube defects in sibs of children with other malformations *Lancet* ii:144–145.

Freda V.J. and Gorman J.G. 1962 Antepartum management of RH hemolytic disease *Bull Sloane Hosp Wom* 8:147–158.

Freeman H.E., Klein R.E., Townsend J.W., and Lechtig A. 1980 Nutrition and cognitive development among rural Guatemalan children *Am J Publ Health* 70:1277–1286.

French F.E. and Bierman J.M. 1962 Probabilities of fetal mortality *Publ Health Rep* 77:835–847.

French F.E., Devitt R.E., and Kenny S. 1962 Thalidomide and congenital abnormalities *Lancet* i:430.

Freudenberg N. 1984 Citizen action for environmental health: Report on a survey of community organizations *AJPH* 74:444–448.

Fried P.A. 1982 Marihuana use by pregnant women and effects on offspring: An update. *Neurobehav Toxicol Teratol* 4:451–454.

Friedlaender M. 1815 *De l'Education Physique de l'Homme* Paris, pp 25–113.

Friedman E.A. and Neff R.K. 1977 *Pregnancy Hypertension* PSG Publishing Co, Littleton, MA, pp 106–114.

Friedman E.A. and Rutherford J.W. 1956 Pregnancy and lupus erythematosus *Obstet Gynecol* 8:601–610.

Friedman E.A. and Sachtleben M.R. 1965 Relation of maternal age to the course of labor *Am J Obstet Gynecol* 91:915–924.

Frisancho A.R., Matos J., and Bollettino L.A. 1984 Influence of growth status and placental function on birth weight of infants born to young still-growing teenagers *Am J Clin Nutr* 40:801–807.

Frisch R.K., Revelle R., and Cook S. 1973 Components of weight at menarche and the initiation of the adolescent growth spurt in girls. Estimated total body water, lean body weight and fat. *Hum Biol* 45:469–483.

Fryers T. 1984 *The Epidemiology of Severe Intellectual Impairment: The Dynamics of Prevalence* Academic Press, London.

Gal P. and Sharpless M.K. 1984 Fetal drug exposure: Behavioral teratogenesis *Drug Int Clin Pharm* 18:186–201.

Gal I. 1972 Risks and benefits of the use of hormonal pregnancy test tablets *Nature* 240:241–242.

Gal I., Kirman B., and Stern J. 1967 Hormonal pregnancy tests and congenital malformation *Nature* 216:83.

Gale A.H. 1945 A century of changes in the mortality and incidence of the principal infections of childhood *Arch Dis Child* 20:2–21.

Galler J.R. 1979 The effects of intergenerational and postnatal malnutrition on the behavioral development of rats In J. Brozek *Behavioral Effects of Energy and Protein Deficits* US Government Printing Office, pp 22–38.

Gallus G., Mandelli C., Marchi M., and Radaelli G. 1986 On surveillance methods for congenital malformation *Stat Med* 5:565–571.

Gayle H.D., Yip R., Frank M.J., Nieburg P., and Binkin N.J. 1988 Validation of maternally reported birth weights among 46,637 Tennessee WIC Program Participants *Pub Health Rep* 103:143–147.

Geber M. and Dean R.E. 1957 The state of development of newborn African children *Lancet* i:1216.

Geber M. and Dean R.E. 1964 Le development psychomoteur et somatique des jeunes enfants africains en Ouganda *Courier* 14:425.

Gebre-Medhin M. and Gurovsky S. 1976 Association of maternal age and parity with birth weight, sex ratio, stillbirths and multiple births *J Trop Ped* 22:99–102.

Gebre-Medhin M., Sterky G., and Taube A. 1978 Observations on intrauterine growth in urban Ethiopia *Acta Paediatr Scand* 67:781–789.

Generoso W.M., Rutledge J.C., Cain K.T. et al. Exposure of female mice to ethylene oxide within hours after mating leads to fetal malformation and death. National Toxicology Program NIEHS and the Office of Health and Environmental Research, U.S. Department of Energy.

Genesis 3:16 The Bible, King James Version.

Genot M.T., Golan H.P., Porter P.J., and Kass E.H. 1970 Effect of administration of tetracycline in pregnancy on the primary dentition of the offspring *J Oral Med* 25:75–79.

George A.K. and Weiler S.J. 1981 Sexuality in middle and late life: The effects of age, cohort, and gender *Arch Gen Psychiatry* 38:919–923.

Germain M.A., Webster W.S., and Edwards M.J. 1985 Hyperthermia as a teratogen: Parameters determining hyperthermia-induced head defects in the rat *Teratology* 31:265–272.

German J. 1968 Mongolism, delayed fertilization and human sexual behaviour *Nature* 217:516–518.

German J. 1984 The embryonic stress hypothesis of teratogenesis *Am J Med* 76:293–301.

German J.L., Demayo A.P., and Bearn A.G. 1962 Inheritance of an abnormal chromosome in Down's syndrome (mongolism) with leukemia *Am J Hum Genet* 14:31–42.

Geronimus A.R. 1986 The effects of race, residence, and prenatal care on the relationship of maternal age to neonatal mortality *AJPH* 76:1416–1421.

Ghosh S. and Daga S. 1967 Comparison of gestational age and weight as standards of prematurity *Pediatrics* 71:173–175.

Gibbs L.M. and Levine M. 1982 *Love Canal: My Story* State University Press, Albany.

Gibson J. and McKeown T. 1952 Observations on all births (23,970) in Birmingham, 1947 VI. Birthweight, duration of gestation, and survival related to sex *Br J Soc Med* 6:152–158.

Giles, J.P., Cooper L.Z., and Krugman S. 1965 The rubella syndrome *J Pediatr* 66:434–437.

Gilmore D.H. and McNay M.B. 1985 Spontaneous fetal loss rate in early pregnancy *Lancet* i:107.

Gilstrap L.C., Cunningham F.G., and Whalley P.J. 1981 Acute pyelonephritis in pregnancy: An anterospective study *Obstet Gynecol* 57:409–413.

Godal T., Lofgren M., and Negassi K. 1972 Immune response to *M. leprae* of healthy leprosy contacts *Int J Lepr* 40:234–250.

Goetsch C. 1962 An evaluation of aminopterin as an abortifacient *Am J Obstet Gynecol* 83:1474–1477.

Goldberg M.F., Edmonds L.D., and Oakley G.P. 1979 Reducing birth defect risk in advanced maternal age *JAMA* 242:2292–2294.

Goldhaber M.K., Polen M.R., and Hiatt R.A. 1988 The risk of miscarriage and birth defects among women who use visual display terminals during pregnancy *Am J Indust Med* 13:695–706.

Golding J., Butler N.R., and Newcombe R.G. 1983 Analysis of completed reproductive histories: A cautionary tale *J Epidemiol Comm Health* 37:78–81.

Goldstein H. and Peckham C. 1976 Birthweight, gestation, neonatal mortality and child development In D.F. Roberts and A.M. Thompson, eds. *The Biology of Human Fetal Growth,* Taylor and Francis, London, pp 81–103.

Goldstein I.F. and Landovitz L. 1977 Analysis of air pollution patterns in New York City. I. Can one station represent the large metropolitan area? *Atmospheric Environment* 11:47–52.

Gorsuch R.L. and Key M.K. 1974 Abnormalities of pregnancy as a function of anxiety and life stress *Psychosomat Med* 36:352–362.

Gosden R.G. 1979 Effects of age and parity on the breeding potential of mice with one or two ovaries *J Reprod Fert* 57:477–487.

Gosden R.G. and Fowler R.E. 1979 Corpus luteum function in ageing inbred mice *Experientia* 35:128–130.

Goujon H., Papiernik E., and Maine D. 1984 The prevention of preterm delivery through prenatal care: An intervention study in Martinique *Int J Gynaecol Obstet* 22:339–343.

Gould M. and Stephano J.L. 1987 Electrical responses of eggs to acrosomal protein similar to those induced by sperm *Science* 235:1654–1656.

Gould S.J. 1981 The Mismeasure of Man Norton, New York.

Graham W., Brass W., and Snow R. 1988 Estimating maternal mortality in developing countries *Lancet* i:416–417.

Gravett M.G., Nelson H.P., DeRouen T., Critchlow C., Eschenbach D.A., and Holmes K.K. 1986 Independent associations of bacterial vaginosis and chlamydia trachomatis infection with adverse pregnancy *JAMA* 256:1899–1903.

Green R.H., Balsamo M.R., Giles J.P., Krugman S., and Mirick G.S. 1965 Studies of the natural history and prevention of rubella *Am J Dis Child* 110:348–365.

Greenberg M., Pellitteri O., and Barton J. 1957 Frequency of defects in infants whose mothers had rubella during pregnancy *JAMA* 165:675–678.

Greenland S. and Kleinbaum, D.G. 1983 Correcting for misclassification in two-way tables and matched-pair analysis *Int J Epidemiol* 12:93–97.

Greenland S. and Neutra R. 1980 Control of confounding in the assessment of medical technology *Int J Epidemiol* 9:361–367.

Greenwald P., Barlow J.J., Nasca P.C., and Burnett W.S. 1971 Vaginal cancer after maternal treatment with synthetic estrogens *N Engl J Med* 285:390–392.

Greenwood A., Greenwood B., Snow R. et al. 1987. A prospective survey of the outcome of pregnancy in a rural area of the Gambia, West Africa *Bull WHO* 65:635–643.

Gregg N. 1941 Congenital cataract following German measles in the mother *Trans Ophthal Soc Aust* 3:35–46.

Grennert L., Persson P.H., and Gennser G. 1978 Benefits of ultrasonic screening of a pregnant population *Acta Obstet Gynaecol Scand* 78:4–14.

Grimes D.A. and Cates W., Jr. 1979 Complications from legally-induced abortion: A review *Obstet Gynecol Surv* 34:177–191.

Grimes D.A. and Cates W., Jr. 1979 The comparative efficacy and safety of intraamniotic prostaglandin F2 alpha and hypertonic saline for second-trimester abortion: A review and critique *J Reprod Med* 22:248–254.

Grisso J.A., Roman E., Inskip H., Beral V., and Donovan J. 1984 Alcohol consumption and outcome of pregnancy *J Epid Comm Health* 38:232–235.

Grob G.N. 1978 *Edward Jarvis and the Medical World of Nineteenth-Century America*, University of Tennessee Press, Knoxville.

Gropp A. 1973 Fetal mortality due to aneuploidy and irregular meiotic segregation in the mouse In A. Boué and C. Thibault, eds. *Les Accidents Chromosomiques de la Reproduction* INSERM, Paris, pp 255–268.

Gruenwald P. 1963 Chronic fetal distress and placental insufficiency *Biol Neonat* 5:215–265.

Gruenwald P. 1966a Growth of the human fetus I. *Am J Obstet Gynecol* 94:1112–1119.

Gruenwald P. 1966b Growth of the human fetus II. *Am J Obstet Gynecol* 94:1120–1132.

Gruenwald P. 1969a Growth and maturation of the foetus and its relationship to perinatal mortality. In N.R. Butler and E.D. Alberman, eds. *Perinatal Problems* Livingston, London, pp 141–162.

Gruenwald P. 1969b Stillbirth and early neonatal death In N.R. Butler and E.D. Alberman, eds. *Perinatal Problems* Livingston, London, pp 163–183.

Gruenwald P., Funakawa H., Mitani S., Nishimura H., and Takenchi S. 1967 Influence of environmental factors on foetal growth in man *Lancet* i:1026–1028.

Grufferman S., Wang H.H., DeLong E.R., Kimm S.Y.S., Delzell E.S., and Falletta J.M. 1982 Environmental factors in the etiology of rhabdomyosarcoma in childhood *JNCI* 68:107–113.

Grunwaldt E. and Bates T. 1957 Nonadrenal female pseudohermaphrodism after administration of testosterone to mother during pregnancy: Report of a case *Pediatrics* 20:503–505.

Guillot N. 1852 Klinische Bemerkungen uber Ammen und Sauglinge *J Kinderke* 19:113–125.

Guillot M., Toubas P.L., Mselati J.C., Gamarra E., Moriette G., and Relier J.P.

1979 Embryo-foetopathie coumarinique et maladie des epiphyses ponctuees *Arch Fr Pediatr* 36:63–66.

Gupta R.C., Reddy M.V., and Randerath K. 1982 32P-postlabelling analysis of non-radioactive aromatic carcinogen-DNA adducts *Carcinogenesis* 3:1081–1092.

Gurland B.J. and Gurland R.V. 1979 Methods of research into sex and aging In R. Green and J. Weiner, eds. *Proceeds of NIMH Conference on Methods of Sex Research*, Washington D.C., New York State Government Publication of 1979, pp 67–99.

Haas J.D., Frongillo E.A., Stepick C.D., Beard J.L., and Luis Hartado G. 1980 Altitude, ethnic and sex differences in birthweight and length in Bolivia *Hum Biol* 52:459–477.

Habicht J.-P., Yarbrough C., Lechtig A., and Klein R.E. 1974 Relation of maternal supplementary feeding during pregnancy to birth weight and other sociobiological factors In M. Winick, ed. *Current Concepts in Nutrition, Vol 1: Nutrition and Fetal Development* John Wiley & Sons, New York, pp 127–145.

Hackman E., Emanuel I., van Belle G., and Daling J. 1983 Maternal birth weight and subsequent pregnancy outcome *JAMA* 250:2016–2019.

Hadders-Algra M., Touwen B.C.L., Olinga A.A., and Huisjes H.J. 1985 Minor neurological dysfunction and behavioural development. A report from the Groningen perinatal project *Early Hum Dev* 11:221–229.

Hadders-Algra M., Touwen B.C.L., and Huisjes H.J. 1986 Neurologically deviant newborns: Neurological and behavioural development at the age of six years *Dev Med Child Neurol* 28:569–578.

Hadlock F.P., Deter R.L., and Harrist R.B. 1984 Sonographic detection of abnormal fetal growth patterns *Clin Obstet Gynecol* 27:342–351.

Hahnemann M. 1973 Chromosome studies in induced abortions *Clin Genet* 4:328–332.

Hales B.F., Smith S., and Robaire B. 1986 Cyclophosphamide in the seminal fluid of treated males: Transmission to females by mating and effect on pregnancy outcome *Toxicol Appl Pharmacol* 84:423–430.

Hall J.G. 1976 Embryopathy associated with oral anticoagulant therapy In *Birth Defects: Original Article Series* Vol XII, pp 33–37.

Hall J.G., Pauli R.M., and Wilson K.M. 1980 Maternal and fetal sequelae of anticoagulation during pregnancy *Am J Med* 68:122–140.

Hall M.H., Carr-Hill R.A., Fraser C., and Samphier M.L. 1985 The extent and antecedents of uncertain gestation *Br J Obstet Gynaecol* 92:445–451.

Halling H. 1979 Suspected link between exposure to hexachlorophene and malformed infants *Ann NY Acad Sci* 320:426–435.

Halperin L.R. and Wilroy R.S. 1978 Maternal hyperthermia and neural tube defects *Lancet* ii:212–213.

Hamilton A. 1785 *A Treatise of Midwifery comprehending the whole management of female complaints and the treatment of children in early infancy*, ed 8, C. Eliot, Edinburgh.

Hamilton A. 1929 *Industrial Poisons in the U.S.* Macmillan, New York.

Hamilton A. 1943 *Exploring the Dangerous Trades* Little, Brown & Co., Boston.

Hammes L.M. and Treloar A.E. 1970 Gestational interval from vital records *Am J Pub Health* 60:1496–1505.

Hanshaw J.B., Scheiner A.P., Moxley A.W., Gaev L., Abel V., and Scheiner B. 1976 School failure and deafness after "silent" congenital cytomegalovirus infection *N Engl J Med* 295:468–470.

Hanson J.W. and Smith D.W. 1975 Teratogenicity of anticoagulants *J Pediatr* 87:838.

Hansson A. and Mikklesen M. 1978 The origin of the extra chromosome 21 in Down syndrome *Cytogenet Cell Genet* 20:194–203.

Hansson E., Jansa S., Wande H., Kallen B., and Ostlund E. 1980 Pregnancy outcome for women working in laboratories in some of the pharmaceutical industries in Sweden *Scand J Work Environ Health* 6:131–134.

Harada Y. 1968 Congenital (or fetal) Minamata disease In *Minamata Disease* Study Group of Minamata Disease Kumamoto University, Japan pp 93–117.

Harcourt J.K., Johnson N.W., and Storey E. 1962 *In vivo* incorporation of tetracycline in the teeth of man *Arch Oral Biol* 7:431–437.

Hardy J.B. 1973 Fetal consequences of maternal viral infections in pregnancy *Arch Otolaryngol* 98:218–227.

Hardy J.B. and Mellits E.D. 1972 Does maternal smoking during pregnancy have a long-term effect on the child? *Lancet* ii:1332–1336.

Hardy J.B. and Mellits E.D. 1977 Relationship of low birthweight to maternal characteristics of age, parity, education and body size In D.M. Reed and F.J. Stanley, eds. *The epidemiology of prematurity* Urban & Schwarzenberg, Baltimore pp 105–117.

Harger J.H., Acher D.F., and Marchese S.G. 1983 Etiology of recurrent pregnancy losses and outcome of subsequent pregnancies *Am J Obstet Gynecol* 62:574–581.

Harkonen H. and Holmberg P. 1982 Obstetric histories of women occupationally exposed to styrene *Scand J Work Environ Health* 8:74–77.

Harlap S. 1973 Down's syndrome in West Jerusalem *Am J Epidemiol* 97:225–232.

Harlap S. and Baras M. 1984 Conception waits in fertile women after stopping oral contraceptives *Int J Fertil* 29:73–80.

Harlap S. and Shiono P. 1980 Alcohol, smoking, and incidence of spontaneous abortions in the first and second trimester *Lancet* ii:173–176.

Harlap S., Shiono P., Pellegrin F., Golbus M., Bachman R., Mann J., Schmidt L., and Lewis J.P. 1979a Chromosome abnormalities in oral contraceptive breakthrough pregnancies *Lancet* i:1342.

Harlap S., Shiono P.H., Ramcharan S., Berendes H., and Pellegrin F. 1979b A prospective study of spontaneous fetal losses after induced abortions *N Engl J Med* 301:677–681.

Harlap S., Shiono P., and Ramcharan S. 1980a A life table of spontaneous abortions and the effects of age parity and other variables In I.H. Porter and E.B. Hook, eds. *Human Embryonic and Fetal Death* Academic Press, New York, pp 145–164.

Harlap S., Shiono P., and Ramcharan S. 1980b Spontaneous foetal losses in women using different contraceptives around the time of conception *Int J Epid* 9:49–56.

Harris J.W. 1919 Influenza occurring in pregnant women *JAMA* 12:978–980.

Harris J.A. and Gunstad B. 1936 The measurement of the individuality of women with respect to their capacity for bringing the foetus to term In

C.O. Rosendahl, R.A. Gartner and F.O. Burr, eds. *Botanist and Biometrician* University of Minnesota Press, Minneapolis.

Harrison K. and Warburton D. 1986 Preferential X-chromosome activity in human female placental tissues *Cytogenet Cell Genet* 41:163–168.

Harrod M.J.E. and Sherrod P.S. 1981 Warfarin embryopathy in siblings *Obstet Gynecol* 57:673–676.

Hartley W.J., Alexander G., and Edwards M.J. 1974 Brain cavitation and microencephaly in lambs exposed to prenatal hyperthermia *Teratology* 9:299–304.

Hassold T.J. 1980 A cytogenetic study of repeated spontaneous abortions *Am J Hum Genet* 32:723–730.

Hassold T. 1982 Mosaic trisomies in human spontaneous abortions *Hum Genet* 61:31–35.

Hassold T. and Chiu D. 1985 Maternal age specific rates of numerical chromosome abnormalities with special reference to trisomy *Hum Genet* 70:11–17.

Hassold T. and Jacobs P.A. 1984 Trisomy in man In Campbell A., Roman H., Sander L., eds. *Ann Rev Genet* 18:69–97.

Hassold T., Chen N., Funkhouser, J., Jooss T., Manuel B., Matsuura, J., Matsuyama A., Wilson C., Yamane J.A., and Jacobs P.A. 1980a A cytogenetic study of 1000 spontaneous abortions *Ann Hum Genet* 44:151–178.

Hassold T., Jacobs P., Kline J., Stein Z., and Warburton, D. 1980b Effect of maternal age on autosomal trisomies *Ann Hum Genet* 44:29–36.

Hassold T., Quillen S.D., And Yamane J.A. 1983 Sex ratio in spontaneous abortions *Ann Hum Genet* 47:39–47.

Hassold T., Chiu D., and Yamane J. 1984a Parental origin of autosomal trisomies *Ann Hum Genet* 48:129–144.

Hassold T., Warburton D., Kline J., and Stein Z. 1984b The relationship of maternal age and trisomy among trisomic spontaneous abortions *Am J Hum Genet* 36:1349–1356.

Hassold T., Kumlin E., Takaesu N., and Leppert M. 1985 Determination of the parental origin of sex-chromosome monosomy using restriction fragment length polymorphisms *Am J Hum Genet* 37:965–972.

Hassold T., Benham F., and Leppert M. 1988 Cytogenetic and molecular analysis of sex-chromosome monosomy *Am J Hum Genet* 42:534–541.

Hatch E.E. and Bracken M.B. 1986 Effect of marijuana use in pregnancy on fetal growth *Am J Epidemiol* 124:986–993.

Hatch M. 1983 Paternal risk factors in spontaneous abortion. PhD Dissertation, Columbia University, New York.

Hayashi K., Bracken, M.B., Freeman D.H., and Hellenbrand K. 1982 Hydatidiform mole in the United States (1970–1977): A statistical and theoretical analysis *Am J Epidemiol* 115:67–77.

Hayles A.B. and Nolan R.B. 1957 Female pseudohermaphroditism: Report of case in an infant born of a mother receiving methyltestosterone during pregnancy *Mayo Clin Proc* 32:41–44.

Hebel J.R., Fox N.L., and Sexton M. 1988 Dose-response of birth weight to various measures of maternal smoking during pregnancy *J Clin Epidemiol* 41:483–489.

Heinonen O.P., Slone D., and Shapiro S. 1977 *Birth Defects and Drugs in Pregnancy* Publishing Science Group, Littleton, MA.

Helm P. and Helm S. 1984 Decrease in menarcheal age from 1966–1983 in Denmark *Acta Obstet Gynaecol Scand* 63:633–635.

Hemminki K. 1983 Nucleic acid adducts of chemical carcinogens and mutagens *Arch Toxicol* 52:249–285.

Hemminki K. and Niemi M.-L. 1982 Community study of spontaneous abortions: Relation to occupation and air pollution by sulfur dioxide, hydrogen sulfide, and carbon disulfide *Int Arch Occup Environ Health* 51:55–63.

Hemminki K., Franssila E., and Vainio H. 1980a Spontaneous abortions among female chemical workers in Finland *Int Arch Occup Environ Health* 45:123–126.

Hemminki K., Niemi M.-L., Koskinen K., and Vainio H. 1980b Spontaneous abortions among women employed in the metal industry in Finland *Int Arch Occup Environ Health* 47:53–60.

Hemminki K., Mutanen P., Saloniemi I., and Luoma K. 1981 Congenital malformations and maternal occupation in Finland: Multivariate analysis *J Epidemiol Comm Health* 35:5–10.

Hemminki K., Mutanen P., Saloniemi I., Niemi M.-L., and Vainio H. 1982 Spontaneous abortions in hospital staff engaged in sterilizing instruments with chemical agents *Br Med J* 285:1461–1463.

Hemminki, K., Kyyronen P., Niemi J.-L., Koskinen K., Sallmen M., and Vainio H. 1983a Spontaneous abortions in an industrialized community in Finland *AJPH* 73:32–37.

Hemminki K., Mutanen P., and Saloniemi I. 1983b Smoking and the occurrence of congenital malformations and spontaneous abortions: Multivariate analysis *Am J Obstet Gynecol* 145:61–66.

Hemminki K., Niemi M.-L., Kyyronen P., Kilpikari I., and Vainio H. 1983c Spontaneous abortions and reproductive selection mechanisms in the rubber and leather industry in Finland *Br J Ind Med* 40:81–86.

Hemminki K., Kyyronen P., and Lindbohm M.-L. 1985 Spontaneous abortions and malformations in the offspring of nurses exposed to anaesthetic gases, cytostatic drugs, and other potential hazards in hospitals based on registered information of outcome *J Epidemiol Comm Health* 39:141–147.

Hempelmann L.H., Langham W.H., Richmond C.R., and Voelz G.L. 1973 Manhattan project plutonium workers: A twenty-seven year follow-up study of selected cases *Health Physic* 25:461–479.

Hendershot G.E. 1979 Work during pregnancy and subsequent hospitalization of mothers and infants *Pub Health Rep* 94:425–431.

Hendershot G.E. 1984 Maternal age and overdue conceptions *Am J Pub Health* 74:35–38.

Hendershot G.E., Mosher W.D., Pratt W.E. 1982 [Controversy] Infertility and age: An unresolved issue *Fam Perspect* 14:287–288.

Henderson M. 1967 Differences in duration of pregnancy *Arch Environ Health* 14:904–911.

Henderson S.A. and Edwards R.G. 1968 Chiasma frequency and maternal age in mammals *Nature* 218:22–28.

Hendrickx A.G. and Stone G.W. 1976 Preliminary studies on the embryo-toxicity of hyperthermia in the bonnet monkey (*M. radiata*) *Teratology* 13:24A.

Henry L. 1957 Fecondite et famille: Modeles mathematiques. II. *Population* 16:27–48.

Henry L. 1961 Some data on natural fertility *Eugenics Quart* 8:81–91.

Herbst A.L. 1981 The epidemiology of vaginal and cervical clear cell adenocarcinoma In A.L. Herbst and H.A. Bern, eds. *Developmental Effects of Diethylstilbestrol (DES) in Pregnancy,* Thieme-Stratton Inc., New York, pp 63–70.

Herbst A.L. and Scully R.E. 1970 Adenocarcinoma of the vagina in adolescence. A report of 7 cases including 6 clear-cell carcinomas (so-called mesonephromas) *Cancer* 25:745–757.

Herbst A.L., Ulfelder H., and Poskanzer D.C. 1971 Adenocarcinoma of the vagina: Association of maternal stilbestrol therapy with tumor appearance in young women *N Engl J Med* 284:878–881.

Herbst A.L., Robboy S.J., Scully R.E., and Poskanzer D.C. 1974 Clear-cell adenocarcinoma of the vagina and cervix in girls: An analysis of 170 registry cases *Am J Obstet Gynecol* 119:713–724.

Herbst A.L., Poskanzer D.C., Robboy S.J., Friedlander L., and Scully R.E. 1975 Prenatal exposure to stilbestrol. A prospective comparison of exposed female offspring with unexposed controls *N Engl J Med* 292:334–339.

Herbst A.L., Cole P., Colton T., Robboy S.J., and Scully R.E. 1977 Age-incidence and risk of diethylstilbestrol-related clear cell adenocarcinoma of the vagina and cervix *Am J Obstet Gynecol* 128:43–50.

Herbst A.L., Hubby M.M., Blough R.R., and Azizi F. 1980 A comparison of pregnancy experience in DES-exposed and DES-unexposed daughters *J Reprod Med* 24:62–69.

Herrera M.G., Mora J.O., de Peredes B., and Wagner M. 1980 Maternal weight/height and the effect of food supplementation during pregnancy and lactation In H. Aebi and R. Whitehead, eds. *Maternal Nutrition During Pregnancy and Lactation* Hans Huber Publishers, Bern, pp 252–263.

Hertig A.T. 1967 The overall problem in man In K. Benirschke, ed. *Comparative Aspects of Reproductive Failure* Springer-Verlag, Berlin, pp 11–41.

Hertig A.T. and Rock J. 1973 Searching for early fertilized human ova *Gyn Inv* 4:121–139.

Hertig A.T. and Sheldon W.H. 1943 Minimal criteria required to prove prima facie case of traumatic abortion or miscarriage *Ann Surg* 117:596–606.

Hertig A.T., Rock J., and Adams E.C. 1956 A description of 34 human ova within the first 17 days of development *Am J Anat* 98:435–494.

Hertig A.T., Rock J., Adams E., and Menkin C. 1959 Thirty-four fertilized human ova, good, bad, and indifferent, recovered from 210 women of known fertility. A study of biologic wastage in early human pregnancy *Pediatrics* 23:202–211.

Hess J.H. 1922 Premature infants *JAMA* 79:552–556.

Hetzel B.S. and Pharoah P.O.D., eds. 1971 *Endemic Cretinism* Institute of Human Biology, Papua, New Guinea, Monograph Series No. 2.

Hetzel B.S. and Hay I.D. 1979 Thyroid function, iodine nutrition and fetal brain development *Clin Endocrinol* II:445–460.

Hewitt D. 1961 A possible seasonal effect of parturition *Am J Obstet Gynecol* 82:940–942.

Hickman C.J. and Johnson M.L. 1980 *Dictionary of Biology.* Penguin, London, 7 ed.

Hill A.B. 1965 The environment and disease: Association or causation *Proc R Soc Med* 58:295–300.

Hill A.B., Doll R., Galloway T.McL., and Hughes J.P. 1958 Virus diseases in pregnancy and congenital defects *Br J Prev Soc Med* 12:1–7.

Himmelberger D.U., Brown B.W., and Cohen E.N. 1978 Cigarette smoking during pregnancy and the occurrence of spontaneous abortion and congenital abnormality *Am J Epidemiol* 108:470–479.

Hingson R., Alpert J., Day N., Dooling E., Kayne H., Morelock S., Oppenheimer E., and Zuckerman B. 1982 Effects of maternal drinking and marijuana use on fetal growth and development *Pediatrics* 70:539–546.

Hirsh J., Cade J.F., and Gallus A.S. 1970 Fetal effects of Coumadin administered during pregnancy *Blood* 36:623–627.

Hoffman F., Overzier C., and Uhde G. 1955 Zur Frage der Hormonalen Erzeugung foetaler Zwitterbildung beim Menschen *Geburtshilfe Fraunheilkd* 15:1061–1070.

Hoffman H.J., Stark C.R., Lundin F.E., and Ashbrook J.D. 1974 Analysis of birth weight, gestational age, and fetal viability, U.S. births, 1968 *Obstet Gynecol Survey* 29:651–681.

Hoffman, H.J., Lundin F.E., Bakketeig L.S., and Harley E.H. 1977 Classification of births by weight and gestational age for future studies of prematurity: Some demographic and statistical perceptions based on bivariate distributions In D.M. Reed and F.J. Stanley, eds. *The Epidemiology of Prematurity* Urban & Schwarzenberg, Baltimore and Munich, pp 297–333.

Hoffman H.J. and Bakketeig L.S. 1984 Risk factors associated with the occurrence of preterm birth *Clin Obstet Gynecol* 27:539–552.

Hogberg U. 1985 Maternal mortality in Sweden In Umea University medical dissertations (New series no. 156), Siga Ab-Gallware, Umea, Sweden.

Hogue C.J.R. 1986 Impact of abortion on subsequent fecundity *Clin Obstet Gynaecol* 13:95–103.

Hogue C.J.R., Cates W., and Tietze C. 1982 The effects of induced abortion on subsequent reproduction *Epidemiol Rev* 4:66–94.

Hogue C.J.R., Buechler J.W., Strauss L.T., and Smith J.C. 1987 Overview of the national infant mortality surveillance (NIMS) project: Design, methods, results *Publ Health Rep* 102:126–138.

Holland W.W., Bennett A.E., Cameron I.R., Florey C.V., Leeder S.R., Schilling R.S.F., Swan A.V., and Waller R.E. 1979 Health effects of particulate pollution: Reappraising the evidence *Am J Epidemiol* 110:527–659.

Hollingsworth D.R. and Kotchen J.M. 1981 Gynecologic age and its relation to neonatal outcomes *Birth Defects* 17:91–105.

Holmberg P.C. and Nurminen M. 1980 Congenital defects of the central nervous system and occupational factors during pregnancy: A case-referent study *Am J Ind Med* 1:167–176.

Holmberg P.C., Hernberg S., Kurppa K., Rantala K., and Riala R. 1982 Oral cleft and organic solvent exposure during pregnancy *Int Arch Occup Environ Health* 50:371–376.

Holtzman N.A. and Khoury M.J. 1986 Monitoring for congenital malformations *Ann Rev Publ Health* 7:237–266.

Holzgreve W., Carey J.C., and Hall B.D. 1976 Warfarin-induced fetal abnormalities *Lancet* ii:914–915.

Hook E.B. 1981a Down syndrome: Its frequency in human populations and some factors pertinent to variation in rates In F. de la Cruz and P.S.

Gerald, eds. *Trisomy 21 (Down syndrome)—Research Perspectives* Academic Press, Baltimore, pp 3–67.

Hook E.B. 1981b Rates of chromosome abnormalities at different maternal ages *Obstet Gynecol* 58:282–285.

Hook E.B. 1983 Down syndrome rates and relaxed selection at older maternal ages *Am J Hum Genet* 35:1307–1313.

Hook E.B. 1985 The impact of aneuploidy upon public health: Mortality and morbidity associated with human chromosome abnormalities In V.L. Dellarco, P.E. Voytek, and A. Hollaender, eds. *Aneuploidy*, Plenum Press, New York and London, pp 7–33.

Hook E.B. and Cross P.K. 1982 Paternal age and Down's syndrome genotypes diagnosed prenatally: No association in New York State data *Hum Genet* 62:167–174.

Hook E.B. and Cross P.K. 1985 Cigarette smoking and Down syndrome *Am J Hum Genet* 37:1216–1224.

Hook E.B. and Cross P.K. 1988 Maternal cigarette smoking, Down syndrome in live births, and infant race *Am J Hum Genet* 42:482–489.

Hook E.B. and Hamerton J.L. 1977 The frequency of chromosome abnormalities detected in consecutive newborn studies, differences between study results by sex, and severity of phenotypic involvement In E.B. Hook and I.H. Porter, eds. *Population Cytogenetics* Academic Press, New York, pp 63–79.

Hook E.B. and Warburton D. 1983 The distribution of chromosomal genotypes associated with Turner's syndrome: Livebirth prevalence rates and evidence for diminished fetal mortality and severity in genotypes associated with structural X abnormalities or mosaicism *Human Genetics* 64:24–27.

Hook E.B. and Regal R.R. 1984 A search for a paternal-age effect upon cases of 47, +21 in which the extra chromosome is of paternal origin *Am J Hum Genet* 36:413–421.

Hook E.B., Cross P.K., Lamson S.H., Regal R.R., Baird P.A., and Uh S.H. 1981 Paternal age and Down's syndrome in British Columbia *Am J Hum Genet* 33:123–128.

Horon I.L., Strobino D.M., and MacDonald H.M. 1983 Birth weights among infants born to adolescent and young adult women *Am J Obstet Gynecol* 146:444–449.

Hosemann H.A. 1948 Schwangerschaftdauer und Neugeborenengewicht *Arch Gynak* 176:109–123.

Hsueh A.J.W., Erickson G.F., and Lu K.H. 1979 Changes in uterine estrogen receptor and morphology in aging female rats *Biol Reprod* 21:793–800.

Huggins G., Vessey M., Flavel R., Yeates D., and McPherson K. 1982 Vaginal spermicides and outcome of pregnancy: Findings in a large cohort study *Contraception* 25:219–230.

Huisjes H.J., Touwen B.C.L., Hoekstra J., van Woerden-Blanksma J.T., Bierman-van Eendenburg M.E.C., Jurgens-van der Zee A.D., Fidler V.J., and Olinga A.A. 1980 Obstetrical-Neonatal Neurological Relationship: A Replication Study *Europ J Obstet Gynaec Reprod Biol* 10:247–256.

Hulka J.K. and Schaaf J.H. 1964 Obstetrics in adolescents: A controlled study of deliveries by mothers 15 years of age and under *Obstet Gynecol* 23:678–685.

Hunt V.R., Manson J.M., Lucas-Wallace K. 1979 *Work and the Health of Women* CRC Press, Boca Raton, FL.

Hunter J. 1787 An experiment to determine the effect of extirpating one ovary upon the number of young produced *Philos Trans R Soc* 77:233.

Hunter W.S., Ellert M.S., Nequin L.G., and Suarez W.A. 1979 Is hyperthermia a teratogen? *Br Med J* 1:887–888.

Huszar G. and Naftolin F. 1984 The myometrium and uterine cervix in normal and preterm labor *N Engl J Med* 311:571–581.

Hutchins V., Kessel S.S., and Placek P.J. 1984 Trends in maternal and infant health factors associated with low infant birth weight, United States, 1972 and 1980 *Pub Health Rep* 99:162–172.

Hutchinson J. 1887 *Syphilis* Lea Brothers and Company, Philadelphia.

Hyman H. 1972 *Secondary Analysis of Sample Surveys: Principles, Procedures and Potentialities.* John Wiley & Son, New York.

Hytten R. and Chamberlain G. 1980 *Clinical Physiology in Obstetrics* Blackwell Scientific Publication, Oxford, pp 164–166, 195–196.

Ingall D. and Norins L. 1976 Syphilis In J.S. Remington and J.O. Klein, eds. *Infectious Diseases of the Fetus and Newborn Infant*, W.B. Saunders Co., Philadelphia, pp 414–463.

International Clearinghouse for Birth Defects Monitoring Systems 1982 Annual Report 1980 Swedish National Board of Health and Welfare, Stockholm.

Ishizuka N., Kawashima Y., Nakanishi T., Sugawa T., and Nishikawa Y. 1962 Statistical observations on genital anomalies of newborns following the administration of progestins to their mothers *J Jpn Obstet Gynecol Soc* 9:271–282.

Israel S.L. and Deutschberger J. 1964 Relation of the mother's age to obstetric performance *Obstet Gynecol* 24:411–417.

Istvan J. 1986 Stress, anxiety, and birth outcomes: A critical review of the evidence *Psychological Bull* 100:331–348.

Jackson-Cook C.K., Flannery D.B., Corey L.A., Nance W.E., and Brown J.A. 1985 Nucleolar organizer region variants as a risk factor for Down syndrome *Am J Hum Genet* 37:1049–1061.

Jacobs P.A. 1982 Human population cytogenetics: The first twenty-five years *Am J Hum Genet* 34:689–698.

Jacobs P.A. and Hassold T.J. 1980 The origin of chromosome abnormalities in spontaneous abortion In I.H. Porter and E.B. Hook, eds. In *Human Embryonic and Fetal Death*, Academic Press, New York, pp 289–298.

Jacobs P.A. and Strong J.A. 1959 A case of human intersexuality having a possible XXY sex-determining mechanism *Nature* 183:302–303.

Jacobs P.A., Baikie A.G., Brown W.M.C., MacGregor T.N., Maclean N., and Harnden D.G. 1959 Evidence for the existence of the human "Super Female" *Lancet* ii:423–425.

Jacobs P.A., Harnden D.G., Buckton K.E., Court Brown W., King M.J., McBride J.A., MacGregor T.N., and Maclean N. 1961 Cytogenetic studies in primary amenorrhoea *Lancet* i:1183–1188.

Jacobs P.A., Brunton M., Melvinne M.M., Brittain R.P., and McClemont W.F. 1965 Aggressive behaviour, mental sub-normality and the XYY male *Nature* 208:1351–1352.

Jacobs P.A., Angell R.R., Buchanan I.M., Hassold T.J., Matsuyama A.M., and Manuel B. 1978 The origin of human triploids *Ann Hum Genet* 42:49–57.

Jacobs P.A., Szulman A.E., Funkhouser J., Matsuura J.S., and Wilson C.C. 1982 Human triploidy: Relationship between parental origin of the additional haploid complement and development of partial hydatidiform mole *Ann Hum Genet* 46:223–231.

Jacobson B.D. 1962 Hazards of norethindrone therapy during pregnancy *Am J Obstet Gynecol* 84:962–968.

Jain A.K. 1969 Fecundability and its relation to age in a sample of Taiwanese women *Pop Studies* 23:69–85.

James W.H. 1963 The problem of spontaneous abortion X: the efficacy of psychotherapy *Am J Obstet Gynec* 85:38.

James W.H. 1974 Spontaneous abortion and birth order *J Biosoc Sci* 6:23–41.

James W.H. 1978 Recurrence rates in sibships and concordance rates in twins for anencephaly *Ann Hum Biol* 5:79–81.

Janerich D.T., Flink E.M., and Keogh M.D. 1976 Down's syndrome and oral contraceptive usage *Br J Obstet Gynaecol* 83:617–620.

Janz D. 1975 The teratogenic risk of antiepileptic drugs *Epilepsia* 16:159–165.

Janz D. 1982 On major malformations and minor anomalies in the offspring of parents with epilepsy: Review of the literature In D. Janz, M. Dam, A. Richens, L. Bossi, H. Helge, and D. Schmidt, eds. *Epilepsy, Pregnancy, and the Child,* Raven Press, New York, pp 211–222.

Jarnfelt-Samsioe A., Samsioe G., and Velinder G.-M. 1983 Nausea and vomiting in pregnancy. A contribution to its epidemiology *Gynec Obstet Invest* 16:221–229.

Jaroszewicz A.M. 1973 Clinical assessment of gestational age in the newborn *S Afr Med J* 47:2123–2124.

Jarvis E. *1855 Report of the Commission on Lunacy.* Reprinted 1971 Harvard University Press, Cambridge.

Jeavons P.M. 1982 Sodium valproate and neural tube defects *Lancet* ii:1282–1283.

Jelliffe E. 1968 Low birth-weight and malarial infection of the placenta *Bull World Health Org* 33:69–78.

Jenkins R.L. 1933 Etiology of mongolism *Am J Dis Child* 45:506–519.

Jespersen C.S., Littauer J., and Sagild U. 1977 Measles as a cause of fetal defects *Acta Paediatr Scand* 66:367–372.

Jick H., Porter J., and Morrison A.S. 1977 Relation between smoking and age of natural menopause *Lancet* i:1354–1355.

Jick H., Walker A.M., Rothman K.J., Hunter J.R., Holmes L.B., Watkins R.N., D'Ewart D.C., Danford A., and Madsen S. 1981 Vaginal spermicides and congenital disorders *JAMA* 245:1329–1332.

Jick H., Shiota K., Shepard T.H., Hunter J.R., Stergachis A., Madsen S., and Porter J.B. 1982 Vaginal spermicides and miscarriages seen primarily in the emergency room *Terato Carcino Mutag* 2:205–210.

Jimenez J.M., Tyson J.E., and Reisch J.A. 1983 Clinical measures of gestational age in normal pregnancies *Obstet Gynecol* 61:438–443.

Johnson L.D., Driscoll S.G., Hertig A.T., Cole P.T., and Nickerson R.J. 1979 Vaginal adenosis in stillborns and neonates exposed to diethylstilbestrol and steroidal estrogens and progestins *Obstet Gynecol* 53:671–679.

Johnston I., Lopata A., Speirs A., Hoult I., Kellow G., and du Plessis Y. 1981 In vitro fertilization: The challenge of the eighties *Fertil Steril* 36:699–706.

Johnston I., Lopata A., Speirs A., Gronow M., Martin M., and Oliva K. 1983 Current Status of an in vitro fertilization programme and early pregnancy diagnosis In H.M. Beier and H.R. Lind, eds. *Fertilization of the Human Egg In Vitro* Springer-Verlag, Berlin, pp 271–281.

Johnstone F.D., Beard R.J., Boyd I.E., and McCarthy T.G. 1976 Cervical diameter after suction termination of pregnancy *Br Med J* 1:68–69.

Johnstone F. and Inglis L. 1974 Familial trends in low birth weight *Br Med J* 3:659–661.

Jones A.H., Fantel A.G., Kocan R.A., and Juchau M.R. 1977 Bioactivation of procarcinogens to mutagens in human fetal and placental tissues *Life Sci* 21:1831–1836.

Jones K.L., Smith D.W., Streissguth A.P., and Myrianthopoulus N.C. 1974 Outcome in offspring of chronic alcoholic women *Lancet* i:1076–1078.

Jongbloet P.H. 1971 Month of birth and gametopathy *Clin Genet* 2:315–330.

Jongbloet P.H., Poestkoke A.J., Hamers A.J., and van Erkelens-Zwetz J.H. 1978 Down syndrome and religious groups *Lancet* ii:1310.

Jost A. 1955 Modalities in the action of gonadal and gonad-stimulating hormones in the foetus *Mem Soc Endocrinol* 4:237–248.

Juberg R.C. and Mowrey P.N. 1983 Origin of nondisjunction in trisomy 21 syndrome: All studies compiled, parental age analysis and international comparisons *Am J Med Genet* 16:111–116.

Jurgens-Van Der Zee A.D., Bierman-Van Eendenburg M.E.C., Fidler V.J., Olinga A.A., Visch J.H., Towen B.C.L., and Huisjes H.G. 1979 Preterm birth, growth retardation and acidemia in relation to neurological abnormality of the new born *Early Hum Dev* 3:141–154.

Kajii T. 1965 Thalidomide experience in Japan *Ann Paediat* 205:341–354.

Kajii T. and Ferrier A. 1978 Cytogenetics of aborters and abortuses *Am J Obstet Gynecol* 131:33–38.

Kajii T. and Ohama K. 1979 Inverse maternal age effect in monosomy X *Hum Genet* 51:147–151.

Kajii T., Ohama K., Niikawa N., Ferrier A., and Avirachan S. 1973 Banding analyses of abnormal karyotypes in spontaneous abortion *Am J Hum Genet* 25:539–547.

Kajii T., Ohama K., and Mikamo K. 1978 Anatomic and chromosomal anomalies in 944 induced abortuses *Hum Genet* 43:247–258.

Kajii T., Ferrier A., Niikawa N., Takahara H., Ohama K., and Avirachan S. 1980 Anatomic and chromosomal anomalies in 639 spontaneous abortuses *Hum Genet* 55:87–98.

Kallen B. and Winberg J. 1968 A Swedish register of congenital malformations *Pediatrics* 41:765–776.

Kallen B., Hag S., and Klingberg M. 1984 Birth defects monitoring systems: Accomplishments and goals In H. Kalter, ed. *Issues Rev Teratol* Vol 2, Plenum Press, New York, pp 1–22.

Kalter H. and Warkany J. 1983 Congenital malformations: Etiologic factors and their role in prevention *N Engl J Med* 308:424–431, 491–497.

Kaltreider D.F. and Johnson J.W.C. 1976 Patients at high risk of low birth weight delivery *Am J Obstet Gynecol* 124:251–256.

Kamiguchi Y. and Mikamo K. 1986 An improved, efficient method for analyzing human sperm chromosomes using zona-free hamster ova *Am J Hum Genet* 38:724–740.

Kaminski M. and Papiernik E. 1974 Multifactorial study of the risk of prematurity at 32 weeks of gestation: II. A comparison between an empirical prediction and a discriminant analysis *J Perinat Med* 2:37.

Kaminski M., Goujard J., and Rumeau-Rouquette C. 1973 Prediction of low birthweight and prematurity by a multiple regression analysis with maternal characteristics known since the beginning of the pregnancy *Int J Epidemiol* 2:195–204.

Kaminski M., Rumeau-Rouquette C., and Schwartz D. 1976 Consummation d'alcool chez les femmes enceintes et issue de la grossesse *Rev Epidemiol Sante Publique* 24:27–40.

Kaminski M., Rumeau C., and Schwartz D. 1978 Alcohol consumption in pregnant women and the outcome of pregnancy *Alcoholism: Clin Exp Res* 2:155–163.

Kaminski M., Franc M., Lebouvier M., du Mazaubrun C., and Rumeau-Rouquette C. 1981 Moderate alcohol use and pregnancy outcome *Neurobehav Toxicol Teratol* 3:173–181.

Kane S.H. 1967 Advancing age and the primigravida *Obstet Gynecol* 29:409–414.

Kanner L. 1964 A history of the care and study of the mentally retarded Charles C Thomas, Springfield, IL.

Kao J., Brown W.A., Schmid B., Goulding E.H., and Fabro S. 1981 Teratogenicity of valproic acid: *In vivo* and *in vitro* investigations *Teratog Carcinog Mutag* 1:367–383.

Karn M.N., Lang-Brown H., MacKenzie H., and Penrose L.S. 1951 Birth weight, gestational time and survival in sibs *Ann Eugen* 15:306–322.

Karn M.N. and Penrose L.S. 1951 Birthweight and gestation time in relation to maternal age, parity and infant survival *Ann Eugen* 16:147–164.

Kass E.H. 1960 The role of asymptomatic bacteriuria in the pathogenesis of pyelonephritis In E.L. Quinn and E.H. Kass, eds. *Biology of Pyelonephritis* Little, Brown & Co., Boston, pp 399–412.

Katz A. 1953 Arstidvariationen av prematurfrekvensen *Nord Med* 26:1637–1638.

Kaufman D.W., Slone D., Rosenberg L., Miettinen O.S., and Shapiro S. 1980 Cigarette smoking and age at natural menopause *Am J Public Health* 70:420–422.

Kaufman M.H. and Bain I.M. 1984 Influence of ethanol on chromosome segregation during the first and second meiotic divisions in the mouse egg *J Exp Zool* 230:315–320.

Keet M.P., Jaroszewicz A.M., and Lombard C.J. 1986 Follow-up study of physical growth of monozygous twins with discordant within-pair birth weights *Pediatrics* 77:336–344.

Keirse M.J.N.C. 1979 Epidemiology of preterm labor In M.J.N.C. Keirse, A.B.M. Anderson, and J.B. Gravenhorst, eds. *Human Parturition* Leiden University Press, Leiden, pp 219–234.

Keirse M.J.N.C., Rush R.W., Anderson A.B., and Turnbull A.C. 1978 Risk of pre-term delivery in patients with previous pre-term delivery and/or abortion *Br J Obstet Gynaecol* 85:81–85.

Keller C.A. and Nugent R.P. 1983 Seasonal patterns in perinatal mortality and preterm delivery *Am J Epidemiol* 118:689–698.

Kelsey J.L., Dwyer T., Holford T.R., and Bracken M.B. 1978 Maternal smoking and congenital malformations: An epidemiological study *J Epidemiol Comm Health* 32:102–107.

Kendall M.G. 1979 The World Fertility Survey: Current Status and Findings *Population Rep,* Series M, No. 3, July.

Kennett R. and Pollak M. 1983 On sequential detection of a shift in the probability of a rare event *JAMA* 78:389–395.

Kerber I.J., Warr O.S., III, and Richardson C. 1968 Pregnancy in a patient with a prosthetic mitral valve associated with a fetal anomaly attributed to warfarin sodium *JAMA* 203:223–225.

Kessel S.S., Villar J., Berendes M.D., and Nugent P. 1984 The changing pattern of low birth weight in the United States *JAMA* 251:1978–1982.

Kessler-Harris A. 1984 Protection for women: Trade unions and labor laws In Chavkin W., ed. *Double Exposure: Women's Health Hazards on the Job and at Home* Monthly Review Press, New York, pp 139–154.

Khera K.S. 1984 Adverse effects in humans and animals of prenatal exposure to selected therapeutic drugs and estimation of embryo-fetal sensitivity of animals for human risk assessment: A review In Kalter H., ed., *Issues and Reviews in Teratology* Vol 2, Plenum Press, New York pp 399–507.

Khoury M.J., Marks J.S., McCarthy B.J., and Zaro S.M. 1985 Factors affecting sex differential in neonatal mortality: The role of respiratory distress syndrome *Am J Obstet Gynecol* 151:777–782.

Khoury M.J. and Holtzman N.A. 1987 On the ability of birth defects monitoring to detect new teratogeny *Am J Epidemiol* 126:136–143.

Kiely J. 1983 A comparative epidemiology study of fetal death during labor, including an analysis of the effect of health care services. PhD Dissertation, Columbia University, New York.

Kiely J., Paneth N., Stein Z., and Susser M. 1981 Cerebral palsy and newborn care. II. Mortality and neurologic handicap in low birth weight infants *Dev Med Child Neurol* 23:650–659.

Kiely J.L., Paneth N., and Susser M. 1983 The epidemiology of fetal death in labor (abstract) *Am J Epidemiol* 118:433–434.

Kiely J.L., Paneth N., and Susser M. 1986 An assessment of the effects of maternal age and parity in different components of perinatal mortality *Am J Epidemiol* 123:444–454.

Kilham L. and Ferm V.H. 1976 Exencephaly in fetal hamsters following exposure to hyperthermia *Teratology* 14:323–326.

Kincaid-Smith P. 1972 Quartan malarial nephrotic syndrome *Lancet* ii:89.

King C.R., Magenis E., and Bennett S. 1978 Pregnancy and the Turner syndrome *Obstet Gynecol* 52:617–624.

King L.S. 1963 *The Growth of Medical Thought* University of Chicago Press, Chicago.

Klebanoff M.A., Graubard B.I., Kessel S.S., and Berendes H.W. 1984a Low birth weight across generations *JAMA* 252:2423–2427.

Klebanoff M.A., Nugent R.P., and Rhoads G.G. 1984b Coitus during pregnancy: Is it safe? *Lancet* ii:914–917.

Kleinebrecht J., Michaelis H., Michaelis J., and Keller S. 1979 Fever in pregnancy and congenital anomalies *Lancet* i:1403.

Kleinman J.C. 1982 Indirect standardization of neonatal mortality for birth weight *Int J Epidemiol* 11:146–154.

Kleinman J.C. and Kopstein A. 1987 Smoking during pregnancy, 1967–80 *Am J Publ Health* 77:823–825.

Kline J. 1977 The epidemiology of spontaneous abortion: An analysis of selected factors PhD dissertation, Columbia University, New York.

Kline J. 1978 I. An epidemiological review of the role of gravidity in spontaneous abortion *Early Hum Develop* 1:337–344.

Kline J. 1984 Environmental exposures and spontaneous abortion In E. Gold, ed. *The Changing Risk of Disease in Women: An Epidemiological Approach* D.C. Heath, Lexington, MA, pp 127–138.

Kline J. 1986 Maternal occupation. Effects on spontaneous abortions and malformations In Z.A. Stein and M.C. Hatch, eds. *Reproductive Problems in the Workplace* Hanley & Belfus Philadelphia *Occupational Medicine* 1:381–403.

Kline J., Stein Z., Strobino B., Susser M., and Warburton D. 1977a Surveillance of spontaneous abortions: Power in environmental monitoring *Am J Epidemiol* 106:345–350.

Kline J., Stein Z., Susser M., and Warburton D. 1977b Smoking: A risk factor for spontaneous abortion *N Engl J Med* 297:793–796.

Kline J., Shrout P., Stein Z., Susser M., and Weiss M. 1978a II. An epidemiological study of the role of gravidity in spontaneous abortion *Early Hum Develop* 1:345–356.

Kline J., Stein Z., Susser M., and Warburton D. 1978b Induced abortion and spontaneous abortion: No connection *Am J Epidemiol* 107:290–298.

Kline J., Stein Z., Susser M., and Warburton D. 1978c Spontaneous abortion and the use of sugar substitutes (saccharin) *Am J Obstet Gynec* 130:708–711.

Kline J., Shrout P., Stein Z., Susser M., and Warburton D. 1980a Drinking during pregnancy and spontaneous abortion *Lancet* ii:176–180.

Kline J., Stein Z., Susser M., and Warburton D. 1980b Environmental influences on early reproductive loss in a current New York City study In I.H. Porter and E.B. Hook, eds. *Human Embryonic and Fetal Death* Academic Press, New York, pp 225–240.

Kline J., Stein Z., Susser M., and Warburton D. 1980c New insights into the epidemiology of chromosomal disorders: Their relevance to the prevention of Down's syndrome In P. Mittler, ed. *Frontiers of Knowledge in Mental Retardation*, Vol. II, University Park Press, Baltimore, pp 131–141.

Kline J., Stein Z., Susser M., and Warburton D. 1980d Socioeconomic differences in spontaneous abortions In Society for Epidemiologic Research Abstracts *Am J Epidemiol* 112:439.

Kline J., Stein Z., Susser M., and Warburton D. 1980e Spontaneous abortion studies: Role in surveillance In P.F. Infante and M.S. Legator, eds. *Proceedings of a Workshop on Methodology for Assessing Reproductive Hazards in the Workplace* U.S. Department of Health and Human Services, Washington, DC, pp 279–292.

Kline J., Lansky-Kiely M., Santana S., Saxena B., and Stein Z. 1981a Estimates of very early fetal loss. In *Abstracts of the Ninth Meeting of the International Epidemiological Association*, Edinburgh, Scotland.

Kline J., Levin B., Stein Z., and Warburton D. 1981b Epidemiologic detection of low dose effects on the developing fetus *Environ Health Perspect* 42:119–126.

Kline J., Stein Z., Strobino B., and Hatch M. 1982 The role of spontaneous abortion studies in environmental research *Environmental Protection Agency Tech Rep* R807355.

Kline J., Levin B., Shrout P., Stein Z., Susser M., and Warburton D. 1983 Maternal smoking and trisomy among spontaneously aborted conceptions *Am J Hum Genet* 35:421–431.

Kline J. and Stein Z. 1984 Spontaneous abortion (miscarriage) In M. Bracken, ed. *Perinatal Epidemiology* Oxford University Press, London, pp 23–51.

Kline J., Stein Z., Susser M., and Warburton D. 1985 Fever during pregnancy and spontaneous abortion *Am J Epidemiol* 121:832–842.

Kline J. and Stein Z. 1985a Very early pregnancy In R.L. Dixon, ed. *Reproductive Toxicology* Raven Press, New York, pp 251–265.

Kline J. and Stein Z. 1985b Environmental causes of aneuploidy: Why so elusive? In V.L. Dellarco, P.E. Voytek, and A. Hollaender, eds. *Aneuploidy: Etiology and Mechanism,* Plenum Press, New York, pp 149–164.

Kline J., Stein Z., Susser M., and Warburton D. 1986 Induced abortion and the chromosomal characteristics of subsequent miscarriages (spontaneous abortions) *Am J Epidemiol* 123:1066–1079.

Kline J. and Stein Z. 1987 Epidemiology of chromosomal anomalies in spontaneous abortions: Prevalence, manifestation and determinants In M.J. Bennett and D.K. Edmonds, eds. *Spontaneous and Recurrent Abortions,* Blackwell Scientific Publications, Oxford and London, pp 29–50.

Kline J., Stein Z., and Hutzler M. 1987 Cigarettes, alcohol and marijuana: Varying associations with birthweight *Int J Epidemiol* 10:47–51.

Knill-Jones R.P., Moir D.D., Rodrigues L.V., and Spence A.A. 1972 Anaesthetic practice and pregnancy *Lancet* i:1326–1328.

Knill-Jones R.P., Newman B.J., and Spence A.A. 1975 Anaesthetic practice and pregnancy *Lancet* ii:807–809.

Knobloch H. and Pasamanick B. 1962 Mental subnormality: Medical progress *N Engl J Med* 266:1045–1051, 1092–1096, 1155–1161.

Knox E.G. 1971 Epidemics of rare diseases *Br Med Bull* 27:43–47.

Koppe J.G., Kloostermann G.J., de Roever-Bonnet H., Eckert-Stroink J.A., Loewer-Sieger D.H., and de Bruijne J.I. 1974 Toxoplasmosis and pregnancy, with a long-term follow-up of the children *Europ J Obstet Gynaecol* 4:101–110.

Koppe J.G., Loewer-Sieger D.H., and de Roever-Bonnet H. 1986 Results of 20-year follow-up of congenital toxoplasmosis *Lancet* i:254–255.

Kondo K., Imagawa M., Iwasa S., Kitada C., Konishi E., Suzuki N., Yamato M., Nukano R., Yoshitake S., and Ishikawa E. 1984 A specific and sensitive sandwich enzyme immunoassay for human chorionic gonadropin using antibodies against the carboxyl-terminal portion of the beta-subunit *Clin Chim Acta* 138:229–235.

Korenbrot C.G., Aalto L.H., and Laros R.K., Jr. 1984 The cost effectiveness of stopping preterm labor with beta-adrenergic treatment *N Engl J Med* 310:691–695.

Kosenow W. and Pfeiffer R.A. 1960 Mikromelie, Haemangiom an Duo-
denalstenose: Wissenschaftliche Ausstellung Nr., 39,59. Tagung der
Deutschen Gesellschaft fur Kinderheilkunde, Kassel, 26–28.

Kramer M.S. 1987a Intrauterine growth and gestational duration determinants
Pediatrics 80:502–511.

Kramer M.S. 1987b Determinants of low birth weight: Methodological assessment and meta-analysis *Bull WHO* 65:663–737.

Kramer M.S., McLean F.H., Boyd M.E., and Usher R.H. 1988 The validity of
gestational age estimation by menstrual dating in term, preterm and postterm gestations *JAMA* 260:3306–3308.

Kronick J., Phelps N.E., McCallion D.J., and Hirsch J. 1974 Effects of sodium
warfarin administered during pregnancy in mice *Am J Obstet Gynecol*
118:819–823.

Kruger H. and Arias-Stella J. 1970 The placenta and the newborn infant at high
altitude *Am J Obstet Gynecol* 106:586–591.

Kuhn T.S. 1970 *The Structure of Scientific Revolutions* (2 ed.) University of Chicago
Press, Chicago.

Kuleshov N.P. 1976 Chromosome anomalies of infants dying during the perinatal period and premature newborn *Hum Genet* 31:151–160.

Kuleshov N.P., Alekhin N.I., Egolina N.A., and Karethikov N.A. 1975 Frequency of chromosome abnormalities among infants who died during the
perinatal period *Genetika* 11:107–113.

Kullander S. and Kallen B. 1971 A prospective study of smoking and pregnancy
Acta Obstet Gynaecol Scand 50:83–94.

Kullander S. and Kallen B. 1976 A prospective study of drugs and pregnancy II.
Anti-emetic drugs *Acta Obstet Gynaecol Scand* 55:105–111.

Kunin C.M., Deutscher R., and Paquin A. 1964 Urinary tract infection in children: An epidemiological, clinical and laboratory study *Medicine* 43:91–
130.

Kunze J. 1980 Neurological disorders in patients with chromosomal anomalies
Neuropediat 11:203–249.

Kurent J.E. and Sever J.L. 1977 Infectious diseases In J.G. Wilson and F.C.
Fraser, eds. *Handbook of Teratology* Vol 1, Plenum Press, New York, pp
225–259.

Kurppa K., Holmberg P.C., Hernberg S., Rantala K., Riala R., and Nurminen T.
1983 Screening for occupational exposures and congenital malformations. Preliminary results from a nationwide case-referent study *Scand J
Work Environ Health* 9:89–93.

Kurtzke J.F., Beebe G.W., and Normal J.E. Jr. 1979 Epidemiology of multiple
sclerosis in U.S. Veterans. I. Race, sex and geographic distribution
Neurology 29:1228–1235.

Kushner B.J. 1982 Strabismus and amblyopia associated with regressed reti-
nopathy of prematurity *Arch Ophthamol* 100:256–261.

Kutscher A.H., Zegarelli E.V., Tovell H.M.M., and Hochberg B. 1963 Discoloration of teeth induced by tetracycline administered antepartum *JAMA*
184:586–587.

Kuzma J.W. and Sokol R.J. 1982 Maternal drinking behavior and decreased
intrauterine growth *Alcohol Clin Exp Res* 6:396–402.

Kwast B.E. and Liff J.M. 1988 Factors associated with maternal mortality in Addis Ababa, Ethiopia *Int J Epidemiol* 17:115–121.

Lagakos S.W., Wessen B.J., and Zelen M. 1986 An analysis of contaminated well water and health effects in Woburn, Massachusetts *J Am Statis Assn* 81:583–596.

Lambert B.E. 1988 Radiation induced cancer risk *Lancet* i:1045–1046.

Lammer E.J., Chen D.T., Hoar R.M., Agnish N.D., Benke P.J., Braun J.T., Curry, C.J., Fernhoff P.M., Grix A.W., Jr., Lott I.T., Richard J.M., and Sun S.C. 1985 Retinoic acid embryopathy *N Engl J Med* 313:837–841.

Lamson S.H., Cross P.K., Hook E.B., and Regal R. 1980 On the inadequacy of quinquennial data for analyzing the paternal age effect on Down's syndrome rates *Hum Genet* 55:49–51.

Lancaster H.O. 1951 Deafness as an epidemic disease in Australia *Br Med J* 2:1429–1432.

Lancaster P.A.L., Johnston W.I.H., Wood C., Saunders D.M. et al. 1985 High incidence of preterm births and early losses in pregnancy after in vitro fertilisation *Br Med J* 291:1160–1163.

Lancet 1982 Valproate and malformations Editorial ii:1313–1314.

Lancet 1985 Urinary tract infection Editorial ii:90–112.

Lancet 1986 Gestational Assessment Editorial i:1474–1476.

Lancet 1988 Congenital abnormalities in infants of diabetic mothers Editorial i:1313–1318.

Landesman-Dwyer S. and Emmanuel I. 1979 Smoking during pregnancy *Teratology* 19:119–126.

Landsdown A.B.G., Pope W.O.B., Halsey M.J., and Bateman P.E. 1976 Analysis of fetal development in rats following maternal exposure to subanesthetic concentrations of halothane *Teratology* 13:299–304.

Langhoff-Roos J., Lindmark G., Gustavson K.-H., and Gebre-Medhin M. 1987 Relative effect of parental birth weight on infant birth weight at term *Clinic Genet* 32:240–248.

Langner T.S. and Michael S.T. 1963 *Life Stress and Mental Health* Collier-Macmillan, London.

Lathrop G.D., Wolfe W.H., Albanese R.A., and Moynahan P.M. 1984 An epidemiologic investigation of health effects in Air Force personnel following exposure to herbicides: Baseline morbidity study results United States Air Force School of Aerospace Medicine, San Antonio, Texas.

Laurence K.M., James N., Miller M.H., Tennant G.B., and Campbell H. 1981 Double-blind randomised controlled trial folate treatment before conception to prevent recurrence of neural-tube defects *Br Med J* 282:1509–1511.

Lauritsen J.G. 1975 The significance of oral contraceptives in causing chromosome anomalies in spontaneous abortions *Acta Obstet Gynaecol Scand* 54:261–264.

Lauritsen J.G. 1976 Aetiology of spontaneous abortion. A cytogenetic and epidemiological study of 288 abortuses and their parents *Acta Obstet Gynaecol Scand* Suppl 52:1–29.

Lauritsen J.G. 1977 Genetic aspects of spontaneous abortion *Dan Med Bull* 24:169–189.

Lauritsen J.G., Kristensen T., and Grunnel N. 1976 Depressed mixed lymphocyte culture reactivity in mothers with recurrent spontaneous abortion *Am J Obstet Gynecol* 125:35–39.

Lawrence J.N.P. 1962 PUQFUA, an IBM 704 code for computing plutonium body burdens *Health Physics* 8:60–66.

Lawson D.H. and Miller A.W.F. 1973 Screening for bacteriuria in pregnancy, a critical reappraisal *Arch Intern Med* 132:904–908.

Layde P.M., Edmonds L.D., and Erickson J.D. 1980 Maternal fever and neural tube defects *Teratology* 21:105–108.

Lazar P., Gueguen S., Boué J., and Boué A. 1973 Epidemiologie des avortements spontanes precoces: A propos de 1469 avortements caryotypes. In A. Boué and C. Thibault, eds. *Les Accidents Chromosomiques de la Reproduction*, Institute Nationale de la Sante et de la Recherche Medicale, Paris, pp 317–332.

Lechat M.F., De Wals P., and Weatherall J.A.C. 1985 European economic community's concerted action on congenital anomalies: The Eurocat project In *Prevention of Physical and Mental Congenital Defects, Part B: Epidemiology, Early Detection and Therapy, and Environment Factors*, Alan R. Liss, New York, pp 11–15.

Lechtig A., Habicht J.P., Delgado H., Klein R.E., Yarbrough C., and Martorell R. 1975 Effect of food supplementation during pregnancy on birthweight *Pediatrics* 56:508–520.

Leck I. 1974 Causation of neural tube defects: Clues from epidemiology *Br Med Bull* 30:158–163.

Leck I. 1975 Causation of malformations *Lancet* ii:1097.

Leck I. 1977 Correlations of malformation frequency with environmental and genetic attributes in man In Wilson J.G. and Fraser F.C., eds. *Handbook of Teratology* Vol 3, Plenum Press, New York, pp 243–323.

Leck I. 1978 Maternal hyperthermia and anencephaly *Lancet* i:671–672.

Leck I. 1983 Fetal malformations In *Obstetrical Epidemiology* Barron S.L. and Thomson A.M., eds. Academic Press, London, pp 263–318.

Leck I.M. and Miller E.L.M. 1962 Incidence of malformations since the introduction of thalidomide *Br Med J* 2:16–20.

Lee G. and Kline J. 1988 Clustering of spontaneous abortions and stillbirths in families: A case control study (abstr) *Am J Epidemiol* 128:936.

Lee K.S., Paneth N., Gartner L.M., and Pearlman M. 1980 The very low-birth-weight rate: Principal predictor of neonatal mortality in industrialized populations *J Pediatr* 97:759–764.

Lemoine P., Harousseau H., Borteyru J.P., and Menuet J.C. 1968 Les enfants de parents alcooliques. Anomalies observees. A propos de 127 cas *Quest Medical* 21:476–482.

Lenke R.R. and Levy H.L. 1980 Maternal phenylketonuria and hyperphenylalaninemia: An international survey of the outcome of untreated and treated pregnancies *N Engl J Med* 202:1202–1208.

Lenz W. 1962 Thalidomide and congenital abnormalities *Lancet* i:45.

Lenz W. 1964 Chemicals and malformations in man In *Second International Conference on Congenital Malformations 1963* M. Fishbein, ed. International Medical Congress, New York, pp 263–276.

Lenz W. 1965 Epidemiology of congenital malformations *Ann NY State Acad Sci* 123:228–236.

Lenz W. and Knapp K. 1962 Thalidomide embryopathy *Arch Environ Health* 5:100–105.

Lejeune J., Gautier M., and Turpin R. 1959 Etude des chromosomes somatiques de neuf enfants mongoliens *C.R. Seanc Acad Sci* 248:1721–1722.

Leridon H. 1973 Demographies des echecs de la reproduction. In Boué A. and Thibault C., eds. *Chromosomal Errors in Relation to Reproductive Failure* INSERM, Paris, pp 13–27.

Leridon H. 1976 Facts and artifacts in the study of intra-uterine mortality: A reconsideration from pregnancy histories *Pop Studies* 30:319–336.

Leridon H. 1977 *Human Fertility: The Basic Concepts,* University of Chicago Press, Chicago.

Leslie R.D.G., John P.N., Pyke D.A., and White J.M. 1978 Haemoglobin A in diabetic pregnancy *Lancet* ii:958–959.

Levin A.A., Schoenbaum S.C., Monson R.R., Stubblefield P.G. and Ryan K.J. 1980 Association of induced abortion with subsequent pregnancy loss *JAMA* 243:2495–2499.

Levin B. 1986 Empirical Bayes estimation in heterogeneous matched binary samples with systematic aging effects In J. Van Ryzin, eds. *Adaptive Statistical Procedures and Related Topics* Institute of Mathematical Statistics, Lecture Notes—Monograph Series, 8:179–194.

Levin B. and Kline J. 1985 The cusum test of homogeneity with an application in spontaneous abortion epidemiology *Statist Med* 4:469–488.

Levin B. and Shrout P.E. 1981 On extending Bock's model of logistic regression to the analysis of categorical data *Commun Statist Theor Meth* A10 2:125–147.

Levine A. 1982 *Love Canal: Science, politics, and people* Lexington Books, Lexington, MA.

Lewis D.W. 1964 Tetracycline discoloration of teeth: Review and case reports *J Can Dent Assoc* 30:496–506.

Liberatos P., Link B., and Kelsey J. 1988 The measurement of social class in epidemiology *Epidemiol Rev* 10:87–121.

Lilienfeld A.M., Parkhurst E., Patton R., and Schlesinger E.R. 1951 Accuracy of supplemental medical information on birth certificates *Publ Health Reports* 66:191–198.

Lilienfeld A.M. and Lilienfeld D.E. 1977 What else is new? An historical excursion *Am J Epidemiol* 105:169–179.

Lind T. 1976 Techniques for assessing fetal development and well-being In D.F. Roberts and A.M. Thomson, eds. *The Biology of Human Fetal Growth* Halsted Press, New York, 24:1–13.

Lindbohm M.L., Hemminki K., and Kyyronen P. 1985 Spontaneous abortions among women employed in the plastic industry *Am J Indust Med* 8:579–586.

Lindhout D. and Schmidt D. 1986 In-utero exposure to valproate and tube defects *Lancet* i:1392–1393.

Linn S., Schoenbaum S.C., Monson R.R., Rosner B., and Ryan K.J. 1982 Delay in conception for former "pill" users *JAMA* 247:629–632.

Linn S., Schoenbaum S.C., Monson R.R., Rosner B., Stubblefield P.G., and Ryan
    K.J. 1982 No association between coffee consumption and adverse out-
    comes of pregnancy *N Engl J Med* 306:141–145.
Linn S., Schoenbaum S.C., Monson R.R., Rosner R., Stubblefield P.G., and Ryan
    K.J. 1983 The association of marijuana use with outcome of pregnancy
    Am J Publ Health 73:1161–1164.
Lippman A. and Farookhi R. 1986 The Montreal pregnancy study: An investiga-
    tion of very early pregnancies *Can J Pub Health* 77 (suppl):157–163.
Lippman-Hand A. and Vekemans M. 1983 Balanced translocations among cou-
    ples with two or more spontaneous abortions: Are males and females
    equally likely carriers? *Hum Genet* 63:252–257.
Little R.E. 1977 Moderate alcohol use during pregnancy and decreased infant
    birthweight *Am J Publ Health* 67:1154–1156.
Little R.E. 1986 Birthweight and gestational age: Mother's estimates compared
    with state and hospital records *Am J Publ Health* 76:1350–1351.
Little R.E. 1987 Mother's and father's birthweight as predictors of infant birth-
    weight *Pediatr Perinat Epidemiol* 1:19–31.
Little R.E. and Sing C.H. 1987 Genetic and environmental influences on human
    birth weight *Am J Hum Genet* 40:512–526.
Little R.E., Asker R.L., Sampson P.D., and Renwick J.H. 1986 Fetal growth and
    moderate drinking in early pregnancy *Am J Epidemiol* 123:270–278.
Liu H.C., Jones H.W., and Rosenwaks Z. 1988 The efficiency of human re-
    production after in vitro fertilization and embryo transfer *Fertil Steril*
    49:649–653.
Lobb T. 1747 *A Compendium of the Practice of Physick* London, p 90.
Longo L.D. 1982 Some health consequences of maternal smoking: Issues with-
    out answers In *Birth Defects: Original Article Series* Vol 18, Alan R. Liss,
    New York, pp 13–31.
Lopata A. 1983 Concepts in human in vitro fertilization and embryo transfer
    Fertil Steril 40:289–301.
Lorden B. 1971 Procedures for reacting to a change in distribution *Ann Math
    Stat* 42:1897–1908.
Louik C., Mitchell A.A., Werler M.M., Hanson J.W., and Shapiro S. 1987 Mater-
    nal exposure to spermicides in relation to certain birth defects *N Engl J
    Med* 317:474–478.
Love G.J. and Kinch R.A. 1965 Factors influencing the birthweight in normal
    pregnancy *Am J Obstet Gynecol* 91:342–349.
Lowe C.R. 1959 Effect of mothers' smoking habits on birth weight of their
    children *Br Med J* 2:673–676.
Lubchenco L.O., Hansman C., Dressler M., and Boyd E. 1963 Intrauterine
    growth as estimated from liveborn birth-weight data at 24 to 42 weeks of
    gestation *Pediatrics* 32:793–800.
Lumey L.H. 1988 Obstetric performance of women after in utero exposure to
    the Dutch famine (1944–1945). Ph.D. Dissertation, Columbia University,
    New York.
Lumey L.H., Stam G.A., Menkveld H., and Koppe J.G. 1988 A cohort study of
    survival of women after in utero and neonatal exposure to the Dutch
    famine of 1944–45 *XI European Congress of Perinatal Medicine*, Rome, April
    pp 1–3.

Lundstrum R. 1962 Rubella during pregnancy *Acta Pediat Suppl* 133:1–110.

Lunn J.E. 1959 A survey of mongol children in Glasgow *Scot Med J* 4:368–372.

MacCluer J.W. 1980 Inbreeding and human fetal death In I.H. Porter and E.B. Hook, eds. *Human Embryonic and Fetal Death,* Academic Press, New York, pp 241–260.

MacDonald P., Alexander D., Catz C., and Edelman R. 1983 Summary of a workshop on maternal genitourinary infections and the outcome of pregnancy *J Infect Dis* 147:596–605.

Macfarlane A. 1987 Altitude and birth weight: Commentary *J Pediat* 111:842–844.

Macfarlane A. and Mugford M. 1984 *Birth Counts: Statistics of Pregnancy and Childbirth.* Her Majesty's Stationery Office, London.

Maclean N., Mitchell J.M., Harnden D.G., Williams J., Jacobs P.A., Buckton K.A., Baikie A.G., Court Brown W.M., McBride J.A., Strong J.A., Close H.G., and Jones D.C. 1962 A survey of sex-chromosome abnormalities among 4514 mental defectives *Lancet* i:293–296.

MacMahon B. 1962 Prenatal-X-ray exposure and childhood cancer *J Natl Cancer Inst* 28:1173–1191.

MacMahon B., Trichopoulos D., Cole P., and Brown J. 1982 Cigarette smoking and urinary estrogens *N Engl J Med* 307:1062–1065.

Machin G.A. 1974 Chromosome abnormality and perinatal death *Lancet* i:549–551.

Machin G.A. and Crolla J.A. 1974 Chromosome constitution of 500 infants dying during the perinatal period: With an appendix concerning other genetic disorders among these infants *Human Genet* 23:183–198.

Macnaughton M.C. 1961 Pregnancy following abortion *J Obstet Gynecol* 68:789–792.

MacRae K.D. 1982 Sodium valproate and neural tube defects *Lancet* ii:1283.

Madore C., Hawes W.E., Many F. and Hextor A.C. 1981 A study on the effects of induced abortion on subsequent pregnancy outcome *Am J Obstet Gynecol* 139:516–521.

Magenis R.E. and Chamberlin J. 1981 Parental origin of nondisjunction In F.F. de la Cruz and P.S. Gerald, eds. *Trisomy 21 (Down Syndrome)—Research Perspectives* University Park Press, Baltimore, pp 77–93.

Magnus P. 1984a Further evidence for a significant effect of fetal genes on variation in birth weight *Clin Genet* 26:289–296.

Magnus P. 1984b Causes of variation in birth weight: A study of offspring of twins *Clin Genet* 25:15–24.

Magnus P., Berg K., Bjerkedal T., and Nance W.E. 1984 Parental determinants of birth weight *Clin Genet* 26:397–405.

Magnus P., Berg K., and Bjerkedal T. 1985 No significant difference in birth weight for offspring of birth weight discordant monozygotic female twins *Early Hum Develop* 12:55–59.

Mall F.P. 1917 On the frequency of localized anomalies in human embryos and infants at birth *Am J Anat Phila* 22:27–72.

Mall F.P. and Meyer A.W. 1921 Studies on abortuses: A survey of pathologic ova in the Carnegie embryological collection *Cont Embryol Carnegie Inst* No. 56, pp 51–107.

Mamelle N., Laumon B., and Lazar P. 1984 Prematurity and occupational activity during pregnancy *Am J Epidemiol* 119:309–322.

Mamelle N. and Munoz F. 1987 Occupational working conditions and preterm birth: A reliable scoring system *Am J Epidemiol* 126:150–152.

Manson M.M., Logan W.P.D., and Loy R.M. 1960 Rubella and other virus infections during pregnancy *Ministry of Health Reports on Public Health and Medical Subjects* Her Majesty's Stationery Office, London 101:1–101.

Mantel N. 1979 Perinatal mortality by birth order *Br Med J* 2:1147.

Marbury M.C., Linn S., Monson R., Schoenbaum S., Stubblefield P.G., and Ryan K.J. 1983 The association of alcohol consumption with outcome of pregnancy *Am J Publ Health* 73:1165–1168.

Marbury M.C., Linn S., Monson R.R., Wegman D.H., Schoenbaum S.C., Stubblefield P.G., and Ryan K.J. 1984 Work and pregnancy *J Occup Med* 26:415–421.

March H.C. 1950 Leukemia in radiologists in a twenty-year period *Am J Med Sci* 220:282–286.

Marmol J.G., Scriggins A.L., and Vollman R.F. 1969 Mothers of mongoloid infants in the collaborative project *Am J Obstet Gynecol* 104:533–543.

Marrs R.P., Saito H., Yee B., Sato F., and Brown J. 1984 Effects of variation of in vitro culture techniques upon oocyte fertilization and embryo development in human in vitro fertilization procedures *Fertil Steril* 41:519–523.

Martin R., Balkan W., Burns K., Rademaker A., Lin C., and Rudd N. 1983 The chromosome constitution of 1000 human spermatozoa *Hum Genet* 63:305–309.

Martin R.H. 1985 Chromosomal abnormalities in human sperm In V.L. Dellarco, P.E. Voytek, and A. Hollaender, eds. *Aneuploidy.* Plenum Press, New York, pp 91–102.

Martin R.H., Mahadevan M.M., Taylor P.J., Hildebrand K., Long-Simpson L., Peterson D., Yamamoto J., and Fleetham J. 1986 Chromosomal analysis of unfertilized human oocytes *J Reprod Fertil* 78:673–678.

Martin R.H. and Rademaker A.W. 1987 The effect of age on the frequency of sperm chromosomal abnormalities in normal men *Am J Hum Genet* 41:484–492.

Martin T.R. and Bracken M.B. 1987 The association between low birth weight and caffeine consumption during pregnancy. *Am J Epidemiol* 126:813–821.

Martin T. and Mulhern B. 1980 Foetal warfarin syndrome *Ir Med J* 73:393–394.

Masson G.M., Anthony F., and Chau E. 1985 Serum chorionic-gonadotropin (hCG), Schwangerschafts-protein-1 (SP1), progesterone and estradiol levels in patients with nausea and vomiting of pregnancy *Br J Obstet Gynaecol* 92:211–215.

Masters W.H. and Johnson V.E. 1966 *Human Sexual Responses* Little, Brown & Co., Boston (Ch 16, The Aging Male).

Masters W.H. and Johnson V.E. 1970 *Human Sexual Inadequacy* Little, Brown & Co., Boston, pp 316–334.

Matsuura J., Chiu D., Jacobs P.A., and Szulman A.E. 1984 Complete hydatidiform mole in Hawaii: An epidemiological study *Genet Epidemiol* 1:271–284.

Mattei J.F., Ayme S., Mattei M.G., and Girauld F. 1980 Maternal age and origin of non-disjunction in trisomy 21 *J Med Genet* 17:368–372.

Mattison D.R. 1982 The effects of smoking on fertility from gametogenesis to implantation *Environ Res* 28:410–433.

Mattison D.R. and Thorgeirsson S.S. 1978 Smoking and industrial pollution, and their effects on menopause and ovarian cancer *Lancet* i:187–188.

Maudlin I. and Fraser L.R. 1978 Maternal age and the incidence of aneuploidy in first-cleavage mouse embryos *J Reprod Fert* 54:423–426.

Maurer R.R. and Foote R.H. 1971 Maternal aging and embryonic mortality in the rabbit *J Reprod Fertil* 25:329–341.

Mauriceau F. 1674 *The Accomplisht Midwife* (trans. H. Chamberlen), p. 85.

Mauriceau F. 1683 *The Diseases of Women with Child, and in Child-Bed* (trans. H. Chamberlen), T. Cox and J. Clarke, London, p 20.

Mazess R.B. 1965 Neonatal mortality and altitude in Peru *Am J Phys Anthrop* 23:209–214.

McBride W.G. 1961 Thalidomide and congenital abnormalities *Lancet* ii:1358.

McBride W.G. 1963 The teratogenic action of drugs *Med J Aust* 2:689–693.

McBurney R.D. 1947 The undernourished full term infant: A case report *West J Surg Obstet Gynecol* 55:363–370.

McCance R.A. and Widdowson E.M. 1974 Review lecture: The determinants of growth and form *Proc Roy Soc Lond (Biol)* 185:1–17.

McConnachie P.R. and McIntyre J.A. 1984 Maternal antipaternal immunity in couples predisposed to repeated pregnancy losses *Am J Reprod Immunol* 5:145–150.

McCormick M. 1985 The contribution of low birthweight to infant mortality and childhood morbidity *N Engl J Med* 312:82–90.

McCredie J. 1974 A hypothesis of neural crest injury as the pathogenesis of congenital malformations *Med J Aust* 1:159–163.

McCullough R.E., Reeves J.T., and Liljegren R.L. 1977 Fetal growth retardation and increased infant mortality at high altitude *Arch Environ Health* 32:36–39.

McCurdy S. 1988 Women's choices of health agents in Tanzania. In Z. Stein and M. Wright, eds., Third Workshop on Poverty Health and the State, Columbia University, New York.

McDonald A.D. 1961 Maternal health in early pregnancy and congenital defect. Final report on a prospective inquiry *Br J Prev Soc Med* 15:154–166.

McDonald A.D., Cherry N.M., Delorme C., and McDonald J.C. 1986 Visual display units and pregnancy: Evidence from the Montreal survey *J Occup Med* 28:1226–1231.

McDonald A.D., McDonald J.C., Armstrong B., Cherry N.M., Nolin A.D., and Robert D. 1988 Prematurity and work in pregnancy *Brit J Industr Med* 45:56–62.

McDonald E., Pollitt E., Mueller W., Hsueh A.M., and Sherwin R. 1981 The Bacon Chow study: Maternal nutrition supplementation and birth weight of offspring *Am J Clin Nutr* 34:2133–2144.

McFadyen I.R., Campbell-Brown M., Abraham R., North W.R.S., and Haines A.P. 1984 Factors affecting birthweights in Hindus, Moslems and Europeans *Br J Obstet Gynaecol* 91:968–972.

McGregor I.A., Wilson E., and Billewicz W.Z. 1983 Malaria infection of the placenta in The Gambia, West Africa; its incidence and relationships to stillbirth, birthweight and placental weight *Trans Roy Soc Trop Med Hyg* 77:223–244.

McIntyre J.A. and Faulk W.P. 1979 Maternal blocking factors in human pregnancy are found in plasma not serum *Lancet* ii:821–823.

McIntyre J.A., Faulk W.P., Nichols-Johnson V.R., and Taylor C.G. 1986 Immunologic testing and immunotherapy in recurrent spontaneous abortion *Obstet Gynecol* 67:169–175.

McKeown T. and Gibson J.R. 1951 Observations on all births (23,970) in Birmingham, 1947, II. *Br J Soc Med* 5:98–112.

McKeown T. and Record R.G. 1952 Observations on foetal growth in multiple pregnancy in man *J Endocrinol* 8:386–401.

McKeown T. and Record R.G. 1953 The influence of placental size on foetal growth according to sex and order of birth *J Endocrinol* 10:73–81.

McKeown T. and Record R.G. 1954 The influence of pre-natal environment on correlation between birth weight and parental height *Am J Hum Genet* 6:457–463.

McKeown T. and Record R.G. 1960 Malformations in a population observed for five years after birth In G.E.W. Wolstenholme and C.M. O'Connor, eds. *CIBA Foundation Symposium on Congenital Malformations*, Churchill, London, p 2.

McKeown T., Marshall T., and Record R.G. 1976 Influences on fetal growth *J Reprod Fertil* 47:167–181.

McKinlay S.M., Bifano N.L., and McKinlay J.B. 1985 Smoking and age at menopause in women *Ann Intern Med* 103:350–356.

McLaren A. 1965 Genetic and environmental effects on foetal and placental growth in mice *J Reprod Fertil* 9:79–98.

McLaren A. and Michie D. 1960 Control of pre-natal growth in mammals *Nature* 187:363–365.

McLaren A. and Michie D. 1963 Nature of the systemic effect of litter size on gestation period in mice *J Reprod Fertil* 6:139–141.

McLean D. and Paneth N. 1989 The reliability of birth certificate data: Completion practices and completion rates in New York City Pediatr Perinat Epidemiol (Abstr) 3:88.

Medawar P.B. 1953 Some immunological and endocrinological problems raised by evolution of viviparity in vertebrates In Society for Experimental Biology. *Evolution* Academic Press, New York, pp 320–388.

Meirik O., Kallen B., Gauffin U., and Ericson A. 1979 Major malformations in infants born of women who worked in laboratories while pregnant *Lancet* ii:91.

Menken J. and Larsen U. 1986 In *Aging, Reproduction and the Climacteric* L. Mastroianni and A. Paulsen, eds. Plenum Press, New York, pp 147–166.

Menken J., Trussell J., and Larsen U. 1986 Age and infertility *Science* 233:1389–1394.

Menser M. 1978 Does hyperthermia affect the human fetus? *Med J Aust* 2:550.

Menzel S., Bjune G., and Kronvall G. 1979 Lymphocyte transformation test in healthy contacts of patients with leprosy. I. Influence of exposure to leprosy within a household *Int J Lepr* 47:138–152.

Menzel S., Bjune G., and Kronvall G. 1979 II. Influence of consanguinity with the patient, sex, and age *Int J Lepr* 47:153–160.

Meredith H.V. 1970 Body weight at birth of viable human infants: A worldwide comparative treatise *Hum Biol* 42:217–264.

Metcalf M.G. 1979 Incidence of ovulatory cycles in women approaching the menopause *J Biosoc Sci* 11:39–48.

Meyer B.A. and Daling J.R. 1985 Activity level of mother's usual occupation and low infant birth weight *J Occup Medicine* 27:841–847.

Meyer M.B. 1977 The effects of maternal smoking and altitude on birth weight and gestation In D.M. Reed and F.J. Stanley, eds. *The Epidemiology of Prematurity*, Urban & Schwarzenberg, Baltimore, pp 81–104.

Meyer M.B., Jonas B.S., and Tonascia J.A. 1976 Perinatal events associated with maternal smoking during pregnancy *Am J Epidemiol* 103:464–476.

Michaels R.H. and Mellin G.W. 1960 Prospective experience with maternal rubella and the associated congenital malformations *Pediatrics* 26:200–209.

Miettinen O.S. 1976 Estimability and estimation in case-reference studies *Am J Epidemiol* 103:226–235.

Mikkelsen M. 1977 Origin of acrocentric trisomies in spontaneous abortuses *Hum Genet* 40:73–78.

Mikkelsen M., Poulsen H., Grinsted J., and Lange A. 1988 Nondisjunction in trisomy 21. Study of chromosomal heteromorphisms in 110 families *Ann Hum Genet* 44:17–28.

Miller E., Hare J.W., Cloherty J.P., Dunn P.J., Gleason R.E., Soeldner J.S., and Kitzmiller J.L. 1981 Elevated maternal hemaglobin A_{1c} in early pregnancy and major congenital anomalies in infants of diabetic mothers *N Engl J Med* 304:1331–1333.

Miller E., Cradock-Watson J.E., and Pollock T.M. 1982 Consequences of confirmed maternal rubella at successive stages of pregnancy *Lancet* ii:781–784.

Miller H.C. and Hassanein K. 1971 Diagnosis of impaired fetal growth in newborn infants *Pediatrics* 48:511–522.

Miller H.C. and Merritt T.A. 1979 *Fetal Growth in Humans*. Year Book Medical Publishers, Chicago.

Miller H.C., Hassanein K., and Hensleigh P. 1977 Effects of behavioral and medical variables on fetal growth retardation *Am J Obstet Gynaecol* 127:643–648.

Miller J.F., Williamson E., Glue J., Gordon Y.B., Grudzinskas J.G., and Sykes A. 1980 Fetal loss after implantation *Lancet* ii:554–556.

Miller N.T. 1886 Die fruhgeborenen und die eigenthumlichkeiten ihrer krankheiten *Jb Kinderheilk* 25:179.

Miller P., Smith D.W., and Shepard T.H. 1978 Maternal hyperthermia as a possible cause of anencephaly *Lancet* i:519–520.

Miller R.W. 1971 Cola-colored babies. Chlorobiphenyl poisoning in Japan *Teratology* 4:211–212.

Miller R.W. and Blot W.J. 1972 Small head size after in-utero exposure to atomic radiation *Lancet* ii:784–787.

Miller R.W. and Mulvihill J.J. 1976 Small head size after atomic irradiation *Teratology* 14:355–358.

Mills J.L. 1982 Malformations in infants of diabetic mothers *Teratology* 25:385–394.

Mills J.L., Harley E.E., Reed G.F., and Berendes H.W. 1982 Are spermicides teratogenic? *JAMA* 248:2148–2151.

Mills J.L., Graubard B.I., Harley E.E., Rhoads G.G., and Berendes H.W. 1984 Maternal alcohol consumption and birth weight: How much drinking during pregnancy is safe? *JAMA* 252:1875–1879.

Mills J.L., Knopp R.H., Simpson J.L. et al. 1988 National Institute of Child Health and Human Development Diabetes in Early Pregnancy Study. Lack of relation of increased malformation rates in infants of diabetic mothers to glycemic control during organogenesis *N Engl J Med* 318:671–676.

Milner R.D.G. and Richards B. 1974 An analysis of birth weight by gestation age of infants born in England and Wales, 1967–71 *J Obstet Gynaecol Br Commonwealth* 81:956–967.

Mitchell A.A., Rosenberg L., Shapiro S., and Slone D. 1981 Birth defects related to bendectin use in pregnancy I. Oral clefts and cardiac defects *JAMA* 245:2311–2314.

Modan B., Baidatz D., Mart H., Steinitz R., and Levin S.G. 1974 Radiation–induced head and neck tumours *Lancet* i:277–279.

Moore K.L. 1973 *The Developing Human.* W.B. Saunders, Philadelphia.

Mora J.O., de Paredes B., Wagner M. et al. 1979 Nutritional supplementation and the outcome of pregnancy: I. Birth weight *Am J Clin Nutr* 32:455–462.

Morbidity and Mortality Weekly Report 1982 Unexplained immunodeficiency and opportunistic infections in infants—New York, New Jersey, California 31:665–666.

Morgagni G.B. 1762 *De sedibus, et causis morborum, per anatomen indigatis, libri quinque* (trans. B. Alexander, 1769), Millar and Cadell, London.

Morishima H.O., Pedersen H., and Finster M. 1978 The influence of maternal psychological stress on the fetus *Am J Obstet Gynecol* 131:286–290.

Morishima H.O., Yeh N.M., and James L.S. 1979 Reduced uterine blood flow and fetal hypoxemia with acute maternal stress: Experimental observation in the pregnant baboon *Am J Obstet Gynecol* 134:270–275.

Morrison I. 1975 The elderly primigravida *Am J Obstet Gynecol* 121:465–470.

Morton H. 1984 Early pregnancy factor (EPF): A link between fertilization and immunomodulation *Aust J Biol Sci* 37:393–407.

Morton H., Rolfe B., Clunie G.J.A., Anderson M.J., and Morrison J. 1977 An early pregnancy factor detected in human serum by the rosette inhibition test *Lancet* i:394–397.

Morton N.E. 1955 The inheritance of human birth weight *Ann Hum Genet* 20:125–134.

Morton N.E. 1977 Genetic aspects of prematurity In Reed D.M. and Stanley F.J., eds. *Epidemiology of Prematurity*, Urban & Schwarzenberg, Baltimore and Munich, pp 213–230.

Mosher W.D. 1988 Fecundity and infertility in the United States *Am J Publ Health* 78:181–182.

Mosher W.D. 1982 Infertility trends among U.S. couples: 1965–76 *Fam Plan Perspect* 14:22–27.

Moustakides G. 1986 Optimal stopping times for detecting changes in distribution *Ann Stat* 14:1379–1387.

Mowbray J.F. and Underwood J.L. 1985 Immunology of abortion *Clin Exp Immunol* 60:1–7.

Mowbray J.F., Gibbings C.R., Sidgwick A.S., Ruszkiewics M., and Beard R.W. 1983 Effects of transfusion in women with recurrent spontaneous abortion *Transpl Proceed* 15:896–899.

Mowbray J.F., Liddell H., Underwood J.L., Gibbings C., Reginald P.W., and Beard R.W. 1985 Controlled trial of treatment of recurrent spontaneous abortion by immunization with paternal cells *Lancet* i:941–943.

Mueller W.H. 1984 The use of anthropometric surveys for studies on the genetics of growth In C. Susanne, ed. *Genetic and Environmental Factors During the Growth Period*, Plenum Publishing, New York pp 49–59.

Mulcahy R. and Knaggs J.F. 1968 Effect of age, parity, and cigarette smoking on outcome of pregnancy *Am J Obstet Gynecol* 101:844–849.

Murphy J.F., Dauncey M., Newcombe R., Garcia J., and Elbourne D. 1984 Employment in pregnancy: Prevalence, maternal characteristics, perinatal outcome *Lancet* i:1163–1166.

Murphy M.L. 1960 Teratogenic effects of tumour-inhibiting chemicals in the foetal rat In *Ciba Foundation Symposium on Congenital Malformations* G.E.W. Wolstenholme and C.M. O'Connor, eds. Little, Brown & Co., Boston, pp 78–114.

Myrianthopoulos N.C. 1978 An approach to the investigation of maternal factors in congenital malformations In N.E. Morton and C.S. Chung, eds. *Genetic Epidemiology*. Academic Press, New York, pp 363–379.

Myrianthopoulos N.C. and Chung C.S. 1974 Congenital malformations in singletons: Epidemiology survey *Birth Defects Original Article Series*, X, p 11.

Naegele F.C. 1812 *Erfahrung und Abhandlung des Weiblichen Geschlechtes.* Mannheim.

Naeye R.L. 1979a The duration of maternal cigarette smoking, fetal and placental disorders *Early Hum Dev* 3:229–237.

Naeye R.L. 1979b Coitus and associated amniotic fluid infections *N Engl J Med* 301:1198–1199.

Naeye R.L. 1980a Abruptio placentae and placenta previa: Frequency, perinatal mortality, and cigarette smoking *Obstet Gynecol* 55:701–704.

Naeye R.L. 1980b Seasonal variations in coitus and other risk factors, and the outcome of pregnancy *Early Hum Dev* 4:61–68.

Naeye R.L. 1981a Maternal nutrition and pregnancy outcome In J. Dobbing ed. *Maternal Nutrition in Pregnancy—Eating for Two?* Academic Press, London, pp 89–102.

Naeye R.L. 1981b Nutritional/nonnutritional interactions that effect the outcome of pregnancy *Am J Clin Nutr* 34:727–731.

Naeye R.L. and Blanc W. 1965 Pathogenesis of congenital rubella *JAMA* 194:1277–1283.

Naeye R.L. and Blanc W.A. 1970 Relation of poverty and race to antenatal infection *N Engl J Med* 282:555–560.

Naeye R.L. and Peters B.S. 1978 Amniotic fluid infections with intact membranes leading to perinatal death: A prospective study *Pediatrics* 61:171–177.

Naeye R.L. and Peters E.C. 1982 Working during pregnancy: Effects on the fetus *Pediatrics* 69:724–727.

Naeye R.L., Ladis B., and Drage J.S. 1976 Sudden infant death syndrome: A prospective study *Am J Dis Child* 130:1207–1210.

Nahmias A.J., Josey W.E., Naib Z.M., Freeman M.G., Fernandez R.J., and Wheeler J.H. 1971 Perinatal risk associated with maternal genital herpes simplex virus infection *Am J Obstet Gynecol* 110:825–837.

Nance W.E., Kramer A.A., Corey L.A., Winter P.M., and Eaves L.J. 1983 A causal analysis of birth weight in the offspring of monozygotic twins *Am J Hum Genet* 35:1211–1223.

National Center for Health Statistics: Vital Statistics of the United States 1972 Vol 1—Natality. U.S. Government Printing Office, Washington, D.C., 1976.

National Center for Health Statistics: Catalog of public use data tapes DHHS Pub No. (PHS) 81-1213. 1980 Public Health Service, U.S. Government Printing Office, Washington D.C.

National Center for Health Statistics: Advance report, final natality statistics 1980 *Monthly Vital Statistics Report,* Vol 31, No 8 (suppl).

National Center for Health Statistics: Advance report of final natality statistics, 1982.

National Center for Health Statistics 1986 Advanced final natality statistics 1983 *Monthly Vital Statistics Report,* Vol 35, No 4.

National Research Council, Committee on the Biological Effects of Ionizing Radiations (BEIR) 1980 *The Effects on Populations of Exposure to Low Levels of Ionizing Radiation: 1980* National Academy Press, Washington, D.C., pp 482–485.

National Research Council, Subcommittee on Vitamin A Deficiency Prevention and Control 1986 Report of a workshop, *Methodologies for Conducting Field Trials of Vitamin A Supplementation* National Academy Press, Washington, D.C.

Nau H., Zierer R., Spielmann H., Neubert D., and Gnasau C. 1981 A new model for embryotoxicity testing: Teratogenicity and pharmacokinetics of valproic acid following constant-rate administration in the mouse using human therapeutic drug and metabolite concentrations *Life Sciences* 29:2803–2814.

Naus J. 1965 The distribution of the size of the maximum cluster of points on a line *J Am Stat Assoc* 60:532–538.

Naylor A.F. 1974 Sequential aspects of spontaneous abortion: Maternal age, parity, and pregnancy compensation artifact *Soc Biol* 21:195–204.

Naylor A.F. and Warburton D. 1974 Genetics of obstetrical variables: A study from the Collaborative Perinatal Project *Clin Genet* 6:351–369.

Naylor A.F. and Warburton D. 1979 Sequential analysis of spontaneous abortion: II. Collaborative study data show that gravidity determines a very substantial rise in risk *Fertil Steril* 31:282–286.

Neel J.V. 1985 The feasibility and urgency of monitoring human population for the genetic effects of radiation and the Hiroshima Nagasaki experience *Basic Life Sci* 33:393–413.

Neilson J.P. and Hood V.D. 1980 Ultrasound in obstetrics and gynaecology *Br Med Bull* 36:249–255.

Neligan G.A., Ballabriga A., Beutnagel H. et al. 1970 Working party to discuss nomenclature based on gestational age and birthweight *Arch Dis Child* 45:730.

Nellhaus G. 1958 Artificially induced female pseudohermaphroditism *N Engl J Med* 258:935–938.

Nelson W.J. 1967 Categorization by weight and gestational age of the infant at birth *J Pediat* 71:309–310.

Neugut R. 1981 Epidemiological appraisal of the literature on the fetal alcohol syndrome in humans *Early Hum Dev* 5:411–429.

Neugut R. 1986 The epidemiology of nausea and vomiting of pregnancy PhD Dissertation, Columbia University, New York.

Neutel C.I. and Buck C. 1971 Effect of smoking during pregnancy on the risk of cancer in children *JNCI* 47:59–63.

NY State J Med 1950 The Certificate of Birth Editorial 806.

Newcombe H.B., Kennedy J.M., Axford S.J., and James A.P. 1959 Automatic linkage of vital records *Science* 130:954–959.

Newman G. 1906 *Infant Mortality* Methuen, London.

Newton R.W., Webster P.A.C., Binu P.S., Maskrey N., and Phillips A.B. 1979 Psychosocial stress in pregnancy and its relation to the onset of premature labour *Br Med J* 2:411–413.

Newton R.W. and Hunt L. 1984 Psychosocial stress in pregnancy and its relation to low birth weight *Br Med J* 288:1191–1194.

New York State, Office of Public Health 1981 *Love Canal: A special report to the Governor and Legislature.* New York State Department of Health, Health Communications Group.

Niebuhr E. 1974 Triploidy in man: Cytogenetical and clinical aspects *Humangenetik* 21:103–125.

Niikawa N., Merotto E., and Kajii T. 1977 Origin of acrocentric trisomies in spontaneous abortuses *Hum Genet* 40:73–78.

Nishimura H. 1970 Incidence of malformation in abortions In C.F. Fraser and V.A. McKusick, eds. *Proceedings of 3rd International Conference on Congenital Malformations The Hague 1969* Excerpta Medica, Amsterdam, pp 275–283.

Nisula B.C. 1985 Measuring early pregnancy loss: Laboratory and field methods *Fertil Steril* 44:366–374.

Norbeck J.S. and Tilden V.P. 1983 Life stress, social support, and emotional disequilibrium in complications of pregnancy: A prospective, multivariate study *J Health Soc Behav* 24:30–46.

Nordstrom S., Beckman L., and Nordenson I. 1979 Occupational and environmental risks in and around a smelter in northern Sweden V. Spontaneous abortion among female employees and decreased birth weight in their offspring *Hereditas* 90:291–296.

North A.F. 1966 Small-for-date neonates. I. Maternal, gestational, and neonatal characteristics *Pediatrics* 38:1013–1019.

Nortman D. 1974 Parental age as a factor in pregnancy outcome and child development *Reports on Population and Family Planning*, Population Council, New York, pp 1–51.

Notake Y. and Suzuki S., eds. 1977 *Biological and Clinical Aspects of the Fetus* University Park Press, Baltimore and London; Igaku Shoin Ltd., Tokyo.

Nuchpakdee M. 1978 Spared brain growth in human intrauterine growth retardation. DrPH Dissertation, School of Public Health, Columbia University, New York.

Nuckolls K.B. 1967 Psychosocial Assets, Life Crisis and the Prognosis of Pregnancy PhD Dissertation, University of North Carolina, Chapel Hill.

Nuckolls K.B., Cassel J., and Kaplan B.H. 1972 Psychosocial assets, life crisis and the prognosis of pregnancy *Am J Epidemiol* 95:431–441.

Oakley A., Chalmers I., and Elbourne D. 1986 The effects of social interventions in pregnancy (Les effets des interventions sociales pendant la grossesse). In E. Papiernik, G. Breart, and N. Spira, eds. *Prevention of Preterm Birth. New goals and new practices in prenatal care (Prevention de la Naissance Prematuree. Nouveaux objectifs et nouvelles pratiques des soins prenataux).* Colloque INSERM, Paris, 138:329–361.

Odell S.D. and Griffin J. 1987 Pulsatile secretion of human chorionic gonadotropin in normal adults *N Engl J Med* 317:1688–1691.

Ohama K., Kusumi I., and Ihara T. 1977 Trisomy 17 in two abortuses *Jpn Hum Genet* 21:257–260.

Ohama K., Kusami I., and Fujiwara A. 1986 Chromosome abnormalities in 1355 induced abortuses *Hirosh J Med Sci* 35:135–141.

Olsen J., Rachootin P., Schiodt A.V., and Damsbo N. 1983 Tobacco use, alcohol consumption and infertility *Int J Epidemiol* 12:179–184.

Omer H., Friedlander D., Palti Z., and Shekel I. 1986 Life stresses and premature labor: Real connection or artifactual findings? *Psychosom Med* 48:362–369.

O'Neill C. 1984 Thrombocytopenia is an initial maternal response to fertilization in mice *J Reprod Fertil* 73:559–566.

O'Neill C., Gidley-Baird A.A., Pike I.L., Porter R.N., Sinosich M.J., and Saunders D.M. 1984 Maternal blood platelet physiology and luteal phase endocrinology as a means of monitoring pre- and post-implantation embryo viability following in vitro fertilization *J Vitro Fertil Embryo Transfer* 2:87–93.

O'Neill C., Pike I.L., Porter R.N., Gidley-Baird A.A., Sinosich M.J., and Saunders D.M. 1985 Maternal recognition of pregnancy prior to implantation: Methods for monitoring embryonic viability in vitro and in vivo *Ann NY Acad Sci* 442:429–439.

Oster J. 1956 The causes of mongolism *Dan Med Bull* 3:158–164.

Otake M. and Schull W.J. 1984 In utero exposure to A-bomb radiation and mental retardation; A reassessment *Br J Radiol* 57:409–414.

Ouelette E.M., Rossett H.L., Rosman N.P., and Weiner L. 1977 Adverse effects on offspring of maternal alcohol abuse during pregnancy *N Engl J Med* 297:528–530.

Ounsted M. 1965 Maternal constraint of foetal growth in man *Develop Med Child Neurol* 7:479–491.

Ounsted M. 1968 The regulation of foetal growth In J.P.H. Jonxis et al., eds. *Aspects of Prematurity and Dysmaturity* Leiden, pp 167–188.

Ounsted M. 1974 Familial trends in low birthweight *Br Med J* 4:163.

Ounsted M. 1986 Transmission through the female line of fetal growth constraint *Early Hum Dev* 13:339–341.

Ounsted M. and Ounsted C. 1968 Rate of intra-uterine growth *Nature* 220:599–600.

Ounsted M. and Ounsted C. 1973 On fetal growth rate: Its variations and their consequences *Clin Dev Med* 46, S.I.M.P., Heineman, London, pp 46–47.

Owen L.N. 1963 The effects of administering tetracyclines to young dogs with particular reference to localization of the drugs in the teeth *Arch Oral Biol* 8:715–727.

Oxford English Dictionary, suppl. 1982 Clarendon Press, London.

Paigen B. 1981 Assessing the problem—Love Canal *Proceedings, Conference on Hazardous Waste* Society for Occupational and Environmental Health.

Paneth N. 1986 Recent trends in preterm delivery rates in the United States (Taux de naissances prematurees aux Etats-Unis) In E. Papiernik, G. Breart, and N. Spira, eds. *Prevention of Preterm Birth: New goals and new practices in prenatal care* (Prevention de la Naissance Prematuree: Nouveaux objectifs et nouvelles pratiques des soins prenataux) Colloque INSERM, Paris, 138:15–30.

Paneth N., Kiely J.L., Stein Z., and Susser M. 1981 Cerebral palsy and newborn care. III. Estimated cohort prevalence rates of cerebral palsy under different rates of mortality and impairment of low birthweight infants *Dev Med Child Neurol* 23:801–807.

Paneth N., Wallenstein S., Kiely J.L., and Susser M.W. 1982a Social class indicators and mortality in low birth weight infants *Am J Epidemiol* 110:364–375.

Paneth N., Kiely J.L., Wallenstein S., Marcus M., Pakter J., and Susser M.W. 1982b Newborn intensive care and neonatal mortality in low birthweight infants: A population study *N Engl J Med* 307:149–155.

Pantelakis S.N., Papadimitriou G.C., and Doxiadis S.A. 1973 Influence of induced and spontaneous abortions on the outcome of subsequent pregnancies *Am J Obstet Gynecol* 116:799–805.

Papaevangelou G., Urettos A.S., Papadalos C., and Alexiou D. 1973 The effect of spontaneous and induced abortion on prematurity and birthweight *J Obstet Gynaecol Br Commonw* 80:418–422.

Papiernik E. 1982 Can preterm births be prevented? *Lancet* i:1412.

Papiernik E., Bouyer J., Dreyfus J., Collin D., Winisdorffer G., Guegen S., Lecomte M., and Lazar P. 1985 Prevention of preterm births: A perinatal study in Haguenau, France *Pediatrics* 76:154–158.

Parkman P.D., Buescher E.L., and Artenstein M.S. 1962 Recovery of rubella virus from army recruits (27750) *Soc Exp Biol Med* 111:225–230.

Parkin J.N. 1971 The assessment of gestational age in Ugandan and British newborn babies *Dev Med Child Neurol* 13:784–788.

Parkinson C.E., Wallis S., and Harvey D. 1981 Effects of behavioral and medical variables on fetal growth retardation *Dev Med Child Neurol* 1:1060.

Pascoe J.M., Loda F.A., Jeffries V., and Earp J.A. 1981 The association between mother's social support and provision of stimulation to their children *J Dev Behav Pediatr* 2:15–19.

Pascoe J.M., Chessare J., Baugh E., Urich L., and Ialongo N. 1987 Help with prenatal household tasks and newborn birth weight: Is there an association? *J Dev Behav Pediatr* 8:207–212.

Paul A.A., Muller E.M., and Whitehead R.G. 1979 The quantitative effects of maternal dietary energy intake on pregnancy and lactation in rural Gambian women *Trans R Soc Trop Med Hyg* 73:686–692.

Pauli R.M., Madden J.D., Kranzler K.J., Culpepper W., and Port R. 1976 Warfarin therapy initiated during pregnancy and phenotypic chondrodysplasia punctata *J Pediatr* 88:506–508.

Peart A.F.W. and Nagler F.P. 1954 Measles in the Canadian Arctic, 1952 *Can J Public Health* 40:146–156.

Pebley A.R., Huffman L., Chowdhury A.K.M., and Stupp O.W. 1985 Intrauterine mortality and maternal nutritional status in rural Bangladesh *Popul Studies* 39:425–440.

Peckham C.H., 1938a Statistical studies in prematurity I. The incidence of prematurity and the effect of certain obstetric factors *J Pediatr* 13:474–483.

Peckham C.H. 1938b Statistical studies on prematurity II. The mortality of prematurity and the effect of certain obstetric factors *J Pediatr* 13:484–496.

Peckham C.S. 1974 Clinical and serological assessment of children exposed in utero to confirmed maternal rubella *Br Med J* 1:259–261.

Peckham C.S. and Marshall W.C. 1983 Infection in pregnancy In S.L. Barron and A.M. Thomson, eds. *Obstetrical Epidemiology*, Academic Press, London, pp 209–262.

Pelkonen O., Jouppila P., and Karki N.T. 1977 Effect of cigarette smoking on 3, 4-benzpyrene and N-methylaniline metabolism in human fetal liver and placenta *Toxicol Appl Pharmacol* 23:399–407.

Pellestor F. and Sele B. 1988 Assessment of aneuploidy in the human female by using cytogenetics of IVF failures *Am J Hum Genet* 42:274–283.

Penrose L.S. 1933 The relative effects of paternal age and maternal age in mongolism *J Genet* 27:219–224.

Penrose L.S. 1951 Data on the genetics of birth weight *Ann Eugen* 16:378–381.

Penrose L.S. 1954a Some recent trends in human genetics *Caryologia* 6 (suppl):521–530.

Penrose L.S. 1954b Genetical factors affecting the growth of the foetus In *La prophylaxie en gynecologie et obstetrique* Conferences et Rapports du Congres International de Gynecologie et d'Obstetrique. Libraire de l'Universite George SA, Geneva, pp 638–648.

Penrose L.S. 1965 Mongolism as a problem in human biology. 1964 In *The Early Conceptus Normal and Abnormal.* Papers and discussions presented at a Symposium held at Queens College, Dundee, pp 94–107.

Penrose L.S. and Berg J.M. 1968 Mongolism and duration of marriage *Nature* 218:300.

Penrose L.S. and Delhanty J.D. 1961 Triploid cell cultures from a macerated foetus *Lancet* i:1261–1262.

Penrose L.S. and Smith G.F. 1966 *Down's Anomaly.* Churchill, London.

Perkins R.P. 1981 The neonatal significance of selected perinatal events among infants of low birth weight *Am J Obstet Gynecol* 139:546–561.

Peterson W.F. 1969 Pregnancy following oral contraceptive therapy *Obstet Gynec* 34:363–367.

Pettersson F. 1968 *Epidemiology of Early Pregnancy Wastage: Biological and Social Correlates of Abortion. An Investigation Based on Materials Collected within Uppsala County, Sweden,* Svenska Bokforlaget, Stockholm.

Pettifor J.M. and Benson R. 1975 Congenital malformations associated with the administration of oral anticoagulants during pregnancy *J Pediatr* 86:459–462.

Pettigrew A.T., Logan R.W., and Willocks J. 1977 Smoking in pregnancy—effects on birthweight and on cyanide and thiocyanate levels in mother and baby *Br J Obstet Gynaecol* 84:31–34.

Pettitt D.J. 1986 The long-range impact of diabetes during pregnancy: The Pima Indian experience *IDF Bulletin* 31:70–71.

Pettitt D.J. and Bennett P.H. 1988 Long-term outcome of infants of diabetic mothers In E.A. Reece and D. Coustan, eds. *Diabetes Mellitus in Pregnancy: Principles and Practice*. New York, Churchill Livingstone, pp 559–571.

Pettitt D.J., Knowler W.C., Baird H.R., and Bennett P.H. 1980 Gestational diabetes: Infant and maternal complications of pregnancy in relation to third-trimester glucose tolerance in the Pima Indians *Diabetes Care* 3:458–464.

Pettitt D.J., Baird R., Aleck K.A., Bennett P.H., and Knowler W.C. 1983 Excessive obesity in offspring of Pima Indian women with diabetes during pregnancy *N Engl J Med* 308:242–245.

Pettitt D.J., Bennett P.H., Knowler W.C., Baird H.R., and Aleck K.A. 1985 Gestational diabetes mellitus and impaired glucose tolerance during pregnancy: Long-term effects on obesity and glucose tolerance in the offspring *Diabetes* 34 (suppl 2):119–122.

Pettitt D.J., Knowler W.C., Bennett P.H., Aleck K.A., and Baird H.R. 1987 Obesity in offspring of diabetic Pima Indian women despite normal birth weight *Diabetes Care* 10:76–80.

Pettitt D.J., Aleck K.A., Baird H.R., Carraher M.J., Bennett P.H., and Knowler W.C. 1988 Role of intrauterine environment *Diabetes* 37:622–628.

Pfeiffer E., Verwoerdt A. and Wang H. 1968 Sexual behavior in aged men and women *Arch Gen Psychiat* 19:753–758.

Pharoah P.O.D., Buttfield I.H., and Hetzel B.S. 1971 Neurological damage to the fetus resulting from severe iodine deficiency during pregnancy *Lancet* i:308–310.

Pharoah P.O.D., Alberman E., and Doyle P. 1977 Outcome of pregnancy among women in anaesthetic practice *Lancet* i:34–36.

Pharoah P.O.D., Delange F., Fierro-Benitez R., and Stanbury J.B. 1980 Endemic cretinism In J.B. Stanbury and B.S. Hetzel, eds. *Endemic Goiter and Endemic Cretinism: Iodine Nutrition in Health and Disease*. John Wiley & Sons, New York, pp 395–421.

Philippe E. and Boué J.G. 1970 Placenta et aberrations chromosomiques au cours des avortements spontanes *Presse Med* 78:641–646.

Pickering R.M. and Forbes J.K. 1985 Risks of preterm delivery and small-for-gestational age infants following abortion: A population study *Br J Obstet Gynaecol* 92:1106–1112.

Picone T.A., Allen L.H., Olsen P.N., and Ferris M.E. 1982 Pregnancy outcome in North American women: I. Effects of diet, cigarette smoking, stress, and weight gain on placentas, and on neonatal physical and behavioral characteristics *Am J Clin Nutr* 36:1214–1224.

Pirani B.B.K. 1978 Smoking during pregnancy *Obstet Gynecol Surv* 33:1–12.

Pitt D.B. 1957 Congenital malformations and maternal rubella *Med J Aust* 233–239.

Pitt D. and Keir E.H. 1965 Results of rubella in pregnancy: I. *Med J Austr* 2:647–561.

Platt B.S. and Stewart R.J.C. 1971 Reversible and irreversible effects of protein-calorie deficiency on the central nervous system of animals and man *World Rev Nutr Diet* 13:43–85.

Pleet H., Graham J.M., and Smith D.W. 1981 Central nervous system and facial defects associated with maternal hyperthermia at 4 to 14 weeks gestation *Pediatrics* 67:785–789.

Poland B.J., Miller J.T., Jones D., and Trimble B.K. 1977 Reproductive counseling in patients who had a spontaneous abortion *Am J Obstet Gynecol* 127:685–691.

Polani P.E. 1981 Chiasmata, Down syndrome, and nondisjunction: An overview In F.F. de la Cruz and Gerald P.S., eds. *Trisomy 21 (Down syndrome)—Research Perspectives*, University Park Press, Baltimore, pp 111–130.

Polani P.E. and Jagiello G.M. 1976 Chiasmata, meiotic univalents, and age in relation to aneuploid imbalance in mice *Cytogenet Cell Genet* 16:505–529.

Polani P.E. and Crolla J.A. 1989 An experimental test of the production line hypothesis of oogenesis in the female mouse. In S. Wachtel, ed. *Evolutionary Mechanisms in Sex Determination* CRC Press, Boca Raton, Florida.

Polani P.E., Briggs J.H., Ford C.E., Clarke C.M., Berg J.M. 1960 A mongol girl with 46 chromosomes *Lancet* i:721–724.

Polednak A.P., Janerich D.T., and Glebatis D.M. 1982 Birthweight and birth defects in relation to maternal spermicide use *Teratology* 26:27–38.

Pollitt E. and Mueller W. 1982 Maternal nutrition supplementation during pregnancy interferes with physical resemblance of siblings at birth according to infant sex *Early Hum Develop* 7:251–256.

Poma P.A. 1981 Effect of maternal age on pregnancy outcome *J Natl Med Assn* 73:1031–1038.

Pomerance J.J., Gluck L., and Lynch V.A. 1974 Physical fitness in pregnancy: Its effect on pregnancy outcome *Am J Obstet Gynecol* 119:867–876.

Popper K.R. 1961 *The Logic of Scientific Discovery* 2 ed. Harper & Row, New York.

Poswillo D., Nunnerly H., Sopher D., and Keith J. 1974 Hyperthermia as a teratogenic agent *Ann Roy Coll Surg Engl* 55:171–174.

Prechtl H.F.R. 1977 The neurological examination of the full-term newborn infant Clinics in Developmental Medicine, No. 63, 2 ed, Heinemann, London.

Prentice A.M. 1980 Variation in maternal dietary intake, birthweight and breast-milk output in the Gambia In H. Aebi and R. Whitehead, eds. *Maternal Nutrition during Pregnancy and Lactation*, Hans Huber Publishers, Bern, pp 167–182.

Prentice A.M., Whitehead R.G., Roberts S.B., and Paul A.A. 1981 Long-term energy balance in child-bearing Gambian women *Am J Clin Nutr* 34:2790–2799.

Prentice A.M., Whitehead R.G., Watkinson M., Lamb W.H., and Cole T.J. 1983 Prenatal dietary supplementation of African women and birth-weight *Lancet* i:489–492.

Preston-Martin S., Yu M.C., Benton B., and Henderson B.E. 1982 N-nitroso compounds and childhood brain tumors: A case-control study *Cancer Res* 42:5240–5245.

Puffer P.R. and Serrano C.V. 1973 *Patterns of mortality in childhood: Report of the Inter-American investigation of mortality in childhood,* Pan American Health Organization Scientific Publication No. 262, Washington, D.C.

Quételet L.A.J. 1869 *Physique Sociale, ou essi Sur le developpement des facultes de l'homme* Vol 1 & 11, C. Muquardt, Brussels.

Quételet L.A.J. 1870 *Anthropometrie ou mesure des differentes facultes de l'homme,* C. Muquardt, Brussels, pp 346–412.

Raivio K.O., Ikonen E., and Saarikoski S. 1977 Fetal risks due to warfarin therapy during pregnancy *Acta Paediatr Scand* 66:735–739.

Ransome-Kuti O. 1985 Intra-uterine growth, birthweights and maturity of the African newborn *Acta Paediatr Scand* 319 (suppl):95–102.

Ramsey C.N., Abell T.C., and Baker L.C. 1986 The relationship between family functioning, life events, family structure, and the outcome of pregnancy. *J Fam Pract* 22:521–527.

Rao D.C., Morton N.E., and Yee S. 1974 Analysis of family resemblance. II. A linear model for familial correlation *Am J Hum Genet* 26:331–359.

Rasmussen K.M., Mock N.B., and Habicht J.-P. 1985 The biological meaning of low birthweight and the use of data on low birthweight for nutritional surveillance. Cornell Nutritional Surveillance Program. Working Paper Series.

Ravelli G.P., Stein Z.A., and Susser M.W. 1976 Obesity in young men after famine exposure in utero and early infancy *N Engl J Med* 295:349–353.

Record R.G. 1961 Anencephalus in Scotland *Br J Prev Soc Med* 15:93–105.

Record R.G. and McKeown T. 1969 The relation of measured intelligence to birth order and maternal age *Ann Hum Genet* 33:61–69.

Redman C.W.G., Beilin L.J., Bonnar J., and Ounsted M.K. 1976 Fetal outcome in trial of antihypertensive treatment in pregnancy *Lancet* ii:753–755.

Reed T.E. and Kelly E.L. 1958 The completed reproductive performance of 161 couples selected before marriage and classified by ABO blood group *Ann Hum Genet* 22:165–181.

Regal R.R., Cross P.K., Lamson S.H., and Hook E.B. 1980 A search for evidence for a paternal age effect independent of a maternal age effect in birth certificate reports of Down's syndrome in New York State *Am J Epidemiol* 112:650–655.

Rendle-Short T.J. 1962 Tetracycline in teeth and bone *Lancet* i:1188.

Report of Panel II. 1981 Guidelines for reproductive studies in exposed human populations In A. Bloom, ed. *Guidelines for Studies of Human Populations Exposed to Mutagenic and Reproductive Hazards.* March of Dimes Birth Defects Foundation, White Plains, NY, pp 37–110.

Report of a WHO Scientific Group. 1970 Spontaneous and induced abortion *World Health Organization Tech Report Series #461,* Geneva.

Reyes F.I., Koh K.S., and Faiman D. 1976 Fertility in women with gonadal dysgenesis *Am J Obstet Gynecol* 126:668–670.

Reynolds D.W., Stagno S., Stubbs K.G., Dahle A.J., Livingston M.M., Saxon S.S., and Alford C.A. 1974 Inapparent congenital cytomegalovirus infection with elevated cord IgM levels: Causal relation with auditory and mental deficiency *N Engl J Med* 290:291–296.

Rhoads G.G. and Mills J.L. 1986 Can vitamin supplements prevent neural tube defects? Current evidence and ongoing investigations *Clin Obstet Gynecol* 29:569–579.

Ribeira M., Stein Z.A., Susser M.W., Cohen P., and Neugut R. 1982 Prenatal starvation and maternal blood pressure near delivery *Am J Clin Nutr* 36:229–234.

Richman E.M. and Lahman J.E. 1976 Fetal anomalies associated with warfarin therapy initiated shortly prior to conception *J Pediatr* 88:509–510.

Rieger R., Michaelio A., and Green M.M. 1976 *Glossary of Genetics and Cytogenetics: Classic and Molecular* Springer-Verlag, Berlin, pp 30–31.

Risch N., Stein Z., Kline J., and Warburton D. 1986 The relationship between maternal age and chromosome size in autosomal trisomy *Am J Hum Genet* 39:68–78.

Robert E. 1982 Valproic acid and spina bifida: A preliminary report—France *MMWR* 31:565–566.

Robert E. and Guibaud P. 1982 Maternal valproic acid and congenital neural tube defects. *Lancet* ii:937.

Robert E. and Rosa F. 1983 Valproate and birth defects *Lancet* ii:1142.

Roberts C.J. and Lloyd S. 1973 Area differences in spontaneous abortion rates in South Wales and their relation to neural tube defect incidence *Br Med J* 4:20–22.

Roberts C.J. and Powell R.G. 1975 Interrelation of the common congenital malformations. Some aetiological implications *Lancet* ii:848–850.

Roberts L. 1987 Atomic bomb doses reassessed: Research News *Science* 238:1649–1651.

Robinson A., Lubs H.A., Nielsen J., and Sorensen K. 1979 Summary of clinical findings: Profiles of children with 47XXY, 47XXX and 47XYY karyotypes In *Sex Chromosome Aneuploidy: Prospective Studies on Children*. The National Foundation, White Plains, N.Y. *Birth Defects: Original Article Series* 15:261–266.

Robinson M.J., Pash J., Grimwade J., and Campbell J. 1978 Fetal warfarin syndrome *Med J Aust* 1:157.

Robinson W.S. 1950 Ecological correlates and the behavior of individuals *Am Sociol Rev* 15:351–357.

Robson E.B. 1955 Birth weight in cousins *Ann Hum Genet* 19:262–268.

Robson E.B. 1978 The genetics of birth weight In F. Falkner and J.M. Tanner, eds. *Human Growth: I. Principles of Prenatal Growth*. Plenum Press, New York, pp 285–297.

Rocklin R.E., Kitzmiller J.L., and Garvoy M.R. 1982 Maternal-fetal relation. II. Further characterization of an immunologic blocking factor that develops during pregnancy *Clin Immunol Immunopath* 22:305–315.

Roederer J.G. 1753 Pondere et longitudine infantum recens natorum *Commentaries of the Royal Society of Gottingen*, p 410.

Rogan W.J. 1982 PCBs and cola-colored babies: Japan, 1968, and Taiwan, 1979 *Teratology* 26:259–261.

Rogan W.J., Gladen B.C., Hung K.L., Koong S.L., Shih L.Y., Taylor J.S., Wu Ye, Yang D., Ragan N.B., and Hsu C.C. 1988 Congenital poisoning by polychlorinated biphenyls and their contaminants in Taiwan *Science* 241:334–336.

Rolfe B.E. 1982 Detection of fetal wastage *Fertil Steril* 37:655–660.

Roman E.A., Doyle P., Beral V., Alberman E., and Pharoah P. 1978 Fetal loss, gravidity and pregnancy order *Early Hum Dev* 2:131–138.

Rosenberg G.H. 1984 The home is the workplace: hazards, stress, and pollutants in the household In W. Chavkin ed. *Double Exposure: Women's Health Hazards on the Job and at Home* Monthly Review Press, New York, pp 219–245.

Rosenberg P. and Kirves A. 1973 Miscarriages among operating theater staff *Acta Anaesth Scand* 53 (suppl):37–42.

Rosenberg P.H. and Vanttinen H. 1978 Occupational hazards to reproduction and health in anesthetists and paediatricians *Acta Anaesth Scand* 22:202–207.

Rosenfield A. and Maine D. 1985 Maternal mortality—a neglected tragedy. Where is the M. in MCH *Lancet* ii:83–85.

Rossiter C.E. 1985 Maternal mortality *Br J Obstet Gynaecol* (suppl)5:100–115.

Rosso P. 1969 The effect of severe early malnutrition on cellular growth of human brain *Pediatr Res* 3:181–184.

Rosso P. 1981 Nutrition and maternal-fetal exchange *Am J Clin Nutr* 34:744–755.

Rosso P. and Winick M. 1974 Intrauterine growth retardation. A new systematic approach based on the clinical and biochemical characteristics of this condition *J Perinat Med* 2:147–160.

Rosso P., Nelson M., and Winick M. 1974 Changes in cellular RNA content and alkaline ribonuclease activity in rat liver during development *Growth* 37:143–151.

Roth M.P., Stoll C., Taillemite J.L., Girard S., and Boué A. 1983 Paternal age and Down's syndrome diagnosed prenatally: No association in French data *Prenat Diagn* 3:327–335.

Rothenberg P. and Varga P.E. 1981 The relationship between age of mother and child health and development *Am J Publ Health* 71:810–817.

Rothman K.J. 1982 Spermicide use and Down's syndrome *Am J Publ Health* 72:399–401.

Rothman K.J. and Louik C. 1978 Oral contraceptives and birth defects *N Engl J Med* 299:522–524.

Royal College of General Practitioners' Oral Contraception Study. 1976 The outcome of pregnancy in former oral contraceptive users *Br J Obstet Gynaecol* 83:608–616.

Rudak E., Dor J., Mashiah S., Nebel L., and Goldman B. 1984 Chromosome analysis of multipronuclear human oocytes fertilized in vitro *Fertil Steril* 41:538–545.

Rundle A., Coppen A., and Cowie V. 1961 Steroid excretion in mothers of mongols *Lancet* ii:846–848.

Rudolph L. 1986 The worker's perspective In Z.A. Stein and M.C. Hatch, eds. *Reproductive Problems in the Workplace* Hanley & Belfus, Philadelphia. *Occupational Medicine*, 1:487–495.

Rush D. 1974 Examination of relationship between birthweight, cigarette smoking during pregnancy and maternal weight gain *J Obstet Gynaecol Br Commonw* 81:746–752.

Rush D. 1982 Effects of changes in protein and caloric intake during pregnancy on the growth of the human fetus In M. Enkin and I. Chalmer, eds. *Effectiveness and satisfaction in antenatal care* Developmental Med Series,

Nos 81 and 82, Wm. Heinemann Medical Books, London, pp 92–113.

Rush D. 1987 Nutrition, birthweight, and child mortality in India: The use of epidemiology in setting priorities *Ind J Comm Med* 12:61–67.

Rush D. 1988 The national WIC evaluation *Am J Clin Nutr* 48 (2 suppl):389–428.

Rush D., Davis H., and Susser M. 1972 Antecedents of low birthweight in Harlem, New York City *Int J Epidemiol* 1:375–387.

Rush D., Stein Z., and Susser M. 1980 *Diet in pregnancy: A randomized controlled trial of prenatal nutritional supplements* Alan R. Liss, New York. March of Dimes Foundation *Birth Defects: Original Article Series* 16:3.

Rush D., Stein Z., and Susser M. 1980 A randomized controlled trial of prenatal nutritional supplementation in New York City *Pediatrics* 125:567–575.

Rush D., Cassano P., Wilson A.U., Koenigsberger R.J., and Cohen J. 1983 Newborn neurologic maturity relates more strongly to concurrent somatic development than gestational age *Am J Perinatol* 1:12–20.

Rush R.W., Keirse M.J.N.C., Howat P., Baum J.D., Anderson A.B.M., and Turnbull A.C. 1976 Contribution of pre term delivery to perinatal mortality *Br Med J* 2:965–968.

Rush R.W., Davey D.A., and Segall M.L. 1978 The effect of preterm delivery on perinatal mortality *Br J Obstet Gynaecol* 85:806–811.

Russel W.L. 1981 Problems and solutions in the estimation of genetic risks from radiation and chemicals In G.G. Berg and H.D. Maillie, eds. *Measurement of Risks*, Environmental Service Research 21:361–384.

Sabbagha R.E., Barton F.B., and Barton B.A. 1976 Sonar biparietal. I. Analysis of percentile growth differences in two normal populations using same methodology *Am J Obstet Gynecol* 126:479–484.

St. Anne-Dargassies S. 1966 Neurological maturation of the premature infant of 28-41 weeks gestational age In F. Falkner, ed. *Human Development* Saunders, Philadelphia.

Sandler D.P., Everson R.B., Wilcox A.J., and Browder J.P. 1985 Cancer risk in adulthood from early life exposure to parents' smoking *Am J Publ Health* 85:487–492.

Santella R.M., Lin C.D., Cleveland W.L., and Weinstein I.B. 1984 Monoclonal antibodies to DNA modified by a benzo(a)pyrene diol epoxide *Carcinogenesis* 5:373–377.

Sargent C. 1982 The implications of role expectations for birth assistance among Bariba women *Soc Sci Med* 16:1483–1489.

Sargent C. 1985 Obstetrical choice among urban women in Benin *Soc Sci Med* 20:287–292.

Sargent I.L., Wilkins T., and Redman C.W.G. 1988 Maternal immune responses to the fetus in early pregnancy and recurrent miscarriage *Lancet* ii:1099–1104.

Sasaki M., Ikeuchi T., Obara Y., Hayata I., Mori M., and Kohno S. 1971 Chromosome studies in early embryogenesis *Am J Obstet Gynecol* 111:8–12.

Saurel M.J. and Kaminski M. 1983 Pregnant women at work *Lancet* i:475.

Saurel-Cubizolles M.J., Kaminski M., and Rumeau-Rouquette C. 1982 Activite professionnelle des femmes enceintes, surveillance prenatale et issue de la grossesse *J Gyn Obstet Biol Reprod* 11:959–967.

Saurel-Cubizolles M.J., Kaminski M., Llado-Arkhipoff J. et al. 1985 Pregnancy and its outcome among hospital personnel according to occupation and working conditions *J Epidemiol Comm Health* 39:129–134.

Saurel-Cubizolles M.J. and Kaminski M. 1986 Work in pregnancy: Its evolving relationship with perinatal outcome (A review) *Soc Sci Med* 22:431–442.

Scarbrough P.R., Hersh J., Kukolich M.K., Carroll A.J., Finley S.C., Hochhberger R., Wilkerson S., Yen F.F., and Althans B.W. 1984 Tetraploidy: A report of three live-born infants *Am J Med Genet* 19:29–37.

Schardein J.L. 1980 Congenital abnormalities and hormones during pregnancy: A clinical review *Teratology* 22:251–270.

Schaudinn F. and Hoffmann E. 1905 Ueber spirochaete pallida bei syphilis und die Unterschiede dieser Form gegenuber anderen Arten dieser Gattung *Berl Klin Wochenschr* 42:673–675.

Schlesinger E.R. and Allaway N.C. 1955 The combined effect of birth weight and length of gestation on neonatal mortality among single premature births *Pediatrics* 15:698–704.

Schoenbaum S.C., et al. 1980 Outcome of the delivery following an induced or spontaneous abortion *Am J Obstet Gynecol* 136:19–24.

Scholl T.O., Sobe E., Tanfer K., Soefer E.F., and Saidman B. 1983 Effects of vaginal spermicides on pregnancy outcome *Fam Plan Persp* 15:244–250.

Schreinemachers D.M., Cross P.K., and Hook E.B. 1982 Rates of trisomies 21, 18, 13 and other chromosome abnormalities in about 20,000 prenatal studies compared with estimated rates in live births *Hum Genet* 61:318–324.

Schull W.J. and Neel J.V. 1962 Maternal radiation and mongolism *Lancet* i:537–538.

Schull W.J. and Bailey J.K. 1984 Critical assessment of genetic effects of ionizing radiation on pre- and postnatal development In H. Kalter, ed. *Issues Rev Teratol* Vol 2, Plenum Press, New York, pp 325–398.

Schwartz D., MacDonald P.D.H., and Heuchel V. 1980 Fecundability, coital frequency and the viability of ova *Pop Studies* 34:397–400.

Scott A., Moar V., and Ounsted M. 1981 The relative contributions of different maternal factors in small-for-gestational age pregnancies *Europ J Obstet Gynaecol Reprod Biol* 12:157–165.

Scott E.M. and Thomson A.M. 1956 A psychological investigation on primigravidae. IV Psychological factors and the clinical phenomena of labour *J Obstet Gynaecol Br Empire* 63:502–508.

Scott J.R., Rote N.S., and Branch D.W. 1987 Immunologic aspects of recurrent abortion and fetal death *Obstet Gynecol* 70:645–656.

Seeds J.W. 1984 Impaired fetal growth: Ultrasonic evaluation and clinical management *Obstet Gynecol* 64:577–584.

Selevan S.G., Lindbohm M.-L., Hornung R.W., and Hemminki K. 1985 A study of occupational exposure to antineoplastic drugs and fetal loss in nurses *N Engl J Med* 313:1173–1178.

Selikoff I.J., Hammond E.C., and Churg J. 1968 Asbestos exposure, smoking and neoplasia *JAMA* 204:106–112.

Seller M.J. 1981 Recurrence risks for neural tube defects in a genetic counselling clinic population *J Med Genet* 18:245–248.

Seller M.J. 1982 Neural-tube defects: Cause and prevention In A. Matteo, P. Benson, F. Giannelli and M. Seller, eds. *Pediatric Research: A Genetic Approach* Spastics International Medical Publication, The Lavenham Press, Lavenham, Suffolk.

Seller M.J. and Nevin N.C. 1984 Periconceptional vitamin supplementation and the prevention of neural tube defects in south-east England and North-ern Ireland *J Med Genet* 21:325–330.

Seltser R. and Sartwell P. 1965 The influence of occupational exposure to radiation on the mortality of American radiologists and other medical specialists *Am J Epidemiol* 81:2–22.

Selvin S. and Janerich D.T. 1971 Four factors influencing birth weight *Br J Prev Soc Med* 25:12–16.

Selwyn P.A., Schoenbaum E.E., Davenny K., Robertson V.J., Feingold A.R., Shulman J.F., Mayers M.M., Klein R.S., Friedland G.H., and Rogers M.F. 1989 Prospective study of human immunodeficiency virus infection and pregnancy outcomes in intravenous drug users *JAMA* 261:1289–1294.

Semmelweiss I.P. 1861 *The Etiology, the Concept, and the Prophylaxis of Childbed Fever* Trans. Carter K.C. (1983) University of Wisconsin Press, Madison.

Sen S., Talukder G., and Sharma A. 1987 Age-related alterations in human chromosome composition and DNA content in vitro during senescence *Biol Rev* 62:25–44.

Sever J.L., Schiff G.M., and Traub R.G. 1962 Rubella virus *JAMA* 182:663–671.

Sever J.L., Ellenberg J.H., and Edmonds D. 1977 Maternal urinary tract infections In D.M. Reed and F.S. Stanley, eds. *The Epidemiology of Prematurity*, Urban & Schwarzenberg, Baltimore, pp 193–196.

Sever L.E. 1973 Hormonal pregnancy tests and spina bifida *Nature* 242:410–411.

Sexton M. and Hebel R. 1984 A clinical trial of change in maternal smoking and its effect on birth weight *JAMA* 251:911–915.

Shah F.K. and Abbey H. 1971 Effects of some factors on neonatal and post-neonatal mortality. Analysis by a binary variable multiple regression method *Milb Mem Fund Q* 49:33–57.

Shapiro S. and Unger J. 1954 Relation of weight at birth to cause of death and age at death in the neonatal period: United States, Early 1950 *Vital Statistics Special Reports. National Office of Vital Statistics* 39:226–299.

Shapiro S. and Moriyama I.M. 1963 International trends in infant mortality and their implications for the United States *Am J Publ Health* 53:747–760.

Shapiro S. and Unger J. 1965 Weight at birth and survival of the newborn, by geographic divisions and urban and rural areas, United States, early 1950 *Vital and Health Statistics* No 1000, Series 21, No 4. U.S. Superintendent of Documents, U.S. Government Printing Office.

Shapiro S., Jones E.W., and Densen P.M. 1962 A life table of pregnancy terminations and correlations of fetal loss *Milb Memorial Fund Quart* 1:7–45.

Shapiro S., Schlesinger E.R., and Nesbit R.E.L. 1968 *Infant, Perinatal, Maternal and Childhood Mortality in the United States* Harvard University Press, Cambridge, MA.

Shapiro S., Levine H.S., and Abramowicz M. 1971 Factors associated with early and late fetal loss *Adv Plan Parent* 6:45–63.

Shapiro S., Slone D., Heinonen O.P., Kaufman D.W., Rosenberg L., Mitchell A.A., and Helmrich S.P. 1982 Birth defects and vaginal spermicides *JAMA* 247:2381–2384.

Shapiro S., McCormick M.C., Starfield B.H., and Crawley B. 1983 Changes in infant morbidity associated with decreases in neonatal mortality *Pediatrics* 72:408–414.

Sharp J. 1671 The Midwives Book, p 102. Quoted in Eccles A (1982) *Obstetrics and Gynaecology in Tudor and Stuart England* Kent State University Press, Kent, OH.

Shaul W.L. and Hall J.G. 1977 Multiple congenital anomalies associated with oral anticoagulants *Am J Obstet Gynecol* 127:191–198.

Shaul W.L., Emery H., and Hall J.G. 1975 Chondrodysplasia punctata and maternal warfarin use during pregnancy *Am J Dis Child* 129:360–362.

Sheffield L.J., Danks D.M., Mayne V., and Hutchinson L.A. 1976 Chondrodysplasia punctata—23 cases of a mild and relatively common variety *J Pediatr* 89:916–923.

Sherman B.M., West J.H., and Korenman S.G. 1976 The menopausal transition: Analysis of LH, FSH, estradiol and progesterone concentrations during menstrual cycles of older women *J Clin Endocrinol Metab* 42:629–636.

Shepard T.H. 1986 Human teratogenicity *Adv Pediatr* 33:225–268.

Shewhart W.A. 1931 *Economic Control of Quality of Manufactured Product* Van Nostrand, New York.

Shilling S. and Lalich N.R. 1984 Maternal occupation and industry and the pregnancy outcome of U.S. married women, 1980 *Publ Health Rep* 99:152–161.

Shiono P.H. and Klebanoff M.A. 1986 Ethnic differences in preterm and very preterm delivery *Am J Publ Health* 76:1317–1321.

Shiono P.H., Klebanoff M.A., and Berendes H.W. 1986a Congenital malformations and maternal smoking during pregnancy *Teratology* 34:65–71.

Shiono P.H., Klebanoff M.A., Graubard M.A., Berendes H.W., and Rhoads G.G. 1986b Birth weight among women of different ethnic groups *JAMA* 255:48–52.

Shiono P.H., Klebanoff M.A., and Rhoads G.G. 1986c Smoking and drinking during pregnancy. Their effects on preterm birth *JAMA* 255:82–84.

Shiota K. 1982 Neural tube defects and maternal hyperthermia in early pregnancy: Epidemiology in a human embryo population *Am J Med Genet* 12:281–288.

Shuttleworth G.E. 1909 Mongolian imbecility *Br Med J* 2:661–665.

Shwachman H. and Schuster A. 1956 The tetracyclines: Applied pharmacology *Pediatr Clin North Am* 3:295–303.

Shy C.M. 1979 Epidemiologic evidence and the United States air quality standards *Am J Epidemiol* 110:661–671.

Siegel M. and Furst H.T. 1966 Low birth weight and maternal virus diseases *J Am Med Assn* 197:680–684.

Siegel M. and Greenberg M. 1959 Virus diseases in pregnancy and their effects on the fetus *Am J Obstet Gynecol* 77:620–627.

Siegel M. and Greenberg M. 1960 Fetal death, malformation and prematurity after maternal rubella *New Engl J Med* 262:389–393.

Sigler A.T., Lilienfeld A.M., Cohen B.H., and Westlake J.E. 1965a Radiation exposure in parents of children with mongolism (Down's syndrome) *Bull Johns Hopkins Hosp* 117:374–399.

Sigler A.T., Lilienfield A.M., Cohen B.H., and Westlake J.E. 1965b Parental age in Down's syndrome (mongolism) *Pediatrics* 67:631–642.

Silverman J., Kline J., Hutzler M., Stein Z.A., and Warburton D. 1985 Maternal employment and the chromosomal characteristics of spontaneously aborted conceptions *J Occup Med* 27:427–438.

Simon N.V., Levisky J.S., Siegle J.C., and Shearer D.M. 1984 Evaluation of the dating of gestation via the growth adjusted sonographic age method *J Clin Ultrasound* 12:195–199.

Simpson J.L. 1986 Repetitive spontaneous abortion In I.H. Porter, N.H. Hatcher, and A.M. Wiley, eds. *Perinatal Genetics: Diagnosis and Treatment* Academic Press, Orlando, FL, pp 41–69.

Simpson J.L., Mills J.L., Holmes L.B., Ober C.L., Aarons J., Jovanovic L., and Knopp R.H. 1987 The diabetes in early pregnancy study: Low fetal loss rates after ultrasound-proved viability in early pregnancy *JAMA* 258:2555–2557.

Simpson W.J. 1957 A preliminary report of cigarette smoking and the incidence of prematurity *Am J Obstet Gynecol* 73:808–815.

Sindram I.S. 1945 De invloed van ondervoeding op de groei van de vrucht *Ned T Verlosk* 45:30–48.

Singer J.E., Westphal M., and Niswander K. 1968 Relationship of weight gain during pregnancy to birth weight and infant growth and development in the first year of life. A report for the Collaborative Study of Cerebral Palsy *Obstet Gynecol* 31:417.

Singh R.P. and Carr D.H. 1967 Anatomic findings in human abortions of known chromosomal constitution *Obstet Gynecol* 29:806–818.

Skouteli H.N., Dubowtiz L.M.S., Levene N.I., and Miller G. 1985 Predictors for survival and normal neurodevelopmental outcome of infants weighing less than 1001 grams at birth 1985 *Develop Med Child Neurol* 27:588–595.

Skovron M-L. 1982 Sex differences in human reproductive outcomes. DrPH dissertation, Columbia University School of Public Health, New York.

Smart Y.C., Roberts T.K., Fraser I.S., Cripps A.W., and Clancy R.L. 1982 Validation of the rosete inhibition test for the detection of early pregnancy in women *Fertil Steril* 37:779–785.

Smellie W. 1766 *A Treatise on the Theory and Practice of Midwifery* 3 ed. W. Wilson and T. Durham, London.

Smith C.A. 1947 Effects of wartime starvation in Holland on pregnancy and its products *Am J Obstet Gynecol* 53:599–608.

Smith D.W., Clarren S.K., and Harvey M.A.S. 1978 Hyperthermia as a possible teratogenic agent *J Pediatr* 92:878–883.

Smith J.C., Hughes J.M., Pekow P.S., and Rochat R.W. 1984 An assessment of the incidence of maternal mortality in the United States *Am J Publ Health* 74:780–783.

Smith M.E. and Newcombe H.B. 1980 Automated follow-up facilities in Canada for monitoring delayed health effects *Am J Publ Health* 70:1261–1268.

Smith M.F. and Cameron M.D. 1979 Warfarin as teratogen *Lancet* i:727.

Smithells R.W. 1962 Thalidomide and malformations in Liverpool *Lancet* i:1270–1273.

Smithells R.W. and Leck I. 1963 The incidence of limb and ear defects since the withdrawal of thalidomide *Lancet* i:1095–1097.

Smithells R.W., Sheppard S., Schorah C.J., Seller M.J., Nevin N.C., Harris R., Read A.P., and Fielding D.W. 1980 Possible prevention of neural-tube defects by periconceptional vitamin supplementation *Lancet* i:339–340.

Smithells R.W., Sheppard S., Schorah C.J., Seller M.J., Nevin N.C., Harris R., Read A.P., and Fielding D.W. 1981 Apparent prevention of neural tube defects by periconceptional vitamin supplementation *Arch Dis Child* 56:911–918.

Smithells R.W., Nevin N.C., Seller M.J., Sheppard S., Harris R., Read A.P., Fielding D.W., Walker S., Schorah C.J., and Wild J. 1983 Further experience of vitamin supplementation for prevention of neural tube defect recurrences *Lancet* 1:1027–1031.

Smithells R.W., Sheppard S., Wild J., Schorah C.J., Fielding D.W., Seller M.J., Nevin N.C., Harris R., Read A.P., and Walker S. 1985 Neural-tube defects and vitamins: The need for a randomized clinical trial *Br J Obstet Gynaecol* 92:185–189.

Sokol J.R., Miller S.I., and Reed G. 1980 Alcohol abuse during pregnancy: An epidemiological study *Alcohol Clin Exp Res* 4:135–145.

Sommer A., Tarwotjo I., Hussaini G., and Susanto D. 1983 Increased mortality in children with mild vitamin A deficiency *Lancet* ii:585–588.

Sonek M., Bibbo M., and Wied G.L. 1976 Colposcopic findings in offspring of DES-treated mothers as related to onset of therapy *J Reprod Med* 16:65–71.

Sorsa M., Hemminki K., and Vainio H. 1985 Occupational exposure to anticancer drugs: potential and real hazards *Mut Res* 154:135–149.

Speed R.M. 1977 The effects of ageing on the meiotic chromosomes of male and female mice *Chromosoma* 64:241–254.

Speed R.M. and Chandley A.C. 1983 Meiosis in the foetal mouse ovary. II Oocyte development and age-related aneuploidy. Does a production line exist? *Chromosoma* 88:184–189.

Speirs A.L. 1962 Thalidomide and congenital abnormalities *Lancet* i:303–305.

Spiers P.S. 1982 Does growth retardation predispose the fetus to congenital malformation? *Lancet* i:312–314.

Spinnato J.A., Sibai B.M., Shaver D.C., and Anderson G.D. 1984 Inaccuracy of Dubowitz gestational age in low birth weight infants *Obstet Gynecol* 63:491–493.

Spinner N.B., Eunpu D.L., Schmickel R.D., Zackai E., Bunin G., and Emanuel B.S. 1986 The role of cytologic and molecular NOR variants in trisomy 21 *Am J Hum Genet* 39:A133.

Spranger J.W., Opitz J.M., and Bidder U. 1971 Heterogeneity of chondrodysplasia punctata *Humangenetik* 11:190–212.

Srole L., Langner T.S., Michael T.S., Opler M.K., and Rennie T.A. 1962 *Mental Health in the Metropolis: The Midtown Study* Vol 1, McGraw-Hill, New York.

Stanford J.L., Hartge P., Brinton L.A., Hoover R.N., and Brookmeyer R. 1987 Factors influencing the age at natural menopause *J Chron Dis* 40:995–1002.

Stanley O.H. and Chambers T.L. 1982 Sodium volproate and neural tube defects *Lancet* ii:1282.

Stedman R.L. 1968 The chemical composition of tobacco and tobacco smoke *Chem Rev* 68:153–207.

Steele R. and Langworth J.T. 1966 The relationship of antenatal and postnatal factors to sudden unexpected death in infancy *Can Med Assoc J* 94:1165–1171.

Stein A., Campbell E.A., Day A., McPherson K., and Cooper P.J. 1987 Social adversity, low birth weight, and preterm delivery *Br Med J* 295:291–293.

Stein Z. 1985 A woman's age: Childbearing and child rearing *Am J Epidemiol* 121:327–342.

Stein Z. and Hatch M.C., eds. 1986 *Reproduction and the Workplace* Hanley and Belfus, Philadelphia. *Occupational Medicine* Vol 1.

Stein Z. and Hatch M. 1987 Biological markers in reproductive epidemiology: Prospects and precautions *Environ Health Perspectives* 74:67–75.

Stein Z. and Kline J. 1983 Smoking, alcohol and reproduction (editorial) *Am J Publ Health* 73:1154–1156.

Stein Z. and Susser M. 1958a A study of obstetric results in an underdeveloped community: I. (a) The objects, materials and methods of the study; (b) some comparative rates *J Obstet Gynaecol Br Emp* 65:763–768.

Stein Z. and Susser M. 1958b A study of obstetric results in an underdeveloped community: II. The incidence and importance of certain factors with bearing on obstetric death rates *J Obstet Gynaecol Br Emp* 65:769–773.

Stein Z. and Susser M. 1959a A study of obstetric results in an underdeveloped community: III. The role of the hospital in the prevention of obstetric death *J Obstet Gynaecol Br Emp* 66:62–67.

Stein Z. and Susser M. 1959b A study of obstetric results in an underdeveloped community: IV. The causes and prevention of maternal and obstetric deaths *J Obstet Gynaecol Br Emp* 66:68–74.

Stein Z. and Susser M. W. 1971a Social change and the epidemiology of mental retardation In D.A.A. Primrose, ed. *Proceedings of the International Association for Scientific Study of Mental Deficiency*, Polish Medical Publishers, Warsaw, pp 659–663.

Stein Z. and Susser M. 1971b The preventability of Down's syndrome (mongolism) *Publ Health Rep* 86:650–658.

Stein Z. and Susser M. 1972 The Cuban health system: A trial of a comprehensive service in a poor country *Int J Health Serv* 2:551–566.

Stein Z. and Susser M. 1978 Epidemiologic and genetic issues in mental retardation In N.E. Morton and C.S. Chung, eds. *Genetic Epidemiology* Academic Press, New York, pp 415–461.

Stein Z. and Susser M. 1980 Prenatal diet and reproductive loss In I.H. Porter and E.B. Hook, eds. *Human Embryonic and Fetal Death* Academic Press, New York, pp 183–196.

Stein Z., Susser M., Saenger G., and Marolla F. 1975a *Famine and Human Development: The Dutch Hunger Winter of 1944–45,* Oxford University Press, New York.

Stein Z., Susser M., and Sturmans F. 1975b Famine and mortality *Tijdschrift voor Soc Geneeskunde* 53:134–141.

Stein Z., Susser M., Warburton D., Wittes J., and Kline J. 1975c Spontaneous abortion as a screening device: The effect of fetal survival on the incidence of birth defects *Am J Epidemiol* 102:275–290.

Stein Z., Susser M., Kline J., and Warburton D. 1977 Amniocentesis and selective abortion for trisomy 21 in the light of the natural history of pregnancy and fetal survival In E.B. Hook and I.H. Porter, eds. *Population Cytogenetics Studies in Humans,* Academic Press, New York, pp 257–274.

Stein Z., Kline J., Susser E., Shrout P., Warburton D., and Susser M. 1980 Maternal age and spontaneous abortion In I.H. Porter and E.B. Hook, eds. *Human Embryonic and Fetal Death* Academic Press, New York, pp 107–127.

Stein Z., Hatch M., Kline J., Shrout P., and Warburton D. 1981a Epidemiologic considerations in assessing health effects at toxic waste sites In W. Lowrance, ed. *Assessment of Health Effects at Chemical Disposal Sites* William Kaufman, Los Altos, CA, pp 126–145.

Stein Z., Kline J., Levin B., Susser M., and Warburton D. 1981b Epidemiologic studies of environmental exposures in human reproduction In G.C. Berg and H.D. Maillie, eds. *Measurement of Risks* Plenum Publishing Corporation, New York, pp 163–188.

Stein Z., Kline J., and Kharrazi M. 1984a What is a teratogen? Epidemiologic criteria In H. Kalter, ed. *Issues and Reviews in Teratology*, Vol 2, Plenum Publishing Corporation, New York, pp 23–66.

Stein Z., Warburton D., and Kline J. 1984b Epidemiology of chromosome anomalies and other malformations in spontaneous abortion In K. Hemminki, M. Sorsa, and H. Vainio, eds. *Occupational Hazards and Reproduction* Hemisphere Publishing Corporation, Washington, D.C., pp 163–173.

Stein Z., Kline J., and Shrout P. 1984c Power in surveillance In K. Hemminki, M. Sorsa, and H. Vainio, eds. *Occupational Hazards and Reproduction* Hemisphere Publishing Corporation, Washington, D.C., pp 203–208.

Stein Z., Stein W., and Susser M. 1986 Attrition of trisomies as a screening device: An explanation for the association of trisomy 21 with maternal age *Lancet* ii:944–946.

Stene J. 1970 Detection of higher recurrence risk for age-dependent chromosome abnormalities with an application to trisomy G (Down's syndrome) *Hum Heredity* 20:112–122.

Stene J. and Warburton D. 1981 Evidence for smaller probabilities for trisomic mosaicism for acrocentric than for nonacrocentric chromosomes *Am J Hum Genet* 33:484–485.

Stene J., Stene E., Stengel-Rutkowski S., and Murken J.D. 1981 Paternal age and Down's syndrome: Data from prenatal diagnoses (DFG) *Hum Genet* 59:119–124.

Stene J., Stene E., and Mikkelsen M. 1984 Risk for chromosome abnormality at amniocentesis following a child with a non-inherited chromosome aberration *Prenatal Diag* 4:81–95.

Stevenson A.C., Dudgeon N.Y., and McClure H.I. 1959 Observations on the results of pregnancies in women resident in Belfast. II. Abortions, hydatidiform moles and ectopic pregnancies *Ann Hum Genet* 23:395–414.

Stevenson A.C., Mason R., and Edwards K.D. 1970 Maternal diagnostic X-irradiation before conception and the frequency of mongolism in children subsequently born *Lancet* ii:1335–1337.

Stevenson R.E., Burton O.M., Ferlauto G.J., and Taylor H.A. 1980 Hazards of oral anticoagulants during pregnancy *JAMA* 243:1549–1551.

Stewart A., Webb J., and Hewitt D.A. 1958 A survey of childhood malignancies *Br Med J* 1:1445–1508.

Stewart G.D., Hassold T.J., Berg A., Watkins P., Tanzi R., and Kurnit D. 1988 Trisomy 21 (Down syndrome): Studying nondisjunction and meiotic recombination by using cytogenetic and molecular polymorphisms that span chromosome 21 *Am J Hum Genet* 42:227–236.

Stewart G.L., Parkman P.D., Hopps H.E., Douglas R.D., Hamilton J.P., and Meyer H.M., Jr. 1967 Rubella-virus hemagglutination-inhibition test *N Engl J Med* 276:554–557.

Stockard C.L. 1921 Developmental rate and structural expression: An experimental study of twins, double monsters and single deformities, and the interaction among embryonic organs during their origin and development *Am J Anat* 28:115–266.

Stott D.H. 1961 Mongolism related to emotional shock in early pregnancy *Vita Humanae* 4:57–76.

Strandberg M., Sandback K., Axelson O., and Sundell L. 1978 Spontaneous abortions among women in a hospital laboratory *Lancet* i:384–385.

Streeter G.L. 1920 Weight, sitting height, head size, foot length and menstrual age of the human embryo *Contrib Embryol* 11:143–170.

Strobino B.R., Kline J., and Stein Z. 1978 Chemical and physical exposures of parents: Effects on human reproduction and offspring *Early Hum Dev* 1:371–399.

Strobino B.R., Kline J., and Stein Z. 1979 Chemical and physical exposures of parents: Effects on human reproduction and offspring *Birth Defects Reprint Series,* The National Foundation, March of Dimes, White Plains, NY.

Strobino B., Kline J., Stein Z., Susser M., and Warburton D. 1980a Exposure to contraceptive creams, jellies and douches and their effect on the zygote *Am J Epidemiol* 112:434.

Strobino B.R., Kline J., Shrout P., Stein Z., Susser M., and Warburton D. 1980b Recurrent spontaneous abortion: Definition of a syndrome In I.H. Porter and E.B. Hook, eds. *Human Embryonic and Fetal Death* Academic Press, New York, pp 315–329.

Strobino B., Fox H., Kline J., Stein Z., Susser M., and Warburton D. 1986a Characteristics of women with recurrent spontaneous abortions and women with favorable reproductive histories *Am J Publ Health* 76:986–991.

Strobino B., Kline J., Lai A., Stein Z., Susser M., and Warburton D. 1986b Vaginal spermicide exposure and spontaneous abortions of known karyotype *Am J Epidemiol* 123:431–443.

Strobino D.M. 1987 The health and medical consequences of adolescent sexuality and pregnancy: A review of the literature. Risking the Future, Vol II, Ch. 5, National Research Council, National Academy Press, Washington, D.C.

Stubbs S.M., Doddridge M.C., John P.N., Steel J.M., and Wright A.D. 1987 Haemoglobin A and congenital malformation *Diabetic Med* 4:156–159.

Sulaiman N.D., Florey C.V., Taylor D.J., and Ogston S.A. 1988 Alcohol consumption in Dundee primigravidas and its effects on outcome of pregnancy *Br Med J* 296:1500–1503.

Susser E. 1983 Spontaneous abortion and induced abortion: An adjustment for the presence of induced abortion when estimating the rate of spontaneous abortion from cross-sectional studies *Am J Epidemiol* 117:305–308.

Susser E. and Kline J. 1984 Effects of induced abortion on spontaneous abortion rates. In K. Hemminki, M. Sorsa, and H. Vainio, eds. *Occupational Hazards and Reproduction,* Hemisphere Publishing, New York, pp 209–217.

Susser I. 1985 Union Carbide and the community surrounding it: The case of a community in Puerto Rico *Intl J Health Ser* 15:561–583.

Susser M. 1968 *Community Psychiatry: Epidemiologic and Social Themes* Random House, New York.

Susser M. 1971 The public health and social change: Implications for professional education in public health in the United States *Int J Health Serv* 1:60–70.

Susser M. 1973 *Causal Thinking in the Health Sciences: Concepts and Strategies in Epidemiology* Oxford University Press, New York.

Susser M. 1976 Psychiatric registers and community mental health services. In B.H. Kaplan, R.N. Wilson, and A.H. Leighton, eds. *Further Explorations in Social Psychiatry* Basic Books, New York, pp 40–79.

Susser M. 1981 Prenatal nutrition, birthweight, and psychological development: An overview of experiments and quasi-experiments in the past decade *Am J Clin Nutr* 34:784–803.

Susser M. 1984 Causal thinking in practice: Strengths and weaknesses of the clinical vantage point *Pediatrics* 74:842–849.

Susser M. 1985 Epidemiology in the United States after World War II: The evolution of technique *Epidemiol Rev* 7:147–177.

Susser M. 1986 The logic of Sir Karl Popper and the practice of epidemiology *Am J Epidemiol* 124:711–718.

Susser M. 1987 Falsification, verification, and causal inference in epidemiology: Reconsiderations in the light of Sir Karl Popper's philosophy In M. Susser *Epidemiology, Health, & Society,* Oxford University Press, New York, pp 82–93.

Susser M.W. and Stein Z.A. 1982 Third variable analysis: Application to causal sequences among nutrient intake, maternal weight, birthweight, placental weight, and gestation *Stat Med* 1:105–120.

Susser M., Marolla F.M., and Fleiss J. 1972 Birthweight, fetal age and perinatal mortality *Am J Epidemiol* 96:197–204.

Susser M., Hauser W.A., Kiely J.L., Paneth N., and Stein Z. 1985a Quantitative estimates of prenatal and perinatal risk factors for perinatal mortality, cerebral palsy, mental retardation, and epilepsy In J.M. Freeman, ed. *Prenatal and Perinatal Factors Associated with Brain Disorders,* NIH Publication, No. 85-1149, pp 359–439.

Susser M.W., Watson W., and Hopper K. 1985b *Sociology in Medicine* Oxford University Press, New York.

Sutherland G.R., Bauld R., and Bain A.D. 1974 Chromosome abnormality and perinatal death *Lancet* i:752.

Sutherland G.R., Carter R.F., Bauld R., Smith I.I., and Bain A.D. 1978 Chromosome studies at the paediatric necropsy *Ann Hum Genet* 42:173–181.

Swallow J.N. 1964 Discoloration of primary dentition after maternal tetracycline ingestion in pregnancy *Lancet* ii:611–612.

Swan C. and Tostevin A.L. 1964 Congenital abnormalities in infants following infectious diseases during pregnancy, with special reference to rubella: A third series of cases *Med J Austr* 1:645–659.

Szmuness W. 1978 Hepatocellular carcinoma and the hepatitis B virus: Evidence for a causal association *Prog Med Virol* 24:40–69.

Taback M. 1951 Birth weight and length of gestation with relation to prematurity *JAMA* 146:897–901.

Tafari N., Naeye R.L., and Gobezie A. 1980 Effects of maternal undernutrition and heavy physical work during pregnancy on birth weight *Br J Obstet Gynaecol* 87:222–226.

Takahara H., Ohama K., and Fujiwara A. 1977 Cytogenetic study in early spontaneous abortion *Hiroshima J Med Sci* 26:291–296.

Takemori S., Tanaka Y., and Suzuki J. 1976 Thalidomide anomalies of the ear *Arch Otolaryngol* 102:425–427.

Tanner J.M. 1962 *Growth at Adolescence* 2 ed. Blackwell Scientific Publications, London.

Tanner J.M., Lejarraga H., and Turner G. 1972 Within-family standards for birth-weight *Lancet* ii:193–197.

Taussig F.J. 1936 *Abortion: Spontaneous and Induced, Medical and Social Aspects,* C.V. Mosby Co., St. Louis.

Taylor C. and Faulk W.P. 1981 Prevention of recurrent abortion with leucocyte transfusions *Lancet* ii:68–70.

Taylor W.F. 1964 On the methodology of measuring the probability of fetal death in a prospective study *Hum Biol* 36:86–103.

Taylor W.F. 1969 The probability of fetal death In F.C. Fraser and V.A. McKusick, eds. *Congenital Malformations,* Excerpta Medica, New York, pp 307–320.

Tejani N. 1973 Anticoagulant therapy with cardiac valve prosthesis during pregnancy *Obstet Gynecol* 42:785–793.

Tennes K. and Blackard C. 1980 Maternal alcohol consumption, birth weight, and minor physical anomalies *Am J Obstet Gynecol* 138:774–780.

Testart J., Lassalle B., Frydman R., and Belaisch J.C. 1983 A study of factors affecting the success of human fertilization in vitro. I. Influence of semen quality and oocyte maturity on fertilization and cleavage *Biol Reprod* 28:425–431.

Thacker S.B. 1985 Quality of controlled clinical trials. The case of imaging ultrasound in obstetrics: A review *Br J Obstet Gynaecol* 92:437–444.

Thaul S. 1988 Preventing preterm delivery: Testing the effectiveness of a prenatal care intervention for high risk black and hispanic women. PhD dissertation, Columbia University, New York.

Theriault G., Iturra H., and Gingras S. 1983 Evaluation of the association between birth defects and exposure to ambient vinyl chloride *Teratology* 27:359–370.

Thiersch J.B. 1952 Therapeutic abortions with a folic acid antagonist, 4 aminopteroylglutamic acid (4-amino P.G.A.) administered by the oral route *Am J Obstet Gynecol* 63:1298–1304.

Thomson A.M. 1983 Fetal growth and size at birth In S.L. Barron and A.M. Thomson, eds. *Obstetrical Epidemiology,* Academic Press, London, pp 89–142.

Thomson A.M. and Billewicz W.Z. 1961 Height, weight and food intake in man *Br J Nutr* 15:241–252.

Thomson A.M., Billewicz W.Z., and Hytten F.E. 1968 The Assessment of Fetal Growth *J Obstet Gynaec Br Cwlth* 75:903–916.

Thomson A.W., Milton J.I., Campbell D.M., and Horne C.H.W. 1980 Rosette inhibition levels during early human gestation *J Reprod Immunol* 2:263–268.

Tietze C. 1957 Reproductive span and rate of reproduction among Hutterite women *Fertil Steril* 8:89–97.

Tijo J.H. and Levan A. 1956 Chromosome number of man *Hereditas* 42:1–6.

Tinneberg H.R., Staves R.P., and Semm K. 1984 Improvement of the rosette inhibition assay for the detection of early pregnancy factor in humans using the monoclonal antibody, anti-human-lyt-3 *Am J Reprod Immunol* 5:151–156.

Tizard J. 1964 *Community Services for the Mentally Handicapped* Oxford, London.

Tokuhata G.K. 1968 Smoking in relation to infertility and fetal loss *Arch Environ Health* 17:353–359.

Tomatis L. 1979 Prenatal exposure to chemical carcinogens and its effect on subsequent generations *Natl Ca Inst Monogr* 51:159–184.

Tomlin P.J. 1979 Health problems of anaesthetists and their families in the West Midlands *Br Med J* 1:779–784.

Torday J.S., Nielsen H.C., Fencl M. de M., and Avery M.E. 1981 Sex differences in fetal lung maturation *Am Rev Resp Dis* 123:205–208.

Toth P., Keszei K., and Mehes K. 1983 Maternal regulation of fetal growth *Acta Paediatr Hungarica* 24:37–40.

Totterman L.E. and Saxen L. 1969 Incorporation of tetracycline into human foetal bones after maternal drug administration *Acta Obstet Gynaecol Scand* 48:542–549.

Toussie S. 1986 Epidemiologic aspects of immune response in pregnancy: Total and active rosette forming T-cells in liveborn pregnancy and spontaneous abortion. PhD Dissertation, Columbia University, New York.

Tow A. 1937 *Diseases of the Newborn* Oxford University Press, New York.

Trasler J.M., Hales B.F., and Robaire B. 1985 Paternal cyclophosphamide treatment of rats causes fetal loss and malformations without affecting male fertility *Nature* 316:144–146.

Treloar A.E., Boynton R.E., Behn B.G., and Brown B.W. 1967a Variation of the human menstrual cycle through reproductive life *Int J Fertil* 12:77–126.

Treloar A.E., Behn B.G., and Cowan D.W. 1967b Analysis of gestational interval *Am J Obstet Gynecol* 99:34–45.

Trounson A.O., Mohr L.R., Wood C., and Leeton J.F. 1982 Effect of delayed insemination on in-vitro fertilization, culture and transfer of human embryos *J Reprod Fertil* 64:285–294.

Uchida I.A. and Curtis E.J. 1961 A possible association between maternal radiation and mongolism *Lancet* ii:848–850.

Uchida I.A. and Freeman V.C.P. 1985 Trisomy 21 Down Syndrome *Hum Genet* 70:246–248.

Uchida I.A., Holunga R., and Lawler C. 1968 Maternal radiation and chromosomal aberrations *Lancet* ii:1045–1049.

Ulrich M. 1982 Fetal growth patterns in a population of Danish newborn infants *Acta Paediatr Scand* 292(Suppl):5–45.

Udani P.M. 1963 Physical growth of children in different socioeconomic groups in Bombay *Ind J Child Health* 12:593–611.

Underwood P., Hester L.L., Laffitte T., Jr., and Gregg K.V. 1965 The relationship of smoking to the outcome of pregnancy *Am J Obstet Gynecol* 91:270–276.

Underwood P.B., Kesler K.F., O'Lane J.M., and Callagan D.A. 1967 Parental smoking empirically related to pregnancy outcome *Obstet Gynecol* 29:1–8.

Unger C., Weiser J.K., McCullough R.E., Keefer S., and Moore L.G. 1988 Altitude, low birth weight, and infant mortality in Colorado *JAMA* 259:3427–3432.

Unger J. 1965 Weight at birth and its effect on survival of the newborn. Vital and Health Statistics, Series 21, No. 4, U.S.D.H.E.W.

Radiation Effects Research Foundation. 1987 *U.S.-Japan Joint Reassessment of Atomic Bomb Radiation Dosimetry in Hiroshima and Nagasaki* Final Report, Hiroshima, Japan.

U.S. Public Health Service. 1950 *International recommendations on definitions of live birth and fetal death* National Office of Vital Statistics PHS Pub No. 39, Washington, D.C., pp 1–11.

U.S. Public Health Service. 1964 *Smoking and Health* Report of the Advisory Committee to the Surgeon General of the Public Health Service. U.S. Department of Health, Education and Welfare, Public Health Service, Center for Disease Control, PHS Publication No. 1103.

U.S. Public Health Service. 1971 *The Health Consequences of Smoking* A Report of the Surgeon General. U.S. Department of Health, Education and Welfare, DHEW Publication No. (HSM) 71-7513, pp 389–407.

U.S. Public Health Service. 1979 *Smoking and Health* A Report of the Surgeon General. U.S. Department of Health, Education and Welfare, DHEW Publication No. (PHS) 79-50066, Chapter 14.

Ursell P., Byrne J., and Strobino B. 1985 Significance of cardiac defects in the developing fetus: A study of spontaneous abortuses *Circulation* 72:1232–1236.

Usher R., McLean F., and Scott K.E. 1966 Judgment of fetal age. II. Clinical significance of gestational age and an objective method for its assessment *Pediatr Clin North Am* 13:835–848.

Vaisman A.I. 1967 Work in operating theatres and its effect on the health of anaesthetists *Experiment Khirur* 12:44–49.

Vaitukaitis J.L., Braunstein G.D., and Ross G.T. 1972 A radioimmunoassay which specifically measures human chorionic gonadotropin in the presence of human luteinizing hormone *Am J Obstet Gynecol* 113:751–758.

Van Dobben de Bruyn, C.S. 1968 *Cumulative Sum Tests: Theory and Practice,* Hafner Publishing Co., New York.

Van Valen L. and Mellin G.W. 1967 Selection in natural populations. 7. New York babies *Ann Hum Genet* 31:109–127.

Vessey M.P., Doll R., Johnson B., and Peto R. 1974 Outcome of pregnancy in women using an intrauterine device *Lancet* i:495–498.

Vessey M.P., Meisler L., Flavel R., and Yeates D. 1979 Outcome of pregnancy in women using different methods of contraception *Br J Obstet Gynaecol* 86:548–556.

Vessey M.P. and Nunn J.F. 1980 Occupational hazards of anaesthesia *Br Med J* 281:696–698.

Vianna N.J. 1980 Adverse pregnancy outcomes—potential endpoints of human toxicity in the Love Canal preliminary results. In I.H. Porter and E.B. Hook, eds. *Human Embryonic and Fetal Death* Academic Press, New York pp 165–168.

Vianna N. and Polan K. 1984 Incidence of low birthweight in Love Canal residents *Science* 226:1217–1219.

Viegas O.A.C., Scott P.H., Cole T.J., Eaton P., Needham P.G., and Wharton B.A. 1982 Dietary protein energy supplementation of pregnant Asian mothers at Sorrento, Birmingham: II. Selective during third trimester only *Br Med J* 285:592–595.

Villar J. and Belizan J.M. 1982a The relative contribution of prematurity and fetal growth retardation to low birth weight in developing and developed societies *Am J Obstet Gynecol* 143:793–798.

Villar J. and Belizan J.M. 1982b The timing factor in the pathophysiology of the intrauterine growth retardation syndrome *Obstet Gynecol Surv* 37:499–506.

Villar J. and Gonzalez-Cossio T. 1986 Nutritional factors associated with low birth weight and short gestational age *Clin Nutr* 5:78–85.

Villar J., Smeriglio V., Martorell R., Brown C.H., and Klein R.E. 1984 Heterogeneous growth and mental development of intrauterine growth-retarded infants during the first 3 years of life *Pediatrics* 74:783–791.

Villar J., Khoury M.J., Finucane F.F., and Delgado H.L. 1986 Differences in the epidemiology of prematurity and intrauterine growth retardation *Early Hum Dev* 14:307–320.

Villar J., Klebanoff M., Kester E. 1988 Intestinal parasitism and fetal growth retardation *Am Public Health Assoc* (Abstract).

Vincent L. 1961 Some data on natural fertility *Eugenics Quart* 8:81–91.

Vincent P. 1950 La stérilité physiologique des populations *Population* 5:45–64.

Visaria P.M. 1967 Sex ratio at birth in territories with a relatively complete registration *Eugen Quart* 14:132–142.

Vitez M., Korany G., Gonczy E., Rudas T., and Czeizel A. 1984 A semiquantitative score system for epidemiologic studies of fetal alcohol syndrome *Am J Epidemiol* 119:301–308.

von Recklinghausen F.D. 1886 Untersuchungen uber die Spina bifida *Virchows Arch Pathol Anat Physiol* 105:243–330.

Wagenbichler P., Killian W., Rett A., and Schnedl W. 1976 Origin of the extra chromosome No. 21 in Down's syndrome *Hum Genet* 32:13–16.

Wald N., Turner H., and Borges W. 1970 Down's syndrome and exposure to X-irradiation *Ann NY Acad Sci* 171:454–467.

Wald N.J. and Polani P.E. 1984 Neural-tube defects and vitamins: The need for a randomized clinical trial *Br J Obstet Gynaecol* 9:516–523.

Walker B.E. 1984 Transplacental exposure to diethylstilbestrol. In H. Kalter, ed. *Issues and Reviews in Teratology* Vol 2, Plenum Press, New York, pp 157–187.

Walther F.J. and Ramaekers L.H.J. 1982 Neonatal morbidity of S.G.A. infants in relation to their nutritional status at birth *Acta Paediatr Scand* 71:437–440.

Walton A. and Hammond J. 1938 The maternal effects on growth and conformation in Shire horse-Shetland pony crosses *Proc Royal Soc, B* 125:311–335.

Warburton D. 1983 Parental age and X-chromosome aneuploidy In A.A. Sandberg, ed. *Cytogenetics of the Mammalian X-chromosome Part B. X-Chromosome Anomalies and Their Clinical Manifestations* Alan R. Liss, New York, pp 23–36.

Warburton D. 1985a Genetic factors influencing aneuploidy frequency In V. Dellarco, P. Voytek, and A. Hollaender, eds. *Aneuploidy: Etiology and Mechanisms* Plenum Press, New York, pp 133–148.

Warburton D. 1985b Effects of common environmental exposures on spontaneous abortion of defined karyotype In M. Marois, ed. *Prevention of Physical and Mental Congenital Defects, Part C: Basic and Medical Science, Education and Future Strategies,* Alan R. Liss, New York, pp 31–36.

Warburton D. and Byrne J. 1986 Estimates of the prevalence of chromosome anomalies expected in chorionic villus sampling procedures In B. Brambati, G. Simoni and S. Fabro, eds. *Chorionic Villus Sampling: Fetal Diagnosis of Genetic Diseases in the First Trimester* New York, Marcel Dekker, pp 23–30.

Warburton D. and Fraser F.C. 1964 Spontaneous abortion risks in man: Data from reproductive histories collected in a medical genetics unit *Am J Hum Genet* 16:1–24.

Warburton D. and Naylor A.F. 1971 The effect of parity on placental weight and birth weight: An immunological phenomenon? A report of the collaborative study of cerebral palsy *Am J Hum Genet* 23:41–54.

Warburton D. and Strobino B. 1987 Recurrent spontaneous abortion In M.J. Bennett and D.K. Edmonds, eds. *Spontaneous and Recurrent Abortion,* Blackwell Scientific Publications, Oxford.

Warburton D., Yu C., Kline J., and Stein Z. 1978 Mosaic autosomal trisomy in cultures from spontaneous abortions *Am J Hum Genet* 30:609–617.

Warburton D., Susser M., Stein Z., and Kline J. 1979 Genetic and epidemiologic investigation of spontaneous abortion: Relevance to clinical practice The National Foundation, White Plains, NY. *Birth Defects: Original Article Series* XV: 5A:127–136.

Warburton D., Kline J., Stein Z., and Susser M. 1980 Monosomy X: A chromosomal anomaly associated with young maternal age *Lancet* i:167–169.

Warburton D., Stein Z., Kline J., and Susser M. 1980 Chromosome abnormalities in spontaneous abortions: Data from the New York study In I.H. Porter and E.B. Hook, eds. *Human Embryonic and Fetal Death,* Academic Press, New York, pp 261–287.

Warburton D., Stein Z., and Kline J. 1983a Epidemiological approach to human reproductive failure assessment In V.B. Vouk and P.J. Sheehan, eds. *Methods to Assess the Effects of Chemicals on Reproductive Function,* John Wiley & Sons, New York, pp 199–216.

Warburton D., Stein Z., and Kline J. 1983b In utero selection against fetuses with trisomy *Am J Hum Genet* 35:1059–1064.

Warburton D., Kline J., Stein Z., and Strobino B. 1986 Cytogenetic abnormalities in spontaneous abortions of recognized conceptions In I.H. Porter, N.H. Hatcher and A.M. Willey, eds. *Perinatal Genetics: Diagnosis and Treatment* Academic Press, New York, pp 23–40.

Warburton D., Kline J., Stein Z., Hutzler M., Chin A., and Hassold T. 1987a Does the karyotype of a spontaneous abortion predict the karyotype of a subsequent abortion? Evidence from 273 women with two karyotyped spontaneous abortions *Am J Hum Genet* 41:465–483.

Warburton D., Neugut R., Lustenberger A., Nicholas A., and Kline J. 1987b

Lack of association between spermicide use and trisomy *N Engl J Med* 317:478–482.

Ward W.P. and Ward P.C. 1984 Infant birth weight and nutrition in industrializing Montreal *Am Hist Rev* 89:324–345.

Wardenburg P.J. 1932 Das menschliche Auge und seine Erbanlagen The Hague

Warkany J. 1975 A warfarin embryopathy? *Am J Dis Child* 129:287–288.

Warkany J. 1977 History of teratology In J.G. Wilson and F.C. Fraser, eds. *Handbook of Teratology*, Vol 1, Plenum Press, New York, pp 3–45.

Warkany J. 1986 Teratogen update: Hyperthermia *Teratology* 33:365–371.

Warkany J., Monroe B.B., and Sutherland B.S. 1961 Intrauterine growth retardation *Am J Dis Child* 102:249–279.

Warren A.C., Chakravarti A., Wong C., Slaugenhaupt S.A., Halloran S.L., Watkins E.C., Metaxotou C., and Antonarakis S.E. 1987 Evidence for reduced recombination on the nondisjoined chromosomes 21 in Down syndrome *Science* 237:652–654.

Watanabe G. 1979 Environmental determinants of birth defects prevalence In M.A. Klingberg and J.A.C. Weatherall, eds. *Epidemiologic Methods for Detection of Teratogens*, Karger, New York, pp 91–100.

Watkins R.N. 1986 Vaginal spermicides and congenital disorders: The validity of a study *JAMA* 256:3095.

Watson G.I., Slater B.C.S., and McDonald J.C. 1962 Maternal health and congenital deformity *Br Med J* 1:793.

Weatherall J.A.C. and Haskey I.C. 1976 Surveillance of malformations *Br Med Bull* 32:39–44.

Weatherall J.A.C. and White G.C. 1976 A study of survival of children with spina bifida In *Child Health: A Collection of Studies* OPCS Studies on Medical and Population Subjects, No 31, Her Majesty's Stationery Office, London, pp 1–11.

Wedeen R.P. 1984 *Poison in the pot: The legacy of lead*, Southern Illinois University Press, Carbondale.

Weg R.B., ed. 1983 *Sexuality in the Later Years: Roles and Behaviour* Academic Press, New York.

Wehmann R.E., Harman S.M., Birken S., Canfield R.E., and Nisula B.C. 1981 Convenient radioimmunoassay for urinary human choriogonadotropin without interference by urinary human lutropin *Clin Chem* 27:1997–2001.

Weicker V.H., Bachmann K.D., Pfeiffer R.A., and Gliess J. 1962 Thalidomide embryopathie *Dtsch Med Wochenschr* 87:1597–1607.

Weinstock M.A. 1982 Cigarette yield and the outcome of pregnancy PhD Dissertation, Columbia University, New York.

Weiss W. and Jackson E.C. 1969 Maternal factors affecting birthweight In *Perinatal Factors Affecting Human Development*, Scientific Publication No 185, 54, Pan American Health Organization, Washington, D.C.

Weller T.H. and Neva F.A. 1962 Propagation in tissue culture of cytopathic agents from patients with rubella-like illness (27749) *Soc Exp Biol Med* 111:215–225.

Wertheim I., Jagiello G.M., and Ducayen M.B. 1986 Aging and aneuploidy in human oocytes and follicular cells *J Gerontol* 41:567–573.

Westerholm P. and Ericson A. 1987 Pregnancy outcome and VDU-work in a cohort of insurance clerks. IN B. Knave and P-G. Wideback. *Selected Papers: International Scientific Conference on Work with Display Units, Stockholm, Sweden* Elsevier, New York, pp 104–110.

Westrom L. 1980 Incidence, prevalence, and trends of acute pelvic inflammatory disease and its consequences in industrialized countries *Am J Obstet Gynecol* 138:880–892.

Whitehead R.G., Rowland M.G.M., Hutton M., Prentice A.M., Muller E., and Paul A. 1978 Factors influencing lactation performance in rural Gambian mothers *Lancet* ii:178–181.

Whitfield M.F. 1980 Chondrodysplasia punctata after warfarin in early pregnancy. Case report and summary of the literature *Arch Dis Child* 55:139–142.

Whittaker P.G., Taylor A., and Lind T. 1983 Unsuspected pregnancy loss in healthy women *Lancet* i:1126–1127.

Whittle B.A. 1976 Pre-clinical teratological studies on sodium valproate (Epilim) and other anticonvulsants In N.J. Legg, ed. *Clinical and Pharmacological Aspects of Sodium Valproate (Epilim) in the Treatment of Epilepsy*, MCS Consultants, London, pp 105–111.

Whyte A. and Heap R.B. 1983 Early pregnancy factor *Nature* 304:121–122.

Whorton M.D., Krauss R.M., Marshall S., and Milby T.H. 1977 Infertility in male pesticide workers *Lancet* ii:1259–1261.

Wiedemann H.R. 1961 Hinweis auf eine derzeitige Haufung hypo- und aplastischer Fehlbildungen der Gliedmassen *Med Welt* 37:1884–1887.

Wiener G. and Milton T. 1970 Demographic correlates of low birth weight *Am J Epidemiol* 91:260–272.

Wigglesworth J.S. 1964 Experimental growth retardation in the foetal rat *J Path Bacteriol* 88:1–13.

Wilcox A.J. 1983 Intrauterine growth retardation: Beyond birthweight criteria *Early Hum Dev* 8:189–193.

Wilcox A.J. and Gladen B.C. 1982 Spontaneous abortion: The role of heterogeneous risk and selective fertility *Early Hum Develop* 7:165–178.

Wilcox A.J. and Russell I.T. 1983a Perinatal mortality: Standardizing for birthweight is biased *Am J Epidemiol* 118:857–864.

Wilcox A.J. and Russell I.T. 1983b Birthweight and perinatal mortality: I. On the frequency distribution of birthweight *Int J Epidemiol* 12:314–318.

Wilcox A.J. and Russell I.T. 1983c Birthweight and perinatal mortality: II. On weight-specific mortality *Int J Epidemiol* 12:319–325.

Wilcox A.J. and Russell I.T. 1986 Birthweight and perinatal mortality. III. Towards a new method of analysis *Int J Epidemiol* 15:188–196.

Wilcox A.J., Weinberg C.R., Wehmann R.E., Armstrong E.G., Canfield R.E., and Nisula B.C. 1985 Measuring early pregnancy loss: Laboratory and field methods *Fertil Steril* 44:366–374.

Wilcox A.J., Weinberg C.R., Armstrong E.G., and Canfield R.E. 1987 Urinary human chorionic gonadotropin among intrauterine device users: Detection with a highly specific and sensitive assay *Fertil Steril* 47:265–269.

Wilcox A.J., Weinberg C.R., O'Connor J.F., Baird D.D., Schlatterer J.P., Canfield R.E., Armstrong E.G., and Nisula B.C. 1988 Incidence of early loss of pregnancy *New Engl J Med* 319:189–194.

Wild J., Read A.P., Sheppard S., Selles M.J., Smithells R.W., Nevin N.C., Schotah C.J., Fielding D.W., Walker S., and Harris R. 1986 Recurrent neural tube defects, risk factors and vitamins *Arch Dis Child* 61:440–444.

Wilkins L. 1957 *The Diagnosis and Treatment of Endocrine Disorders in Childhood and Adolescence* 2 ed. Charles C Thomas, Springfield, IL, pp 276–283.

Wilkins L., Jones H.W., Holman G.H., and Stempfel R.S., Jr. 1958 Masculinization of the female fetus associated with administration of oral and intramuscular progestins during gestation: Non-adrenal female pseudohermaphrodism *J Clin Endocrinol* 18:559–585.

Williams J.H. 1984 Employment in pregnancy *Lancet* ii:103–104.

Willughby P. 1972 *Observations in midwifery* SR Publishers, Wakefield. p 254.

Wilson J.G. 1973 *Environment and Birth Defects* Academic Press, New York, pp 4–8.

Wilson J.G. 1977 Embryotoxicity of drugs in man In J.G. Wilson and F.C. Fraser, eds. *Handbook of Teratology*, Vol 1, Plenum Press, New York, pp 309–355.

Winikoff B. and Debrovner C.H. 1981 Anthropometric determinants of birth weight *Obstet Gynecol* 58:678–684.

Wise P.M. 1983 Aging of the female reproductive system *Rev Biol Res Aging* 1:195–222.

Wood J.W., Johnson K.G., and Omori Y. 1967a In utero exposure to the Hiroshima atomic bomb. An evaluation of head size and mental retardation: Twenty years later *Pediatrics* 39:385–392.

Wood J.W., Johnson K.G., Omori Y., Kawamoto S., and Keehn R.J. 1967b Mental retardation in children exposed in utero to the atomic bombs in Hiroshima and Nagasaki *Am J Publ Health* 58:1381–1390.

World Health Organization 1950 *Expert Group on Prematurity. Final Report*, Technical Report, Series 27, Geneva.

World Health Organization 1965 Expert Committee on Eclampsia Special Technical Report, No. 302, Geneva.

World Health Organization 1967 Principles for the testing of drugs for teratogenicity: Report of a WHO scientific group *WHO Tech Rep Ser* 364:1–18.

World Health Organization 1970 Spontaneous and induced abortion WHO Technical Report, Series No. 461, Geneva, pp 1–51.

World Health Organization 1977 Recommended definitions, terminology and format for statistical tables related to the perinatal period and use of a new certificate for cause of perinatal deaths (modifications recommended by FIGO as amended October 14, 1976) *Acta Obstet Gynaecol Scand* 56:247–253.

World Health Organization 1978 *Social and Biological Effects on Perinatal Mortality*, Vol 2, Geneva.

World Health Organization, Division of Family Health 1980 The incidence of low birth weight: A clinical review of available information *W Health Stat Q* 33:197.

World Health Organization 1985 *Report of Interregional Meeting on Maternal Mortality*, Geneva, pp 11–15.

World Health Organization 1986 Maternal mortality: Helping women off the road to death *WHO Chron* 40:175–183.

Working party to discuss nomenclature based on gestational age and birthweight 1970 *Arch Dis Child* 45:730.

Wramsby H., Fredga K., and Liedholm P. 1987 Chromosome analysis of human oocytes recovered from preovulatory follicles in stimulated cycles *N Engl J Med* 316:121–124.

Wright J.T., Barrison I.G., Lewis I.G., MacRae K.D., Waterson E.J., Toplis P.J., Gordon M.G., Morris N.F., and Murray-Lyon I.M. 1983 Alcohol consumption, pregnancy, and low birthweight *Lancet* 1:663–665.

Yamamoto M., Takashi I., and Watanabe G. 1977 Determination of prenatal sex ratio in man *Hum Genet* 36:265–269.

Yamamoto M. and Watanabe G. 1979 Epidemiology of gross chromosomal anomalies at the early embryonic stage of pregnancy In M.A. Klingberg et al. *Epidemiologic Methods for Detecting Teratogens* pp 101–106.

Yamamoto M., Shimada T., Endo A., and Watanabe G.I. 1973 Effects of low-dose X irradiation on the chromosomal non-disjunction in aged mice *Natl N Biol* 244:206–208.

Yamazaki J., Wright S.W., and Wright P.M. 1954 Outcome of pregnancy in women exposed to the atomic bomb in Nagasaki *Am J Dis Child* 87:448–463.

Yates J.R.W. and Ferguson-Smith M.A. 1983 No evidence for a paternal age effect on the frequency of trisomy 21 at amniocentesis in 13,300 pregnancies: An analysis of data from a European collaborative study *J Med Genet* 20:457.

Yen S. and MacMahon B. 1968 Epidemiologic features of trophoblastic disease *Am J Obstet Gynecol* 101:126–132.

Yerushalmy J. 1967 The classification of newborn infants by birth weight and gestational age *Pediatrics* 71:164–172.

Yerushalmy J. 1973 Congenital heart disease and maternal smoking habits *Nature* 242:262–263.

Yerushalmy J. and Milkovich L. 1965 Evaluation of the teratogenic effect of meclizine in man *Am J Obstet Gynecol* 93:553–561.

Yerushalmy J., Bierman J.M., Kemp D.H., Connor A., and French F.E. 1956 Longitudinal studies of pregnancy on the island of Kauai, Territory of Hawaii *Am J Obstet Gynecol* 71:80.

Yerushalmy J., van den Berg B., Ehrhardt C.L., and Jacobziner H. 1965 Birth weight and gestation as indices of "immaturity" *Am J Dis Child* 109:43.

Yip R. 1987 Altitude and birth weight *J Pediatr* 111:869–876.

Ylinen K., Aula P., Stenman U.-H., Kesaniemi–Kuokkanen T., and Teramo K. 1984 Risk of minor and major fetal malformations in diabetics with high haemoglobin A values in early pregnancy *Br Med J* 289:345–346.

Ylppo A. 1919 Zur Physiologie, Klinik and zum Schicksal der Fruhgeboren *Zeitschrift fur Kinderheilkunde* 24:1–110.

Zander J. and Muller H.A. 1953 Uber die Methylandrostenediol Behandlung wahrend einer Schwangerschaft *Geburtshilfe Fraunheilkd* 13:216–222.

Zegarelli E.V., Denning C.R., Kutscher A.H., Tuoti F., and di Saint'Agnese P.A. 1961 Discoloration of the teeth in patients with cystic fibrosis of the pancreas: A preliminary report *NY State Dent J* 27:237–238.

Zuckerman B., Alpert J.J., Dooling E., Hingson R., Kayne H., Morelock S., and

Oppenheimer E. 1983 Neonatal outcomes: Is adolescent pregnancy a risk factor? *Pediatrics* 71:489–493.

Zuckerman B.S., Frank D.A., Hingson R., Morelock S., and Kayne H.L. 1986 Impact of maternal work outside the home during pregnancy on neonatal outcome *Pediatrics* 77:459–464.

Author Index

416

Subject Index

Abnormality
  at birth, 70, 75–77
  frequency in miscarriage, 75–78
  frequency in subclinical loss, 77
  frequency measures, 73–78
  incidence, 74–77
  in utero survival, 70–72, 75–77, 91
  pathogenetic mechanisms, 119
  types and definitions, 81–82
Age
  components of the variable, 259
  maternal, 259–94: advancing and
    reproduction, 263–76; at first birth,
    secular changes, 266; birth weight,
    273, 277–79; chromosomally normal
    miscarriage, 270–72, 275; conception
    delay, 269; confounding in
    recurrence studies, 148; fecundability,
    268–70, 275; fertility, animal studies,
    260–63; fertility, humans, 264–67;
    hydatidiform mole, 279; miscarriage,
    270; monosomy X, 279–80; neonatal
    mortality, 273–74, 276, 278–79;
    stillbirth, 273–74, 276; trisomy, 270–
    72, 275, 279, 282–94; trisomy
    recurrence, 156–59; youth and
    reproduction, 276–81
  maternal mortality, 274, 276
  menarche, 276–77
  menopause, 267
  menstruation, 269–70
  paternal: monosomy X, 280; trisomy,
    287–89
Agent Orange, malformations, 328, 330
Alcohol
  birth weight, 215
  chromosomally aberrant and normal
    miscarriage, 130–31
  dose, 28
  Fetal alcohol syndrome, 8, 28
  miscarriage, 129–31
  social class, 129
Altitude, birth weight, 215–16, 225

Aminopterin, malformations, 7
Androgenic hormones, masculinization, 7,
  11, 33, 311
Anesthetics, miscarriage, 143–44
Aneuploidy, definition, 82
Anticonvulsants, malformations, 37–39
Artificial insemination, maternal age and
  conception, 269
Association
  consistency on replication, 14–16
  specificity of, 18–30
  statistical and biologic coherence, 31–39
  strength of, 10–14
  time order, 9–10
Atomic bomb, 28, 137, 140, 335
Attributable risk
  birth weight, 253–56
  definition, 336
  infant mortality, 253–56

Baird, Dugald, 237
Ballantyne, William, 166
Bernard, Claude, 309
Billewicz, William, 238
Bills of Mortality, 312
Biochemical pregnancy loss, 47, 55–56,
  67–68
Biological markers, 5–6, 334
Birth cohort, 259
Birth rate, definition, 264
Birth registration, World Health
  Organization, 181
Birth weight. See also Intrauterine growth
  adult height, 235, 238
  Alaskan Eskimos, 245
  alcohol, 215
  altitude, 215–16, 225
  animal models, 237
  appropriate norms, 226
  Argentina, 246
  attributable risk for infant mortality,
    253–55
  Bombay, 246

424

Prenatal supplementation, Guatemala, 247
Prerecognition phase of pregnancy,
    definition, 47
Preterm delivery. *See also* Gestational age
    chromosomally normal miscarriage, 150
    cigarette smoking, 194–95
    complications of pregnancy, 205–6
    definitions, 178–82
    diethylstilbestrol, 238–39
    Dutch Famine, 200–201
    establishing categories, 178–82
    establishing dates, 175–78
    ethnicity, 193–94
    in vitro fertilization, 206
    induction of labor, 206
    infection, 201, 203–4
    less developed countries, 246
    maternal age, 277
    maternal disorders, chronic, 206
    measles, 250
    morbidity, 211
    nutrition, 200–201, 247
    occupation, 195–97
    placental problems, 205
    preeclamptic toxemia, 205
    psychosocial stress, 197–200
    race, 193–94
    recurrence, 205, 239
    recurrence and miscarriage, 150–52
    risk factors, 191–207
    seasonality, 202
    sexual activity, 202
    social class, 192, 247
    starvation, 247
Prevalence, definition, 74–77
Psychosocial stress, preterm delivery, 197–
    200
Puerperal sepsis, maternal mortality, 242

Quételet, Adolphe Lambert, 165

Race
    birth weight, 223
    chromosomally aberrant and normal
        miscarriage, 124–25
    developmental age, 188
    intrauterine growth, 223
    miscarriage, 123–26
    preterm delivery, 193–94
Recall bias, studies of occupation, 143
Recurrence
    birth weight, 231–40
    causal factors, 147
    cervical incompetence, 147, 152
    chromosomally normal miscarriage, 150
    definition, 146
    intrauterine growth, 239–40
    methods of study, 147–49
    miscarriage, 149–50
    preterm delivery, 205, 239
    trisomy, 156–62

Refinement
    of the exposure variable, 24–30
    of the outcome variable, 19–24
Registries, surveillance, 310–14, 327
Reporting bias, 16
Reproductive outcome
    expected frequencies, table, 333
    surveillance, 307–8, 331–33
Response rates, 16
    studies of anesthetics and miscarriage,
        143
Rh incompatibility, 98, 152
Risk factor. *See* Factor
Rubella
    epidemiologic insight in discovery, 309–
        10
    malformations, 8
    misclassification of exposure, 12–13
    pathogenesis, 21
    secular change, 313

Seasonality
    miscarriage, 247
    preterm delivery, 202
Secular change
    age at menarche, 276
    maternal age and fertility, 265–66
    rubella, 313
    thalidomide, 32, 310
Semmelweis, Ignaz, 242
Sensitivity, definition, 323
Sets technique, monitoring, 321
Sex
    birth weight, 221
    in utero survival, 95
    intrauterine growth, 212, 221
    postnatal growth, 212, 222
Sexual activity, preterm delivery, 202
Sisterhood method, maternal mortality,
    243
Smellie, William, 242
Social class
    alcohol, 129
    birth weight, less developed countries,
        246
    chromosomal aberration, 124–25
    chromosomally normal miscarriage, 125
    cigarette smoking, 126
    miscarriage, 123–26
    preterm delivery, 192
    preterm delivery, less developed
        countries, 246–47
Specificity of association
    alcohol and karyotype, 130–31
    causal criteria, 18–30
    smoking and karyotype, 128–29
Specificity-in-the-cause, 18–19
Specificity-in-the-effect, 18
Sperm
    chromosomal aberration, 86–87
    meiosis, 118–19